AF598034

Methods in Molecular Biology™

Series Editor
John M. Walker
School of Life Sciences
University of Hertfordshire
Hatfield, Hertfordshire, AL10 9AB, UK

For further volumes:
http://www.springer.com/series/7651

Psychoneuroimmunology

Methods and Protocols

Edited by

Qing Yan

PharmTao, Santa Clara, CA, USA

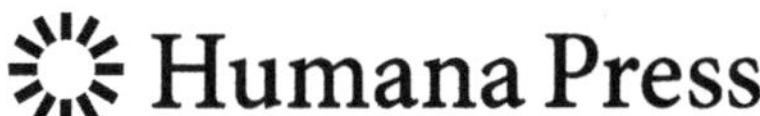

Editor
Qing Yan
PharmTao
Santa Clara, CA, USA

ISSN 1064-3745 ISSN 1940-6029 (electronic)
ISBN 978-1-62703-070-0 ISBN 978-1-62703-071-7 (eBook)
DOI 10.1007/978-1-62703-071-7
Springer New York Heidelberg Dordrecht London

Library of Congress Control Number: 2012944178

Printed on acid-free paper

Humana Press is a brand of Springer
Springer is part of Springer Science+Business Media (www.springer.com)

Preface

Psychoneuroimmunology (PNI) has developed rapidly in the last four decades. As a multidisciplinary area, PNI may provide a scientific basis for mind–body relationships toward the development of personalized and systems medicine. Although it is still an emerging field, it already has profound influences across all of the biomedical community. The biopsychosocial model is becoming the central theme for understanding health and diseases. Such understanding would contribute to more accurate diagnosis and better therapeutics in personalized medicine.

This book has several features that readers may find helpful to their work. First of all, it focuses on translational medicine by applying PNI approaches in clinical practice. One of the major challenges in current bioscience is the translation of basic scientific discoveries into better clinical outcomes. This book is written in response to this challenge by highlighting the clinical implications of PNI.

We hope that these approaches may help trigger some breakthroughs and advancement toward the realization of personalized and mind–body medicine, which is also the second feature of the book. That is, many of the methods and protocols described in the book are geared toward the development of integrative and individualized therapeutics in multiple dimensions from drugs to behaviors.

The third feature is that this book provides both practical methods and comprehensive resources that can be used for solving complicated problems of complex systems. A wide range of theoretical and experimental approaches are introduced with problem-solving objectives, from laboratory tests to computational analysis.

The fourth feature is that this book integrates the advancement of science with innovative technologies. While the first part of the book describes basic concepts and important topics in PNI, the second and third parts illustrate how the concepts and technologies can be applied for disease understanding and improving clinical interventions.

Part I of the book introduces basic and novel concepts in PNI, especially the relationship between stress and immunity, one of the most important topics in PNI. In this part, the association between stress and immunity is discussed in details from different aspects and various levels, including how immune cells respond to stress, the roles of neuroendocrine receptors, as well as the influences of job stress and life experiences. Some mechanisms of potential interventions are also described, such as the effects of physical activity.

This part explains how PNI may provide the scientific basis for the practice of mind–body medicine as well as personalized and systems medicine (see Chap. 1). Some relevant topics and concepts are discussed, such as biopsychosocial models, translational medicine, and systems biology. The close relationships among stress, depression, and inflammation are explored, as well as the clinical implications in diseases including obesity, cardiovascular disease, diabetes, arthritis, skin diseases, infectious diseases, and sleep disorders. Integrative interventions in multiple dimensions for modulating stress responses and promoting healthier behaviors are also proposed, such as drug therapies, diets, nutritional supplements, meditation, and other behavioral and mind–body strategies.

Evidences have shown that life experience has fundamental biological relevance with impacts on all adaptive systems such as the endocrine, immune, and nerve systems, with profound meanings on health and diseases (see Chap. 2). Even though experience is often ignored in the research of PNI, it deserves more attention for understanding the dynamic interplay between mind, body, behavior, and environment. Such exploration may allow meaningful and relevant interpretation and predictions in PNI.

Specifically, meta-analyses of the association between psychosocial job stress and immune parameters in blood, saliva, and urine have found that stresses such as high job demands, low job control, and economic recession are related to disrupted immune responses (see Chap. 3). At the molecular and cellular levels, studies of the neuroendocrine receptor activity by immune cells and neuroimmune responses may provide insights into the pathophysiological mechanisms of health and disease (see Chap. 4).

Integrative and multidimensional interventions have been found helpful for relieving stress and relevant diseases. For example, regular exercise may be associated with stress reduction and better mood (see Chap. 5). Epidemiological evidences have shown the relationships between physical activity and mental health. The inflammatory response has been considered a central mechanism underlying such correlations.

Part II of this book focuses on the clinical implications of these concepts and methods in the translation of PNI into the understanding of various disease states and development of personalized therapeutics. Because biomarkers play critical roles in the practice of personalized medicine, translational implications of potential biomarkers in various disorders are discussed in details in this part.

Among the potential PNI biomarkers, inflammatory markers deserve special attention as they play a pivotal role linking various health conditions and disorders including depression, obesity, cancer, cardiovascular diseases, Alzheimer's disease, and HIV (see Chap. 6). Applications of systems biology approaches would enable the insights into the correlations among various systems for the identification of the basic elements of the psychophysiological framework. The understanding of the cytokine networks, immune–brain–behavior interactions, and systemic pathways among different disorders may contribute to the transition from the disease-centered medicine to patient-centered medicine.

Specifically, cytokines are the central players in the neuroinflammatory cascades related to the neurodegenerative process in Parkinson's disease (PD) and other neurological disorders (see Chap. 7). With great promise as serological biomarkers in PD, cytokines have potential applications in diagnosis, prognosis, drug discovery, and analysis of treatment responses. On the basis of cytokine panel profiles, subclassification or risk stratification in PD can be defined, which is meaningful for the development of personalized interventions. The major cytokine multiplex assay platforms can be useful tools for biomarker discovery in PD and its cognitive comorbidities (see Chap. 7). In another example, complex disorders like Gulf War illness (GWI) can be distinguishable by measuring the co-expression of multiple markers, such as using a three-way multivariate projection model with 12 markers of endocrine and immune functions (see Chap. 8).

Depressed heart failure (HF) patients often have worse clinical outcomes than the non-depressed counterparts. PNI principals can be applied to elucidate the mechanisms such as cytokine activation connecting the comorbid disorders (see Chap. 9). In cancers, recent studies have found that the prognosis not only depends on the biological features of tumors, but also on the immune status of cancer patients that is under a psychoneuroendocrine control. The therapeutic approach based on PNI for the treatment of cancer should try to reestablish the neuroimmune conditions (see Chap. 10).

In addition, the impact of immune activation on the central nervous system (CNS) is especially important for aged individuals. Effective treatments must reduce inflammatory activity and preserving microglia's neuroprotective function at the same time. Discovering factors of neuroinflammation may contribute to potential preventative therapies for maintaining normal microglia activity in the aged brain (see Chap. 11).

Furthermore, immune functions have been associated with autism spectrum disorders (ASD), e.g., some genes related to immune regulation are changed in ASD. Many systemic and cellular immune abnormalities have been found in individuals with ASD and their families, such as changes in cytokine and chemokine production with increasing impairment in behaviors. Understanding of the interactions between the nervous and immune system during early neurodevelopment may have important therapeutic implications (see Chap. 12).

Part III of this book introduces various cutting-edge technologies models for PNI studies, from experimental approaches to data analysis and decision support. These technologies include the utilizations of mouse models, the chromium release whole blood assay, imaging techniques, vaccine models, as well as translational bioinformatics.

Specifically, mouse models have extensive applications in PNI studies. Immunobehavioral phenotyping is a first-line approach for exploring the neuroimmune system and its reactions. Behavioral tests are frequently used to examine neuroimmune activation in mice (see Chap. 13). The murine MRL model with high validity in revealing principal pathogenic circuits has been considered indispensable in understanding the brain-immune links (see Chap. 14). In addition, mouse models have been useful for examining the effects of the complex biology of cytokines such as IL-2 on multiple systems. Models such as congenic IL-2 knockout mice can be applied to investigate neuroimmunological processes in neurological diseases such as Alzheimer's disease and schizophrenia, as well as autoimmune diseases such as multiple sclerosis (see Chap. 15).

Natural killer (NK) cells are sensitive barometers of the effects of stressors on the immune system. A chromium (51Cr) release whole blood bioassay can be used to measure the target cell killing capacity of NK cells (see Chap. 16). Positron emission tomography (PET) imaging is a tool for measuring brain metabolism and target molecules. By detecting brain variables, PET imaging can be combined with other experimental and clinical model systems for PNI research (see Chap. 17).

In addition, vaccination models are very useful for the examination of the effects of psychosocial factors on immunity (see Chap. 18). Such protocols can help elucidate the association between stress and the vaccination response. These models can be applied for promoting vaccine responses in at risk populations by assisting decisions on the choice of vaccination, timing of assessments, and the available outcome measures (see Chap. 19).

Furthermore, translational bioinformatics provides a powerful method to bridge the gaps between various knowledge domains in PNI and systems biology (see Chap. 20). Translational bioinformatics methods at various systems levels are introduced. These methods can facilitate pattern recognition and expedite the discovery of systemic biomarkers for clinical trials and outcome assessments. Methods and applications of data integration, data mining, and decision support in PNI are also discussed.

By covering topics from fundamental concepts to advanced technologies, this book can be used by biomedical students and professionals at all levels who are interested in integrative studies in psychology, psychiatry, neuroscience, immunology, PNI, molecular biology, genetics, bioinformatics, bioengineering, biochemistry, physiology, pathology, microbiology, pharmacology, toxicology, systems biology, drug discovery, and clinical medicine. Written by leading experts in the field, this book intends to provide a practical, state-of-the-art, and holistic view for the translation of PNI into better preventive and personalized medical practice.

I would like to thank all of the authors for sharing their profound thoughts and experiences, and for making valuable contributions to this exciting new field. I also thank the series editor, Dr. John Walker, for his help with the editing.

Qing Yan
Santa Clara, CA, USA

Contents

Contributors

PAUL ASHWOOD • *Department of Medical Microbiology and Immunology and the M.I.N.D. Institute, University of California at Davis, Davis, CA, USA*
ZACHARY BARNES • *Department of Medicine, University of Miami, Miami, FL, USA*
TRACY BAYNARD • *Department of Kinesiology and Community Health, University of Illinois, Urbana, IL, USA*
NEIL A. BLEVINS • *Department of Pathology, College of Medicine, University of Illinois, Urbana, IL, USA*
GORDON BRODERICK • *Department of Medicine, Division of Pulmonary Medicine, University of Alberta, Edmonton, AB, Canada*
VICTORIA E. BURNS • *School of Sport and Exercise Sciences, University of Birmingham, Birmingham, UK*
MILO CAREAGA • *Department of Medical Microbiology and Immunology and the M.I.N.D. Institute, University of California at Davis, Davis, CA, USA*
ROMANO ENDRIGHI • *Psychobiology Group, Department of Epidemiology and Public Health, University College London, London, UK*
MARY ANN FLETCHER • *Department of Medicine, University of Miami, Miami, FL, USA; Miami Veterans Affairs Medical Center Miami, FL, USA*
GREGORY G. FREUND • *Department of Pathology, College of Medicine, University of Illinois at Urbana Champaign, Urbana, IL, USA*
MICHAEL GALLAGHER • *Department of Family Medicine, University of Calgary, Calgary, AB, Canada*
MARK HAMER • *Psychobiology Group, Department of Epidemiology and Public Health, University College London, London, UK*
JONAS HANNESTAD • *Department of Psychiatry, Yale University School of Medicine, New Haven, CT, USA*
SHAWN HAYLEY • *Department of Neuroscience, Carleton University, Ottawa, ON, Canada*
ZHI HUANG • *Departments of Psychiatry, Neuroscience, and Pharmacology and Therapeutics, McKnight Brain Institute, University of Florida, Gainesville, FL, USA*
JESSICA A. JIMÉNEZ • *Department of Psychiatry, University of California at San Diego, San Diego, CA, USA*
HARLAN P. JONES • *Department of Molecular Biology and Immunology, University of North Texas Health Science Center, Fort Worth, TX, USA*
NANCY G. KLIMAS • *Institute for Neuro-immune Medicine, Nova Southeastern University, Ft. Lauderdale, FL, USA; Miami Veterans Affairs Medical Center Miami, FL, USA*
RACHEL A. KOHMAN • *Department of Psychology, University of Illinois at Urbana-Champaign, Beckman Institute, Urbana, IL, USA*

PAOLO LISSONI • *Institute of Biological Medicine, Milan, Italy*
DARCY LITTELJOHN • *Department of Neuroscience, Carleton University, Ottawa, ON, Canada*
DANIELLE MEOLA • *Departments of Psychiatry, Neuroscience, and Pharmacology and Therapeutics, McKnight Brain Institute, University of Florida, Gainesville, FL, USA*
PAUL J. MILLS • *Department of Psychiatry, University of California San Diego, San Diego, CA, USA*
AKINORI NAKATA • *Division of Applied Research and Technology, National Institute for Occupational Safety and Health, Centers for Disease Control and Prevention, Cincinnati, OH, USA*
JOHN M. PETITTO • *Departments of Psychiatry, Neuroscience, and Pharmacology and Therapeutics, McKnight Brain Institute, University of Florida, Gainesville, FL, USA*
ANNA C. PHILLIPS • *School of Sport and Exercise Sciences, University of Birmingham, Birmingham, UK*
LYDIA POOLE • *Psychobiology Group, Department of Epidemiology and Public Health, University College London, London, UK*
BORIS SAKIĆ • *Department of Psychiatry and Behavioral Neurosciences, McMaster University, Hamilton, ON, Canada*
ELLING ULVESTAD • *Department of Microbiology, The Gade Institute, Haukeland University Hospital, University of Bergen, Bergen, Norway*
SUZANNE D. VERNON • *The CFIDS Association of America, Charlotte, NC, USA*
QING YAN • *PharmTao, Santa Clara, CA, USA; University of Phoenix, Phoenix, AZ, USA*
JASON M. YORK • *Department of Animal Sciences, University of Illinois, Urbana, IL, USA*

Part I

Stress and Immunity: Biopsychosocial Models

Chapter 1

The Role of Psychoneuroimmunology in Personalized and Systems Medicine

Qing Yan

Abstract

Psychoneuroimmunology (PNI) may provide the scientific basis for personalized and systems medicine. The exploration of the extensive interactions among psychological and behavioral factors, the nervous system, the immune system, and the endocrine system may help understand the mechanisms underlying health, wellness, and diseases. PNI theories based on systems biology methodologies may contribute to the identification of patient patterns for establishing psychological and physiological profiles for personalized medicine. A biopsychosocial model will help elucidate the systemic interrelationships between psychosocial and bio-physiological factors for the development of systems medicine. Many evidences have supported the close relationships between stress, depression, inflammation, and disorders including obesity, cardiovascular disease, diabetes, arthritis, skin diseases, infectious diseases, and sleep disorders. As inflammation is a critical connection among different diseases, the elucidation of the associations may contribute to the findings of systemic therapeutic targets. With the understanding of the translational implications of PNI, integrative interventions in multiple dimensions can be applied to modulate stress responses and promote healthier behaviors. These interventions include combination drug therapies, diets, nutritional supplements, meditation, and other behavioral and mind-body strategies.

Key words: Brain, Depression, Inflammation, Immune, Mind-body, Personalized medicine, Psychoneuroimmunology, Stress, Systems biology, Translational medicine

1. Introduction

As an emerging field, psychoneuroimmunology (PNI) may provide the scientific basis for personalized and systems medicine (1, 2). During its fast development in the last 40 years, this multidisciplinary area already has influenced many fields profoundly all across the biomedical research society, including psychology, neuroscience, endocrinology, immunology, pharmacology, and toxicology (3). This rapidly developing field may have insightful meanings for the practice of systems biology in personalized medicine. Systems biology studies the interactions and interrelationships among

Qing Yan (ed.), *Psychoneuroimmunology: Methods and Protocols*, Methods in Molecular Biology, vol. 934, DOI 10.1007/978-1-62703-071-7_1, © Springer Science+Business Media, LLC 2012

biomedical components at various systems levels and dimensions, from molecules to cells, from the human society to the environment (4). The practice of systems biology may contribute to the development of systems medicine. Specifically, PNI studies the bidirectional interactions among psychological and behavioral factors, the nervous system, the immune system, and the endocrine system (5–7). These systems are not isolated but are interactive and cooperative components of the integrated adaptive processes (8). Historical, experimental, and clinical observations have demonstrated that physical and psychological conditions have close impacts on each other. For example, attitudes and social supports can affect the likelihood of diseases and life expectancy (9). Behavioral and life style interventions may improve therapeutic outcomes. On the other hand, physical illness may lead to psychological alterations in mood, behavior, and memory (9).

The exploration of the extensive interactions between the behavior and the physiological systems may help elucidate the mechanisms underlying health, wellness, and diseases. For example, through hardwiring sympathetic and parasympathetic nerves to lymphoid organs, the brain can regulate the immune system directly (10). The balance of cytokines produced by the immune system can be influenced by neuroendocrine hormones including the corticotrophin-releasing hormone or substance P. On the other hand, the immune system can affect the activities of the brain such as sleep and body temperature (10). Such tight functional and anatomical connections enable highly reciprocal influences among these systems. The intricate interactions enable the sense of danger and the adaptive responses, and play critical roles in various diseases. For instance, immune malfunction is one of the major reasons of many age-related disorders, such as cardiovascular disease, cancers, type 2 diabetes, osteoporosis, arthritis, and functional decline (11). Psychological states such as negative emotions can affect these conditions via the promotion of proinflammatory cytokine productions.

An important question that PNI tries to answer is the effects of stress and negative emotions on the immune system. For example, chronic stress has been found to contribute to anxiety and depression (9). The underlying mechanisms of such effects include alterations in the hypothalamic–pituitary–adrenal (HPA) axis, the sympathetic–adrenal–medullary axis, and the immune system (12). At the molecular level, chronic stress and depression have been associated with increased levels of proinflammatory cytokines, glucocorticoids, catecholamines, as well as defects in the serotonergic functions (9, 12). Chronic stress may affect the corticotropin-releasing hormone system and disturb the signaling of the glucocorticoid receptor (13). Glucocorticoid receptors on immune cells may bind to cortisol to alter the function of nuclear factor-κB (NF-κB) (12). Beyond the molecular level, alterations in the HPA axis and the immune system may lead to neurodegenerative changes in hippocampus, prefrontal cortex, and amygdalae (9).

Changes at these different levels may have systemic consequences. The alterations in the release patterns of vasopressin, dopamine, and serotonin may result in changes of emotionality, cognitive functions, and social behaviors. The alterations in gene expression mediated by glucocorticoid hormones and catecholamines may cause malfunctions of the immune system that have various health implications (12). Such changes may result in behavioral changes related to depression, and correlate chronic stress and depression to the age-related disorders such as dementia and Alzheimer's disease (9, 14). Furthermore, distress can slow down the wound healing process, increase susceptibility to infections, and reduce immune responses to vaccines. For example, in women with cervical dysplasia, stress was found to be related to lower HPV-specific immune responses (15). The HPV vaccine's efficacy may be impaired because stress may negatively influence both the antibody and T-cell immunity. Such observations have demonstrated that behavioral interventions will also be important for improving the efficacies of vaccines.

To fully understand such complex interactions among multiple levels from molecules to the brain tissues, from behavioral changes to environmental effects, it is necessary to incorporate interdisciplinary methodologies such as those used in systems biology (1, 13). Such approaches will enable the development of novel intervention strategies for achieving the objectives of predictive, preventive, and personalized medicine. As the key model for health and diseases, a biopsychosocial paradigm will elucidate the systemic interactions between psychosocial and biological factors for the development of systems medicine (2, 4, 16, 17).

In fact, the development in PNI may contribute significantly to reestablish the philosophical connection between holism and reductionism in biomedical science. The currently increased interests in the mind–body connections call for an integrative and holistic framework in biomedicine for a more complete understanding of the interactions among various systems. On the other hand, traditional in vitro approaches are often based on cultured cells that are not influenced by interactions with other types of cells, hormones, and neurotransmitters (9). These factors may contribute to the inconsistent results between laboratory experiments and clinical studies, as well as the barriers to the translation of basic scientific studies into effective clinical therapeutics. Considering these factors, studies in PNI based on systems biology approaches may help rebuild the philosophical balance between holism and reductionism by establishing integrative models of the systemic interactions. Such approaches may help elucidate the correlations between structures and functions at various systems levels, and correlate genotypes with phenotypes, the key issues in personalized medicine (2).

The understanding of the multi-level interactions and the biopsychosocial model will also be beneficial for the transformation from the disease-centered medicine to human-centered medicine (4). Malfunctions of the pathways and systemic changes such as inflammation that commonly occur in multiple diseases rather than one single disease state can be used as preventive and therapeutic targets. With the integration of factors from both the mind and the body, more accurate diagnosis, lower risks of adverse events, and better treatment outcomes can be achieved toward the goals of personalized medicine (2).

2. Incorporating Systemic Psychoneuroimmunology Factors for Personalized Medicine: The Biopsychosocial Model

Based on the biopsychosocial model, personalized medicine should incorporate both behavioral and physiological factors at various systems levels for identifying patient patterns and profiles for the differentiation of patient subgroups. For example, at the molecular level, functional genetic variations need to be explored to study individual responses (see Fig. 1). At the cellular level, cytokine

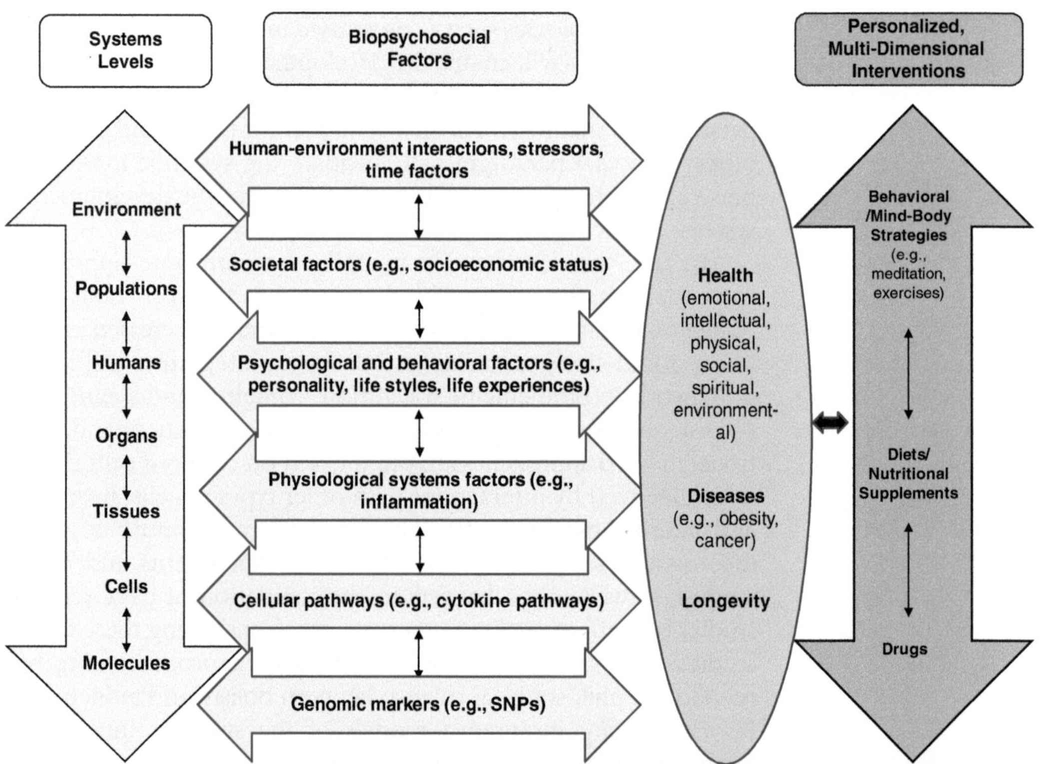

Fig. 1. A systems biology perspective of psychoneuroimmunology for the development of personalized medicine: biopsychosocial factors at various systems levels and potential personalized interventions in multiple dimensions.

networks and signaling pathways are important for systems investigation. Factors and potential biomarkers at these levels will be discussed in more detail in Chapter 6. At the psychological level, differences in personalities and behaviors need to be considered because individual variations in stress reactivity, coping styles, and emotionality are associated with physiological responses including immunity-related states (18). These psychological effects on the immune system can affect disease states. Complex interactions between the different levels in various time dimensions, such as the gene–environment interactions during various periods in the life span, should also be included.

Among all the factors, individual patterns of cognitive and behavioral responses are especially important for understanding the immune processes in different diseases. For instance, bereavement is a stressful state that may induce alterations in the immune responses including the activities of natural killer (NK) cells (19). In such a state, factors such as personality may cause different psychological responses and result in different physiological changes in different persons. Specifically, people with high levels of trait "negative affectivity" are more likely to respond with depression and anxiety, compared with those who do not have such traits (19).

Patterns in different behavioral and physiological stress responses, e.g., the offensive aggressive behavior, have been shown as the best predictor for the individual susceptibility to many diseases related to the immune system (20). For example, although the connection between stress and heart disease was inconsistent, cynical hostility has been shown as a consistent predictor in cardiovascular diseases (21). Such observations demonstrate that personality factors may be more important than the stressful environment itself, as such factors can often be used for the prediction of health outcomes regardless if stressful challenges exist or not.

In fact, causal connections have been established between personality, health, diseases, and longevity (21). Multiple pathways may be involved in the bidirectional interactions between personality and health conditions. For instance, unhealthy behavior patterns such as poor diet habits, smoking, and lack of physical activity may lead to physiological malfunctions and illnesses. Based on such understanding, interventions on personalities may become necessary or even more important than a single medication. Regular treatment of depression may not be useful for preventing heart diseases even though depression has been associated with heart disease, because personality factors may play a more important role (21).

Other factors in multiple dimensions such as time and life experiences should also be considered for an integrative diagnosis and intervention (see Fig. 1). For instance, even though conscientiousness has been shown as a critical predictor of longevity across the full lifespan, simple interventions on un-conscientiousness may not be possible or effective (21). Other factors should also be considered, such as patterns of individual reactions and changes over different timeframes in the lifespan.

Furthermore, different human and socioeconomic factors should be included to fill in the integrative map of personalized medicine (see Fig. 1). Cognitive processes play a key role in the physiological responses to the social world. Many factors have been found to contribute to the association between poorer health and lower socioeconomic status. These factors include higher exposure to indoor allergens such as cockroach and mouse, as well as pollutants including tobacco smoke and diesel-related particles (22, 23). Pollutants such as pharmaceuticals, pesticides, and industrial contaminants may disrupt neuroendocrine pathways to affect the ability to deal with stress and other challenges (24). In another example, social status threat may induce a series of contextual, psychological, and biological responses with health consequences (6). Chronic social threats include discrimination, devaluation, or rejection. According to the social threat conceptual model, the exposure of chronic social threat may lead to a neural sensitivity and disturb the neurohormonal pathways including the HPA axis (6). Such exposure may result in elevated production of proinflammatory cytokines and glucocorticoid alterations. These changes may increase the risks of inflammatory activities and many health disorders. The perceptions of social threat have been considered a mediator of these effects (6).

These observations have indicated that a comprehensive and integrated biopsychosocial model needs to be established to provide a multi-dimensional framework (see Fig. 1). Such a framework should link patterns of genetics, environments, personality, behaviors, health, diseases, and longevity in individuals within different timeframes. To establish such a framework, approaches from systems biology will be needed because a single factor or theory will not meet with such demands. For example, models for a simple HPA response to chronic stress have been found to be inappropriate or insufficient (21). However, "A new wave of theories needs to be developed to incorporate the moderating influences of timing, nature of stress, controllability, and individual psychiatric response" (25). Such theories based on systems biology methodologies (also see Chapter 20) may help identify psychological and physiological patterns in PNI toward the establishment of personalized medicine.

3. Stress and Inflammation: A Systems Biology Perspective

Stress refers to environmental changes that may lead to disturbed homeostasis (9). According to this definition, different individuals may respond to a stressful stimulus or stressors differently. The effects of the stressful stimulus may be varied, as they may cause significant behavioral or physiological changes in one person while little changes may happen to another person. The variability of responses in different individuals may also depend on the coping strategies and the adaptation to stressors. Current studies have shown that stress responses can be beneficial and protective (9). Adaptation is a learned process that may help the individual adjust to future adverse conditions. However, chronic, repetitive, uncontrollable, and continued stress may lead to impaired adaptation. In such conditions, hypercortisolism, hypertension, abnormal immune responses, and psychological alterations may result in pathological alterations in the brain. The changes in the HPA axis may further lead to anxiety, depression, and psychotic disorders (9).

Complex mechanisms at various systems levels including the endocrine and neurotransmitter systems are involved in the immune responses to stress. Stress may result in negative emotions, increase sympathetic hyperactivity, and enhance oxidative stress (6, 7, 16). These mechanisms are mediated via cytokine receptors on endocrine cells and neurons, as well as hormone and neurotransmitter receptors on cells of the immune system. Various molecules are involved in these mechanisms, including catecholamines, glucocorticoids, endorphins, and other neuropeptides (9). Psychosocial stress has been related to higher levels of inflammatory markers including proinflammatory cytokines, the activation of inflammatory pathways such as the NF-κB pathway, and impaired HPA axis regulation of inflammatory signaling pathways (26).

According to the biopsychosocial model, how an individual understands and responds to the environment such as stressors would have profound clinical meanings (17). The brain-immune interactions play critical roles in health, wellness, and diseases. The hyperactivity of the sympatho-adrenal system and the hypersecretion of the glucocorticoids related to chronic stress may cause metabolic alterations that lead to diabetes, fat accumulation, and hypertension. Stressful events and depression may affect food choices, and usually stimulate less healthy choices (27). For example, stress and depression were related with less fresh fruit consumption but higher intake of snack foods in Chinese college students (28). Stress also influences metabolic responses to foods (27). Stress may change the gastroduodenal motility, disturb gastric emptying, and alter intestinal transit and colonic motility (29). For example, acute stress delayed the clearance of triglyceride after an intravenously administered fat emulsion (30). After stimulation with a laboratory stressor, it took averagely 14 % longer time for the clearance of an exogenous fat load, compared with the non-stress controls (30).

The elucidation of the association between stress and inflammation may contribute to the findings of treatments targeting the common inflammatory mechanisms in different diseases. This may help with the practice of personalized medicine, i.e., the treatment of human beings rather than just a single disease. Inflammation may affect a spectrum of central nervous system (CNS) functions including neurotransmitter metabolism, neuroendocrine function, and information processing (2). Inflammation is also the common link among the leading causes of death (31). For example, proinflammatory cytokines including interleukin-6 (IL-6) and IL-1beta are critical elements in a spectrum of disorders such as cardiovascular disease, cancers, type II diabetes, arthritis, osteoporosis, Alzheimer's disease, skin disorders including psoriasis, and functional decline (11). The production of proinflammatory cytokines and other inflammatory markers can be promoted by psychological stress and negative emotions including depression, anxiety, as well as psychiatric diseases such as the post-traumatic stress disorder (PTSD) (32, 33). For instance, chronic stress among caregivers of dementia relatives may lead to significantly higher levels of serum IL-6 (34). Continued proinflammatory cytokine production caused by stress and depression may be related to longer infectious time and slower wound healing (35). Higher IL-6 response is related to the pathogenesis of coronary heart disease via a combination of autocrine, paracrine, and endocrine mechanisms (36).

In another example, life experience is also a critical factor (see Fig. 1). Adults with a history of early-life stress have shown an enhanced inflammatory response to acute stress challenges. Early-life stress, especially childhood maltreatment has been considered a risk factor for systemic inflammation in adulthood. Significantly higher IL-6 concentrations in response to stress challenges were observed among those who experienced moderate–severe childhood maltreatment, compared with the controls without the maltreatment (33). Exposure to early-life stress may also increase chances of adult obesity (37). In the connection between childhood adverse experiences and poor adult physical and mental health, inflammation has been found to be an important mediator.

In summary, the understanding of the associations between stress and inflammation may help explain various health problems. From the systems biology perspective, biological and environmental factors at various levels have been found to account for chronic inflammation and diseases (see Fig. 1). These factors include the increased proinflammatory and decreased anti-inflammatory cytokines at the molecular level, as well as the signaling pathways and the status of T-cell subpopulations at the cellular level (26). At the systems and behavioral level, these factors include stress, dietary intake, adiposity, and the bacterial composition of the gut microbiota (26). Chronic inflammation may become a common target to prevent and treat many different diseases including cardiovascular disease, diabetes, cancer, and depression. The clinical implications of the connections among stress, inflammation, and various diseases will be discussed in more detail in the next section.

4. Psychoneuroimmunology and Translational Medicine: Clinical Implications

Based on the integrative paradigm and biopsychosocial model, PNI can play an important role in translational medicine because it provides the connection between basic scientific research and clinical practice in various areas. Because of its multidisciplinary characteristics, PNI may serve as the foundation for preventive and personalized medicine over the next decade (2).

For instance, PNI can contribute to better nursing care by supporting better caring and empathetic approaches (38, 39). PNI-based framework has been shown helpful for guiding clinical trials among patients with HIV and cancer for the evaluation of nursing care in the processes of reducing stress and promoting coping strategies (40). With the elucidation of the interactions among behaviors, the neuroendocrine system, the immune system, and their effects on clinical outcomes, PNI would allow health practitioners to help their patients prevent infections and improve the healing ability (41). For example, in intensive care units, patients' immune functions are often weakened by physiological and psychological stressors such as trauma, pain, anxiety, fear, and sleep deprivation (41). Physicians and nurses can use the PNI models to help relieve the stresses among those patients.

Many evidences have supported the close relationship between depression, inflammation, and other diseases. Although depression is shown as a psychological problem, it has deep impact on the immune system. For example, those with inflammatory diseases including multiple sclerosis, psoriasis, cancers, rheumatoid arthritis, and cardiovascular disease often have higher incidences of depression (42). People with chronic stress and depression often have elevated levels of inflammatory markers including IL-6, C-reactive protein (CRP), TNF-α, and the endothelial activation marker sICAM-1 (7). Depression may cause promoted proinflammatory pathways and suppressed anti-inflammatory pathways (9). Those who have been administered inflammatory cytokines such as interferon α (IFN-α) (for the treatment of disorders such as hepatitis C and malignant melanoma) are more susceptible to develop depression. Because proinflammatory cytokines are involved in neurotransmitter metabolism, neuroendocrine functions, and synaptic plasticity, they can interact with all of the pathophysiologic domains that are associated with depression (42).

Chronic depression has been found to cause structural alterations at various levels correlated with other diseases. At the molecular and cellular level, activated microglia cause higher production of proinflammatory cytokines that may be involved in neurodegeneration (9). Lower production of neurotrophic factors including BDNF may lead to decreased neuronal repair and increased loss of neurons and astrocytes (9). At the tissue and organ level, lower volumes of the hippocampus, frontal cortex, and amygdalae have been observed in chronically depressed patients. These changes may provide linkages between depression and higher risks of Alzheimer's disease.

A bidirectional relationship has been established between obesity and depression (42). For example, in women with severe or morbid obesity, body mass index (BMI) (for measuring obesity) was positively related to inflammatory markers such as IL-6 and CRP (43). These markers were also closely associated with depression and anxiety. On the other hand, weight loss methods were found to result in lower inflammation, reductions in inflammatory markers especially CRP, as well as improvement in emotional status and lower levels of anxiety (43). These findings have demonstrated that inflammation is an important mediator of psychological features of obese people.

Epidemiological studies have shown that the prevalence rates of obesity and metabolic syndrome are especially high in those with psychiatric disorders such as PTSD (44). Mediated through the neuropeptide Y (NPY) and glucocorticoid systems, stress has been found to increase the susceptibility to obesity and other metabolic syndrome in mice fed with a high caloric diet (44). Changes in the NPY and glucocorticoid systems can also influence behavioral adaptation to stress. Investigation of the relationships between these systems and stress has deep translational meanings for the discovery of more effective prevention and treatment methods for obesity and metabolic syndrome.

Furthermore, psychological stressors have been shown to play crucial roles in the development of coronary artery disease (CAD) via their effects on the immune system (45). Such stressors may alter endothelial functions. Acute psychological stressors may cause leukocytosis, elevated cytotoxicity of NK cells, and decreased proliferative response to mitogens. However, chronic stressors may result in adverse effects and alterations in cardiovascular functions. Both acute and chronic stressors may affect hemostatic factors and acute phase proteins, and result in thrombus formation and myocardial infarction (45). As depression may cause inflammation, the combination of depression and inflammation may form complex mechanisms to affect CAD. Studies have found that both depression and CRP are prognostic risk factors of acute coronary syndromes (46). Patients with either of the risk factors may benefit from similar interventions such as exercises, antidepressants, and healthy diets (7).

Cancer has also been closely related to stress. Stressors may modulate the development of malignancies, and inhibit lymphocyte proliferation and the activity of NK cells (1). However, stress reduction interventions such as relaxation training may prolong the survival of patients with metastatic neoplasms, possibly by modulating the cytotoxic function and the functions of NK cells (1).

In addition, psychological stress is involved in the disease activity in rheumatoid arthritis (RA). Psychological stress may lead to higher cardiovascular activity as well as adrenocorticotropic hormone (ACTH) and cortisol levels, and the elevation in monocyte production of TNF-α among RA patients (47). On the other hand, TNF-α antagonists may counteract the stress stimulation of the inflammatory markers and serve as potential therapeutics for RA. Such understanding would enable the findings of various translational targets in the molecular networks of inflammation and stress.

One of the most significantly influenced organs by emotional factors is the skin. For example, psychological stress is closely correlated with wound healing. Stress has been shown to influence the healing of various wound types, including both acute and chronic wounds, as well as blister wounds and minor skin damages (47). Patients of skin diseases often report a temporal relationship between the occurrence of the disease and stressful life events (1). Emotional stressors have been associated with many cutaneous diseases such as acne, atopic eczema, herpes simplex infections, psoriasis, and vitiligo (1). For example, emotional stressors may be involved in the onset of psoriasis and precipitate flares. Psoriasis patients with stress-related exacerbations often have malfunction in the HPA axis. Such patients responded to experimental stressors with higher blood pressure and heart rate (1). On the other hand, many psychosocial interventions for reducing stress have been shown to be beneficial in the treatment of psoriasis. These interventions include using meditation tapes during phototherapy sessions for faster clearance of psoriasis, and the application of hypnosis sessions (1).

Infections and infectious diseases are another group of disorders that are significantly influenced by stress conditions. Stressors may have deleterious effects on bacterial infections of the skin (1). Recurrent herpetic infection can be precipitated under the influences of psychiatric diseases and life events. The development of human infection with herpes simplex viruses may also be affected by stress (1). However, chronic rather than acute stress has been related to experimental viral infections. Another proof of the connection between infections and psychological factors is that psychosocial interventions have been found to reduce the recurrences of herpes simplex infections (1).

As a dynamic behavioral state, sleep plays an important role in neuroendocrine activities and homeostasis. Sleep may have profound influences on the immune system. For example, sleep disturbances have been associated with decreased activities of NK cells, and enhanced inflammatory markers in depressed patients (7). The problem of insomnia and chronic sleep disturbances have been related to altered levels of proinflammatory cytokines and cellular immune responses. Experimental sleep loss may cause higher levels of inflammatory markers including IL-6, TNF, and CRP (7). The protein NF-κB has been suggested to be a mediator of the inflammatory responses. Poor sleep has been implied as a predictor of cardiovascular disease and risks of other chronic diseases such as arthritis and diabetes (7). The connection between sleep and inflammation may provide translational implications because interventions targeting sleep problems may help inhibit inflammation and prevent a spectrum of chronic diseases.

5. Psychoneuro-immunology, Integrative Interventions, and Mind–Body Medicine

With the understanding of the translational implications of PNI, integrative interventions in multiple dimensions such as psychological and pharmaceutical approaches can be applied to modulate stress responses and promote healthier behaviors (see Fig. 1). Combination therapies can be designed with different mechanisms applied, such as sensory, cognitive, expressive, and physical methods (48). For instance, more adaptive approaches of responding to life challenges and better coping strategies can be trained for dealing with aging disorders (17). To achieve the objectives of personalized medicine, the utilizations of such systemic interactions and feedbacks would promote health and wellness in the emotional, intellectual, physical, social, spiritual, and environmental dimensions (4).

Based on the systems models, drugs can be designed for targeting the common pathways of different diseases, rather than for targeting just a single disease. As mentioned above, this will also help convert the disease-centered drugs to human-centered medicine, the major task of personalized medicine. For instance, targeting inflammatory markers such as IL-1 and IL-6, and targeting cytokine signaling networks such as NF-κB and p38 MAPK pathways may be useful for treating a wide range of diseases including depression, cancer, and cardiovascular disease (2). Such approaches would also enable novel drug combination strategies by using existing drugs for better clinical results while saving the costs from new drug development (4). For example, drugs such as etanercept, infliximab, and anakinra have been traditionally applied for treating rheumatoid arthritis. However, these drugs also have potential effects on disrupted mood status (49). Etanercept administration has been shown to have beneficial effects on depression in psoriasis patients.

In addition to drugs, integrative interventions in multiple dimensions such as diets and behaviors can also be used for targeting the common pathways of inflammation (see Fig. 1). Psychological stress and depression have been associated with inflammation via the same pathways, by influencing food choices and stimulating maladaptive metabolic responses to unhealthy diets (27). Certain diets promote inflammation, including those high in refined starches, sugar, and saturated fats (50). On the other hand, vegetables and fruits have antioxidant and anti-inflammatory properties. Diets may influence inflammatory factors and dietary-related inflammation may enhance depression, while depression can in turn promote inflammation. With such understanding of the diet-immune–stress interactions, systemic interventions using diets can then be applied to inhibit inflammation and reduce stress. For example, the Mediterranean dietary pattern has been found to have protective effects for the prevention of depression (51).

In another example, arachidonic-acid-derived (omega-6) eicosanoids can enhance the production of proinflammatory cytokines (52). Dietary sources of omega-6 eicosanoids include refined vegetable oils, e.g., corn, sunflower, and safflower oils. However, the omega-3 polyunsaturated fatty acids can inhibit the production of arachidonic-acid-derived eicosanoids (53). Higher "omega-6:omega-3" ratios may lead to higher proinflammatory cytokine production. For example, depression has been related to higher omega-6:omega-3 ratios (53). On the other hand, nutritional supplements of omega-3 fatty acid may have beneficial effects on mood, vagal tone, and inflammation (54). Such supplements may suppress the activation of NF-κB and responses to endotoxin to modulate inflammatory responses (27). Dietary sources of omega-3 polyunsaturated fatty acids include fish oil, wheat germ, and flax seeds.

In addition, among the elderly people, those with poor mental and physical health conditions have been found to have decreased circulating levels of alpha-tocopherol, with elevations of the inflammatory markers such as IL-6 and CRP (55). Because nutritional factors such as vitamin E are closely associated with immune functions and life quality, they should be considered as important interventions for targeting both mental and physical disorders.

Moreover, interventions that involve behavioral and mind-body strategies would be effective for relieving depression and reducing inflammation. For example, mindfulness meditation training has been shown to reduce stress. In HIV-1 patients, meditation training was able to buffer the declination of CD4+ T lymphocyte (56). Mindfulness-based cognitive therapy (MBCT) may relieve residual depressive symptoms and prevent depression relapse (57, 58). MBCT is a program that integrates cognitive-behavioral therapy and mindfulness-based stress reduction. The practice of MBCT was also found useful for decreasing anxiety symptoms in those with bipolar disorder, as well as in patients with anxiety disorders (58). Another meditation technique that includes a mindfulness element is compassion meditation, which was found to reduce IL-6 inflammatory responses induced by a psychosocial laboratory stressor (59). Meditation practices have been suggested to influence physiological pathways that are involved in stress and diseases.

Even short-term meditation may significantly improve physiological reactions in heart rate, respiratory amplitude and rate, and skin conductance response (SCR) (60). For example, compared with the relaxation control, 5 days of integrative body–mind training (IBMT) resulted in better regulation of the autonomic nervous system (ANS) by a ventral midfrontal brain system (60). In addition, yogic cognitive-behavioral practices such as meditation, yoga asanas, and pranayama breathing have been found to influence humoral factors, nervous system activity, and cell trafficking (61). Yogic practices have many beneficial effects on health such as delaying aging and relieving chronic illness and stress from disability. Such practices may help improve homeostatic negative feedback loops in molecular and cellular interactions (61). These observations have demonstrated that integrative interventions can be effective for targeting the potential markers for the optimal therapeutic results.

Furthermore, combination interventions have been found effective in the treatment of depression and related health problems. For example, lifestyle modifications, exercises, and weight loss methods were beneficial for relieving symptoms of depression (62, 63). Exercise has anti-inflammatory effects that may lead to decreased body fat and macrophage accumulation in adipose tissue, with the reduction of inflammatory markers (64). In a study examining the effect of laughter on stress, saliva samples were collected from healthy people before and after watching a comic film or a non-humorous control film (65). The study found that the stress score reduced significantly following watching the comic film. These results confirmed that laughter has a stress relief effect.

In conclusion, PNI may play a central role for the translation of the scientific discoveries in various disciplines into personalized medicine. Using systems biology approaches, complex mechanisms involved in the interactions such as inflammation, stress, and diseases can be elucidated. Based on the biopsychosocial model, patient patterns and systemic psychological and physiological profiles can be established for more accurate diagnosis and prognosis. Such approaches will contribute to the identification of systemic targets and the development of integrative interventions for achieving health and wellness in multiple dimensions.

References

1. Tausk F, Elenkov I, Moynihan J (2008) Psychoneuroimmunology. Dermatol Ther 21:22–31
2. Yan Q (2011) Translation of psychoneuroimmunology into personalized medicine: a systems biology perspective. Per Med 8:641–649
3. Prolo P, Chiappelli F, Fiorucci A et al (2002) Psychoneuroimmunology: new avenues of research for the twenty-first century. Ann N Y Acad Sci 966:400–408
4. Yan Q (2011) Toward the integration of personalized and systems medicine: challenges, opportunities and approaches. Per Med 8:1–4
5. Zachariae R (2009) Psychoneuroimmunology: a bio-psycho-social approach to health and disease. Scand J Psychol 50(6):645–651

6. Kemeny ME (2009) Psychobiological responses to social threat: evolution of a psychological model in psychoneuroimmunology. Brain Behav Immun 23:1–9
7. Irwin MR (2008) Human psychoneuroimmunology: 20 years of discovery. Brain Behav Immun 22:129–139
8. Ader R (2000) On the development of psychoneuroimmunology. Eur J Pharmacol 405: 167–176
9. Leonard BE, Myint A (2009) The psychoneuroimmunology of depression. Hum Psychopharmacol 24:165–175
10. Ziemssen T, Kern S (2007) Psychoneuroimmunology—cross-talk between the immune and nervous systems. J Neurol 254(suppl 2):II8–II11
11. Kiecolt-Glaser JK, McGuire L, Robles TF et al (2002) Psychoneuroimmunology: psychological influences on immune function and health. J Consult Clin Psychol 70:537–547
12. Goncharova LB, Tarakanov AO (2007) Molecular networks of brain and immunity. Brain Res Rev 55(1):155–166
13. Touma C (2011) Stress and affective disorders: animal models elucidating the molecular basis of neuroendocrine-behavior interactions. Pharmacopsychiatry 44(suppl 1):S15–S26
14. Kiecolt-Glaser JK (2009) Psychoneuroimmunology psychology's gateway to the biomedical future. Perspect Psychol Sci 4: 367–369
15. Fang CY, Miller SM, Bovbjerg DH et al (2008) Perceived stress is associated with impaired T-cell response to HPV16 in women with cervical dysplasia. Ann Behav Med 35:87–96
16. Alford L (2007) Findings of interest from immunology and psychoneuroimmunology. Man Ther 12:176–180
17. Lutgendorf SK, Costanzo ES (2003) Psychoneuroimmunology and health psychology: an integrative model. Brain Behav Immun 17:225–232
18. Kemeny ME, Schedlowski M (2007) Understanding the interaction between psychosocial stress and immune-related diseases: a stepwise progression. Brain Behav Immun 21:1009–1018
19. Kemeny ME, Laudenslager ML (1999) Introduction beyond stress: the role of individual difference factors in psychoneuroimmunology. Brain Behav Immun 13:73–75
20. Koolhaas JM (2008) Coping style and immunity in animals: making sense of individual variation. Brain Behav Immun 22:662–667
21. Friedman HS (2008) The multiple linkages of personality and disease. Brain Behav Immun 22:668–675
22. Friedman EM, Lawrence DA (2002) Environmental stress mediates changes in neuroimmunological interactions. Toxicol Sci 67:4–10
23. Wright RJ, Subramanian SV (2007) Advancing a multilevel framework for epidemiologic research on asthma disparities. Chest 132(suppl):757S–769S
24. Waye A, Trudeau VL (2011) Neuroendocrine disruption: more than hormones are upset. J Toxicol Environ Health B Crit Rev 14: 270–291
25. Miller GE, Chen E, Zhou ES (2007) If it goes up, must it come down? Chronic stress and the hypothalamic-pituitary-adrenocortical axis in humans. Psychol Bull 133:25–45
26. Haroon E, Raison CL, Miller AH (2012) Psychoneuroimmunology meets neuropsychopharmacology: translational implications of the impact of inflammation on behavior. Neuropsychopharmacology 37:137–162
27. Kiecolt-Glaser JK (2010) Stress, food, and inflammation: psychoneuroimmunology and nutrition at the cutting edge. Psychosom Med 72:365–369
28. Liu C, Xie B, Chou CP et al (2007) Perceived stress, depression and food consumption frequency in the college students of China Seven Cities. Physiol Behav 92:748–754
29. Yin J, Levanon D, Chen JDZ (2004) Inhibitory effects of stress on postprandial gastric myoelectrical activity and vagal tone in healthy subjects. Neurogastroenterol Motil 16:737–744
30. Stoney CM, West SG, Hughes JW et al (2002) Acute psychological stress reduces plasma triglyceride clearance. Psychophysiology 39:80–85
31. Aggarwal BB, Shishodia S, Sandur SK et al (2006) Inflammation and cancer: how hot is the link? Biochem Pharmacol 72:1605–1621
32. Segerstrom SC, Miller GE (2004) Psychological stress and the human immune system: a meta-analytic study of 30 years of inquiry. Psychol Bull 130:1–37
33. Carpenter LL, Gawuga CE, Tyrka AR et al (2010) Association between plasma IL-6 response to acute stress and early-life adversity in healthy adults. Neuropsychopharmacology 35:2617–2623
34. Kiecolt-Glaser JK, Preacher KJ, MacCallum RC et al (2003) Chronic stress and age-related increases in the proinflammatory cytokine IL-6. Proc Natl Acad Sci U S A 100: 9090–9095
35. Glaser R, Kiecolt-Glaser JK (2005) Stress-induced immune dysfunction: implications for health. Nat Rev Immunol 5:243–251

36. Yudkin JS, Kumari M, Humphries SE et al (2000) Inflammation, obesity, stress and coronary heart disease: is interleukin-6 the link? Atherosclerosis 148:209–214
37. D'Argenio A, Mazzi C, Pecchioli L et al (2009) Early trauma and adult obesity: is psychological dysfunction the mediating mechanism? Physiol Behav 98:543–546
38. Langley P, Fonseca J, Iphofen R (2006) Psychoneuroimmunology and health from a nursing perspective. Br J Nurs 15:1126–1129
39. Starkweather A, Witek-Janusek L, Mathews HL (2005) Applying the psychoneuroimmunology framework to nursing research. J Neurosci Nurs 37:56–62
40. McCain NL, Gray DP, Walter JM et al (2005) Implementing a comprehensive approach to the study of health dynamics using the psychoneuroimmunology paradigm. ANS Adv Nurs Sci 28:320–332
41. DeKeyser F (2003) Psychoneuroimmunology in critically ill patients. AACN Clin Issues 14:25–32
42. Shelton RC, Miller AH (2010) Eating ourselves to death (and despair): the contribution of adiposity and inflammation to depression. Prog Neurobiol 91:275–299
43. Capuron L, Poitou C, Machaux-Tholliez D et al (2010) Relationship between adiposity, emotional status and eating behaviour in obese women: role of inflammation. Psychol Med 41:1517–1528
44. Rasmusson AM, Schnurr PP, Zukowska Z, Scioli E et al (2010) Adaptation to extreme stress: post-traumatic stress disorder, neuropeptide Y and metabolic syndrome. Exp Biol Med 235:1150–1162
45. Ho RCM, Neo LF, Chua ANC et al (2010) Research on psychoneuroimmunology: does stress influence immunity and cause coronary artery disease? Ann Acad Med Singapore 39:191–196
46. Frasure-Smith N, Lesperance F, Irwin MR et al (2007) Depression, C-reactive protein and two-year major adverse cardiac events in men after acute coronary syndromes. Biol Psychiatry 62:302–308
47. Motivala SJ, Khanna D, FitzGerald J et al (2008) Stress activation of cellular markers of inflammation in rheumatoid arthritis: protective effects of tumor necrosis factor alpha antagonists. Arthritis Rheum 58: 376–383
48. Bauer-WuSM(2002)Psychoneuroimmunology. Part II: mind-body interventions. Clin J Oncol Nurs 6:243–246
49. Irwin MR, Miller AH (2007) Depressive disorders and immunity: 20 years of progress and discovery. Brain Behav Immun 21:374–383
50. Giugliano D, Ceriello A, Esposito K (2006) The effects of diet on inflammation—emphasis on the metabolic syndrome. J Am Coll Cardiol 48:677–685
51. Sanchez-Villegas A, Delgado-Rodriguez M, Alonso A et al (2009) Association of the Mediterranean dietary pattern with the incidence of depression: the Seguimiento Universidad de Navarra/University of Navarra Follow-up (SUN) cohort. Arch Gen Psychiatry 66:1090–1098
52. van West D, Maes M (2003) Polyunsaturated fatty acids in depression. Acta Neuropsychiatr 15:15–21
53. Pischon T, Hankinson SE, Hotamisligil GS et al (2003) Habitual dietary intake of n-3 and n-6 fatty acids in relation to inflammatory markers among U.S. men and women. Circulation 108:155–160
54. Hibbeln JR, Nieminen L, Blasbalg TL et al (2006) Healthy intakes of n-3 and n-6 fatty acids: estimations considering worldwide diversity. Am J Clin Nutr 83:1483S–1493S
55. Capuron L, Moranis A, Combe N et al (2009) Vitamin E status and quality of life in the elderly: influence of inflammatory processes. Br J Nutr 102:1390–1394
56. Creswell JD, Myers HF, Cole SW et al (2009) Mindfulness meditation training effects on CD4+ T lymphocytes in HIV-1 infected adults: a small randomized controlled trial. Brain Behav Immun 23:184–188
57. Bondolfi G, Jermann F, der Linden MV et al (2010) Depression relapse prophylaxis with mindfulness-based cognitive therapy: replication and extension in the Swiss health care system. J Affect Disord 122:224–231
58. Chiesa A, Serretti A (2010) Mindfulness based cognitive therapy for psychiatric disorders: a systematic review and meta-analysis. Psychiatry Res 187:441–453
59. Pace TW, Negi LT, Adame DD et al (2009) Effect of compassion meditation on neuroendocrine, innate immune and behavioral responses to psychosocial stress. Psychoneuroendocrinology 34:87–98
60. Tang YY, Ma Y, Fan Y et al (2009) Central and autonomic nervous system interaction is altered by short-term meditation. Proc Natl Acad Sci U S A 106:8865–8870
61. Kuntsevich V, Bushell WC, Theise ND (2010) Mechanisms of yogic practices in health, aging, and disease. Mt Sinai J Med 77:559–569

62. Fabricatore AN, Wadden TA, Higginbotham AJ et al (2011) Intentional weight loss and changes in symptoms of depression: a systematic review and meta-analysis. Int J Obes (Lond) 35:1363–1376
63. Barbour KA, Blumenthal JA (2005) Exercise training and depression in older adults. Neurobiol Aging 26(suppl 1):119–123
64. Woods JA, Vieira VJ, Keylock KT (2009) Exercise, inflammation, and innate immunity. Immunol Allergy Clin North Am 29: 381–393
65. Toda M, Kusakabe S, Nagasawa S et al (2007) Effect of laughter on salivary endocrinological stress marker chromogranin A. Biomed Res 28:115–118

Chapter 2

Psychoneuroimmunology: The Experiential Dimension

Elling Ulvestad

Abstract

Accumulating evidence has made clear that experience—the knowledge an individual acquires during a lifetime of sensing and acting—is of fundamental biological relevance. Experience makes an impact on all adaptive systems, including the endocrine, immune, and nerve systems, and is of the essence, not only for the unfolding of an organisms' healthy status, but also for the development of malfunctional traits. Nevertheless, experience is often excluded from empirical approaches. A variety of complex interactions that influence life histories are thereby neglected. Such ignorance is especially detrimental for psychoneuroimmunology, the science that seeks to understand how the exquisite and dynamic interplay between mind, body, and environment relates to behavioral characteristics. The article reviews claims for incorporating experience as a member of good explanatory standing in biology and medicine, and more specifically, claims that experiential knowledge is required to enable meaningful and relevant explanations and predictions in the psychoneuroimmunological realm.

Key words: Experience, Microbiome, Umwelt, Development, Evolution, Function, Psychoneuroimmunology, Immune

1. Introduction

Ideas that the nervous, immune, and endocrine systems work in close concert with each other as well as with external inputs were not in high vogue prior to the 1980s. Scientists were still preoccupied with elaborations of the internal workings of the three adaptive systems, and rarely made cross-over connections. That such an integrative effort would be rewarding was, however, highlighted in a 1981 landmark publication entitled Psychoneuroimmunology (1). The book, edited by Robert Ader, consisted of a collection of reviews on emerging work, and made a fascinating but also a challenging reading.

Qing Yan (ed.), *Psychoneuroimmunology: Methods and Protocols*, Methods in Molecular Biology, vol. 934, DOI 10.1007/978-1-62703-071-7_2, © Springer Science+Business Media, LLC 2012

In the book's foreword, Robert A. Good (2) outlined a research agenda for the integrative efforts that should follow:

> The question that remains is how these three major networks—the nervous system, the endocrine system, and the immunologic system—interact and, how, by understanding these interactions in precise quantitative terms, we can learn to predict and control them (2, p. xix).

In the immediate follow-up article, *Psychosocial factors in infectious disease*, S. Michael Plaut and Stanford B. Friedman (3) additionally stated that psychoneuroimmunology needs to understand how various psychosocial factors of the experiencing subject can modify external challenges. They thus elaborated further on an often observed phenomenon—that not all individuals infected with a certain infectious agent come down with disease—and emphasized that there must be "something more" involved in pathogenesis than just a battle between the infectious agent and the immune system. They made references to results from human studies which demonstrated that the meaning a person attaches to a phenomenon makes an impact on disease outcome, and so claimed that:

> The relevant question is not whether a given disease is caused by a pathogenic agent or by psychological factors, but rather to what extent the disease can be related to each of a number of factors in the history, makeup, and environment of the organism (3, p. 7).

By this claim they highlighted a shift in research focus—not only should scientists investigate why individuals are *susceptible* to illness, they should as well investigate why individuals are *resistant* to disease. The "received view," that infectious agents and psychological stressors are sufficient causes of disease, should therefore be replaced with a more comprehensive and interdisciplinary understanding of causation.

The challenge posed by Plaut and Friedman—that the human organism's life history needs to be included in the explanatory framework—is demanding. For not only did the two researchers claim that the life history should be approached from a scientific viewpoint, it should in addition be approached from the individual's perspective—from the meaning the susceptible person and his adaptive systems attach to precipitating situations. These are hard tasks indeed—for they ask of science more than science is allowed to deliver, the reason being that science in its "craving for generality" actually takes a "contemptuous attitude towards the particular case" (4, p. 18).

This idea can be explicated by way of a dilemma from scientific publishing. On the one hand, editors are reluctant to communicate case reports because cases are subject to a variety of uncontrolled and uncontrollable influences, and so generalization of the individual outcome is a precarious undertaking. On the other hand, editors endorse group-based investigations, because such studies are amenable to strict control and thus generalization. However, as publishers well know—results from group-based investigations lack an important virtue of the case. Individual characteristics and contextual parameters are seldom irrelevant for the outcome, and by treating these as confounders, group-based studies thereby neglect the experiential dimension and thus lose touch with the very individuals they represent.

Even a science that acknowledges the experiential dimension and thus attempts to incorporate experiential parameters in the form of major life events—e.g., divorce, death of a spouse, or serious disease—often fails the task. As highlighted in a critical review, individuals rarely apply the same meaning to a life event (5). Different subjects interpret events differently, and this differential interpretation is a determinant of how individuals respond psychoendocrinologically. The "objective" characteristics of an event, which are foundational in group-based investigations, are thus not objective in a strict sense—they are rather interpreted in an idiosyncratic manner by each different participator.

Knowledge of group characteristics is highly relevant but nevertheless insufficient for understanding the individual, and it thus appears that science needs a theory of the organism that also allows for the emergence of "private" responses. This does not, however, imply that science should become subjective and so comply with the slogan "anything goes." Science's ultimate task is to give objective accounts of nature, also of individual experience. To stay true to its ideal, science should therefore give well grounded *accounts of subjective experience. Subjective accounts of experience*, although important for individual behavior, are nevertheless, at least for the time being, outside the scientific realm.

In the following I will provide an exploration of the challenge posed by Plaut and Friedman. In so doing I will invoke the age old dilemma between the one and the many, and investigate how this applies to the objective perspective taken by an external observer and to the subjective perspective of a participant. The importance of the subject's environment, exemplified by the microbial communities of our intestines, will also be highlighted, as will the role of subjective interpretations of environmental stimuli over the life cycle. These deliberations will hopefully reveal the complexity of the experiential challenges facing psychoneuroimmunology.

2. The Meaning of Perception

A good starter for objective appropriation of subjective experiences can be found in the Estonian zoologist Jakob von Uexküll's (1864–1944) elaborations on the individual organism's dealing with nature. When confronted with contemporary views of the organism, Uexküll noted a discrepancy between what he believed was the animal's world—an active organism that interacts with its surroundings in a meaningful manner, and the scientific conceptualization of it—an animal that mechanically adapts its behavior to a given environment. To rectify this incongruity, he set out to build a new biology in which the animal's perspective was retained (6). And in so doing, he came to emphasize the importance of perception. As he saw it, the animal's perceptual perspective is not something gained by passively receiving inputs in the shape of information; rather, it involves an active interpretation of signals rendered meaningful by the animal's previous experiences.

Upon portraying animals as developmental structures with communicative capabilities, Uexküll also came to notify that environmental stimuli are of unequal importance for different kinds of animals. He thus elaborated a distinction between the animal's environment, i.e., its physical surroundings, and the animal's Umwelt—the meaning-carrying structure that contains a "sign or symbol that members of the same species can understand, but that those of another species cannot comprehend" (7, p. 77). Hence, even though animals of different species may share the same environment, their differing Umwelts make them experience the same environment differently.

By emphasizing the animal's perspective, Uexküll reached a surprising insight—environmental signals are already meaningful as they reach the animal. To see how this may come about, one has to think of the couplings between organisms and their surroundings as emerging from activity played out during two distinct temporalities—one during the evolutionary history of the species, when perceptual abilities are being shaped, and the other during the developmental history of the individual, when the same perceptual capabilities are being structured in relation to external inputs.

Perception of the Umwelt thus consists of a phylogenetic component, which allows for a fairly stereotyped pattern of behavior, and an ontogenetic component that serves to diversify and tailor each organism's behavior to the actual environment (Fig. 1) (8).

Although Uexküll initially received many followers, including the ethologist Konrad Lorentz and the philosopher on human experience Martin Heidegger, his work had vitalistic undertones and was therefore regarded unscientific. His emphasis on the qualitative aspects of animal perception and behavior were therefore soon replaced by more quantitative and mathematically oriented theories, and investigations related to the organism's perceptual couplings to the environment were thereby relayed to the background. However, much of this changed in the 1970s when Uexküll's ideas were revitalized by the emerging field of biosemiotics (9), and not the least by neurophysiologists and immunologists who began to reorient their investigations along similar integrative lines. To achieve the most from universalizing investigations, while at the same time avoiding loss of the individual, it would thus be

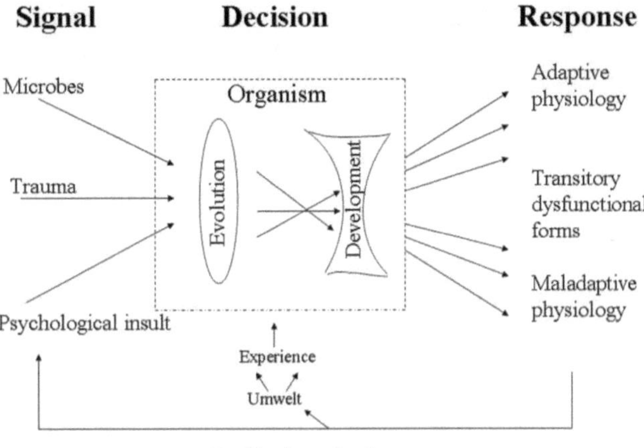

Fig. 1. Each individual is the result of the lineage's adaptive processes during evolutionary time and adaptive processes during developmental time. These two adaptive processes are integrated in every organism. The concave lens depicts the evolutionary resources of the organism, and includes its genetic make-up. The convex lens, in contrast, depicts the developmentally shaped resources of the organism, including the epigenetic make-up and the wirings of the central nervous system, the immune system, and the endocrine system. The Umwelt makes up the context in which the experiences make their impact. Dependent upon how these systems integrate within the organism, the response may turn out as functional or dysfunctional. And, since the organism's responses are in many ways instructive of latter responses, the responses are depicted to feed back to alter both the Umwelt and latter responses to the same or dissimilar challenges.

fruitful to integrate psychoneuroimmunology with the biosemiotic view of the world. But as humans differ from other animals in several respects, the Uexküllian path needs to be adapted to the specific human trajectory and situation.

3. The Human Umwelt

Compared to other mammals and primates, humans differ in several respects. Human life stories are distinguished by having an exceptionally long life span, an extended period of juvenile dependence, and support of reproduction by older postreproductive females as well as by males (10). In contrast to other animals, with the exception of primates, humans also possess specific brain structures that enable them to experience and interpret internal physiological processes (11). When such processes, which may be pain, motion, nausea, thirst or hunger, reach consciousness, they create a subjective experience of own body. Variations in this structure may thus be part of the explanation for the great variation of experience of a given bodily state by different humans (12).

Human beings are also distinguished by having unique psychological characteristics—a capacity for self-reflection, for designing sophisticated symbolic structures, for attaching metaphorical concepts to experiences and for building models and categories with the aid of the imagination. There is thus a creative element in man's dealing with his world—our brains create "a fantasy that coincides with reality" (13, p. 111). And exceptionally—when this reality seems unfit, humans additionally have the capacity to alter the same reality in radical ways during a process termed niche construction (14). Man's Umwelt is thus not only ecological, but also cultural—all the way (15). And as culture is an important part of man's Umwelt, it should not come unexpected that artifacts of culture may act as a selective force, thus feeding back on human beings in a form strong enough to even alter the genome (16). In the same vein, alterations in perception and thought processes feedback on the brain, thus altering neurophysiological and neurochemical activities involved in perception, action, and emotional control (17)—thus *mind matters* in a literal sense.

Man's experiences are not entirely determined by the way the world is—man is himself active in acquisition, selection, interpretation, and organization of the information. And as culture is shaped as a cooperative effort along the generations, the human organism is always and without exception a lived body in which history and biography are woven together with interpersonal meaning as well as individual purpose. While humans create and convey meaning in coexistence with other humans, every person nevertheless interprets experience within his own horizon which only partly coincides with "all the others," even within the same cultural circle or society. Such interpretation does not disappear in reality, even when scientific methodology excludes these elements from the study—and thereby from science (18).

By disregarding experience, science also disregards the effects of culture on human action. Since the meaning of a situation has strong cultural bindings—something regarded as an upsetting event in one culture may go quite unnoticed in another—there are reasons to anticipate a major contribution of culture to variation in psychoneuroimmunological development and function. The habit of including a relatively homogenous group of participants from Western, Educated, Industrialized, Rich, and Democratic (WEIRD) societies in psychoneuroimmunological studies thus effectively precludes the chance of understanding variation across human populations (19). There are even reasons to believe that these WEIRD individuals are amongst the least representative members one could use to generalize across human populations.

4. Restructuring the Explanatory Gap

Human beings come into the world with naturally selected coping mechanisms. And since these mechanisms have evolutionary preconditions, it is a task for science to ask whether or not such preconditions interfere with man's perception of the Umwelt in a true manner.

There are two reasons why this question is important—first, a science that aims to understand humans has to know how humans experience the world and second, a science that aims to understand the world must have an idea of science's own foundations for knowledge acquisition. Exactly such preconditions and preconceptions have been given critical attention by researchers in the phenomenological tradition (20) and their investigations are thus in many ways supplementary to the Uexküllian tradition.

The phenomenological tradition has made huge efforts to understand the human experiential dimension and thus make it accessible to investigation. As the phenomenologist sees it, any biological individual accesses the Umwelt through a *first-person* perspective. For humans, this is the world as they know it, imbued with meaning and emotions. Any human being has access to a wide range of historically situated knowledge that helps him to respond to external challenges in a meaningful way. The knowledge of each generation is different, and knowledge also differs in different parts of the world. Such knowledge is therefore spatiotemporally restricted.

But human beings can also access knowledge that is true irrespective of time and place. To obtain such valued knowledge, man has to "bracket" his first-person perspective on the world. He has to take a God-like perspective, be the spectator who takes a view from nowhere. The *third-person* perspective, which is the foundational view of science, is not easily achieved. To reach the goal of true knowledge, scientists have to act as disinterested, emotionless, and neutral observers, and so have to undergo a long and arduous training to achieve control over their inborn perceptual capabilities. This is a complicated task, as they have to erase some of their developmentally learned presuppositions.

The degree to which the third-person perspective can be achieved varies widely between the sciences. While mathematicians and logicians can be trained to master their subject in a true "disinterested" manner, it is more questionable whether biologists, social scientists, and humanists can achieve the same degree of perfection. And for a simple reason—biological entities, including human beings, are historically situated; they have a history that matters as to what and who they are. That biological entities, including the nervous, immune, and endocrine systems, have a history, does not, however, imply that they elude investigation by a science with universalizing ambitions. But it does imply that science should make more precise which aspects of the historical entities it can reach firm conclusions about and which it cannot.

Although an arduous task, especially since science constantly develops new concepts and exploratory technologies that push the line of demarcation between knowledge and ignorance, it does appear evident, at least for the time being, that science cannot reach the innermost experiences of an individual. Science can for example explore the general effects of major life events, but how each individual experiences a divorce or the loss of a beloved one is a private matter. It thus appears necessary to make an analytic distinction between a *public* first-person perspective, which is amenable for scientific investigations, and a *private* first-person perspective which is not. The private perspective is a specific characteristic of each individual, be it a human being or a perceptual system. And as such, it has no characteristics that can be generalized—it is thus located beyond the realms of science. The public first-person perspective is, on the other hand, accessible from the outside. It includes perceptual traits that are specific for a given species, and is as such co-extensional with the animal's Umwelt.

While the public first-person aspect can be made explicit by means of genetic, environmental, and developmental investigations, the private first-person aspect is an experiential dimension and as such not accessible for scientific investigation. Such experience does not lend itself easily to standardized interpretation; it is always an experience of something for someone, in a unique context. There is thus a gap between what science can explain and what it cannot—and the gap goes straight through the individual, between the private and public aspects of the first-person. Nonetheless, exactly where the line of accessibility should be drawn is a matter on which science should have a saying. The explanatory gap should be made more precise, but prospects for its closing are for the time being dim.

5. Relations: All the Way

Some of the most surprising knowledge coming out of the genomics research programs has been novel insights into man's relations with the environment as well as to himself. Not only have the sequencing efforts yielded rich empirical crops, they have in addition highlighted the importance of different analytic perspectives. The latter is perhaps made most apparent by recent efforts to understand relations between hosts and their microbes.

Ever since the microbiological revolution in the late eighteen hundreds, led by Louis Pasteur and Robert Koch, microbes have been conceptualized as external enemies against which man had to fight a war. Although the perspective has been extremely rewarding in terms of lives saved by vaccines and antibiotics, the war metaphor has been seriously misleading as an aid to understand man's microbial Umwelt. Only about 100 microbial species regularly infect human beings and cause disease, while millions of others either ignore us or they cooperate with us in an evolutionary selected manner, thus making their absence—not their presence—the real problem.

Several new observations derived from investigations of the human genome as well as from the microbial communities that colonize our mucous membranes and skin have made evident that it is no longer possible to conceptualize microbes as simply "external." They are internal and cooperative as well. The sequencing of the human genome made clear that our chromosomes are teemed with microbially derived elements. The genome consists of 45% transposons—DNA sequences that are able to copy and move within chromosomes—of which approximately 8% are retrovirus-like (21). Some of these retroviral integrations have been of great importance for vertebrate physiological development. Although most transposons that accumulate in the genome have no known function, they contribute a large potential substrate for the evolution and development of regulatory networks (22, 23).

The genome also contains bacterially derived DNA, some of which regulates the interaction between the eukaryotic cells and their bacterially derived mitochondrial symbionts. The mitochondria, which have evolved to become an integral part of the host's cells, have transferred some of their genes to the cell's nucleus. And in so doing, they lost the ability to reproduce freely. This loss has, however, been matched by a comparative gain in survival capacity—mitochondria, by their very location, have become shielded off from immune destruction. The importance of keeping the interaction between the eukaryotic cell and its mitochondria tightly regulated is dramatically spelled out during debilitating physical trauma in which mitochondria relocate or become destroyed. This leads to a breakdown of the conditions for cooperation between the host cell and the symbiont, and the host may thus develop a dangerous systemic inflammatory response. The response includes fever, low blood pressure and increased heart rate (24), and is thus analogous to the inflammatory process observed as a result of contaminating bacteria during sepsis.

Another surprising observation that came out of the sequencing of the human genome was the relative paucity of genes. Based on complexity estimates, man was thought to have about 100,000 genes prior to the sequencing. But only about 25,000 genes were detected. Man was as complex as before, so how could the complexity be accounted for by so few genes? One answer has to do with the way the DNA is used for making proteins and regulatory factors, and it has turned out that this process is far more efficient than first thought (25). But this is not the whole story; additional data have since revealed that humans also have access to a plethora of genes not coded for in the genome. And these genes, which are located within bacteria and viruses on the skin and the mucous membranes, by far outnumber the genes in the cellular nucleus. Estimates have indicated that an adult human being is composed of 10^{13} eukaryotic and 10^{14} prokaryotic cells, and human beings can thus be described as super-organisms consisting of 90% prokaryotic and 10% eukaryotic cells. Since every bacterium may be infected with as many as 100 bacteriophages, thus giving an estimate of ten billion viruses in each gram of human feces, there is definitely a plethora of genes availably within the human niche (26, 27).

The community of intestinal microbes, termed the microbiota, which establishes itself shortly after birth, reaches adult levels in early childhood. Although influenced by changes in diet and life events, the microbiota appears to be relatively resilient to alterations caused by stressful life events and antibiotic treatments. Its non-random organization depends on both host genetics and environmental exposure of microbes (28–30), but relatively little is known about the rules of its assembly or how the human body controls microbiota composition (31). Neither is much known about what constitutes a healthy microbiome—the collection of genes in these organisms—nor on how this in turn influences human health. Nevertheless, evidence increasingly converge on the hypothesis that gut microbes may shape the host metabolic and immune systems and thus influence the development of obesity, diabetes, and other inflammatory diseases (32, 33).

It is by now well established that the microbiota regulates the developing immune system (34), and that it likely played a critical role in the evolution of the adaptive immune system (35). There is also accumulating evidence demonstrating that the gut microbiota can modulate brain development and thus behavior. For example, a recent study revealed that mice raised in germ-free conditions have significantly increased motor activity and decreased anxiety as compared to mice with normally colonized intestines (36). Furthermore, when re-colonized with microbes, the developmental deficits in the germ-free pups normalized while re-colonization of adult germ-free mice did not, thus suggesting that there is a developmental window during which the microbiota is critical to brain development.

The mechanisms by which the gut microbiota effectuate changes in synaptic connections, which provide the essential substrate for functional brain networks that underlie perception, cognition, and action, are still not known. But since the microbiota has an effect on immune cells, it seems likely that some of the effects are mediated by signals from these cells. This interpretation is supported by evidence showing that the immune system is capable of modulating brain function both during development and adulthood (37). In addition, the vagus nerve, which plays an important role in the transmission of immune information from gut to brain as well as from brain to gut (38, 39), apparently also plays an important role during development of the microbiota–brain communication.

Given the bidirectional flow of regulatory signals between the microbiota and the brain, it should come as little surprise that psychological stress leads to altered intestinal barrier function (40) and host–microbiota interactions (41). Increasing values of psychological stress also negatively affects the immune system (42), as demonstrated by reduced antibody responses to vaccines (43). There thus appears to be a close connection between the hypothalamic–pituitary–adrenal (HPA)-axis, the autonomic nervous system, the gut, the kidneys, and the immune system, and this connection is mediated via cortisol, neuronal transmitters, cytokines, and hormones (44).

The long-time observation—that infectious disease is too complex to be analyzed exclusively in terms of mechanistic interactions between the immune system and the pathogen—has thus received rich empirical support. Adaptive systems are relational all the way, and to understand a given interaction, we have to understand a whole lot more than the target system. To define immunocompetence singularly in terms of internal molecular and cellular properties of the immune system is, accordingly, misconceived. This way of understanding immunocompetence provides a one-sided and thus insufficient understanding. Immunocompetence should rather be understood as a relational property that transcends the boundaries of the organism. To understand immunocompetence is thus to understand how the individual's immune system relates to the other adaptive systems as well as to the organism's Umwelt. Accordingly, organisms may be immunocompetent despite harboring deficient immune resources. And conversely, immunocompetence may be reduced despite the presence of a well-functioning immune system. It all comes down to how the relations develop.

6. The "Early Origins" Scheme

The relevance of external inputs, in the form of infection or stress, is in many ways dependent upon the internal wirings of the experiencing organism's adaptive systems. And since these wirings are laid down during the developmental process, it follows that development is of tremendous importance for the organism's adaptability. The now obvious idea that development is an integral part of evolutionary biology was, nevertheless, largely ignored by evolutionary biologists from about 1900 to about 1980 (45). The separation of the fields was so extensive that when Mayr (46) in an influential paper discussed cause and effect in biology, he still distinguished between evolutionary and developmental biology as of two separate explanatory fields that differed in methods, explanatory projects, and concepts.

During the making of the "modern synthesis" of evolution in the 1930s, in which Darwin's theory of natural selection was blended with the rediscovered Mendelian genetics, evolution was portrayed as an interplay between mutation and selection, with the former providing a supply of variation and the latter acting as a fitness-based sieve (45). In the case of unicellular organisms, this representation is fairly accurate. But in the case of multicellular organisms, where genes serve as modulators of biochemical and physiological parameters that in turn influence the growth of embryonic tissues, the effects of mutation on fitness are not directly accessible for selection. Since selection works on phenotypes and their functional characteristics, since development is a major determinant on the multicellular organism's phenotype, and since some ontogenetic trajectories are better for reproducing and survival than their competitors, development is important for the pathway taken by natural selection.

Development impinges on evolution because it ties the organism up in a system of references to other living and non-living entities in-between fertilization and death. Hence, organismal life is not simply conforming to a predetermined trajectory but follows a variable path upon which developmental decisions are influential. Genes, the "master modulators" of the modern synthesis, are thus acting more as context sensitive difference makers than as determining factors; genes make regulatory factors, signaling molecules, enzymes, and receptors that interact with each other in highly regulated networks, and these are all strongly modulated by epigenetic processes, including histone modification and DNA-methylation (47). Thus, identical twins with the same genetic make-up may turn out quite different owing to epigenetic processes and developmental plasticity (48).

Epigenetic and developmental processes have been evolutionary selected because they adapt organisms to the environment. But, as has been increasingly recognized, they have maladaptive potential as well. This may occur if environmental signals, for instance such that were required for the establishment of proper DNA transcription or stable patterns of interaction between cells of the adaptive systems, change in salient ways. The so-called hygiene hypothesis, the best-reasoned theory for the epidemic-like recent increase in allergy and autoimmunity, utilizes this explanatory framework. According to the hypothesis, humans of today experience an absence of stimuli from microbes which are important for the functional development of the immune system. This creates an input-deficiency syndrome, thus leading to malfunctional development of the regulatory cells of the immune system (49, 50). Although little is known about why one kind of inflammatory disease develops instead of another, or why it develops in one individual but not in another, compelling evidence indicate that the malfunctioning develops as a consequence of perturbations to the long co-evolutionary relationships between intestinal microbes and their vertebrate hosts (51).

Not only does the hygiene hypothesis tell a story of how the microbial Umwelt affects the maturing immune system, it additionally tells the story of how human beings affect their microbial Umwelt. Man, being an expert niche constructor (14), is capable of changing his environment at an astonishing rate—for better and worse. On the better side, epidemiological data from European countries have taught us that human life expectancy was about 25 years until the mid eighteenth century (52). Up to that time the leading cause of death was infectious diseases in childhood, and so the increasing life expectancy primarily reflected progress in the control of infectious disease; in the mid-nineteenth century by means of hygiene, in the late-nineteenth century by vaccines, and by antibiotics in the mid-twentieth century. The adaptations were thus of cultural type rather than adjustments of immunity by natural selection.

The downside is that the constructed niche gives rise to a mismatch between man's biologically derived response patterns and environmental challenges. The westernization of society has, for example, made food available in large quantities. And along with better housing and health conditions, the struggle for daily survival has almost vanished. But this change has by no means ended life's struggles—man has instead become increasingly susceptible to developmental aberrations and precipitation of various diseases, including coronary heart disease, diabetes, hypertension, as well as cognitive and psychological impairment (53, 54).

7. The Paradox of Deterioration

As of today, individuals in low and middle income countries in Africa have a life expectancy of 49 years, while people in high income European countries may expect to live until they reach the age of 80 years (55). It is still the young that die in Africa—46% of all deaths in Africa are children aged under 15 years, whereas only 20% are 60 years or older. In contrast, only 1% of deaths in high income countries are in children less than 15 years, whereas 84% are aged 60 years and over. This uneven distribution of death is matched by a similar uneven distribution of causes—while infectious disease is still the major cause of death in Africa, people in Western societies die from cardiovascular disease and cancer.

Owing to the remarkable postponement of death that has occurred during the last 100 years, folk increasingly develop degenerative diseases of the adaptive systems, including diabetes, Alzheimer's disease, and immunodeficiency—death rates for people over 65 years of age compared to people aged 25–44 are, for example, 43-fold for cancer and 89-fold for pneumonia and influenza (56). Aging people thus struggle with a loss of integrity, in many ways a truly astonishing phenomenon since it suggests that the adaptive systems, which produce and maintain themselves during development, are unable to perform the seemingly much simpler task of maintaining what is already formed. This paradox of deterioration is a real challenge for scientists that aim to predict and control the psychoneuroimmunological systems. Unfortunately, the paradox' solution provides little theoretical support for the achievement of therapeutic control.

As summarized by Mayr (46), there are two principled kinds of cause in biology—proximate causes that give explanations in terms of developmental and physiological mechanisms, and ultimate causes which provide explanations in terms of evolutionary mechanisms. The two are connected by evolutionary time—the ultimate causes shape the proximate causes. And since natural selection is a progressive force, one would expect evolution to shape developmental systems to near optimal functioning. But, as elaborated by Williams (57), natural selection works on genes that enhance reproduction, not longevity. And the genes responsible for aging may thus be kept in the gene pool by selection on their beneficial effects to the young that possess them and not owing to their detrimental effects in senescence. This phenomenon, termed antagonistic pleiotropy, explains why the selective pressure on machinery responsible for maintenance of genomic and cellular integrity in aging tissues has been insignificant (58).

Since infectious disease has been a major threat to the survival of young children and thus to their reproductive potential, natural selection should be expected to shape the immune system so as to increase its efficiency during the early years of life. And as evidenced by observational data, production of inflammatory mediators by the innate immune system complies well with the antagonistic pleiotropic framework. The importance of a highly active innate immune system has been corroborated by comparative data between African and European populations. The data strongly suggest that individuals of African ancestry have a more active inflammatory response, perhaps owing to a greater burden of infectious disease (59). Furthermore, emerging evidence indicates that pro-inflammatory genotypes are associated with a higher incidence of inflammatory disease in later life, including atherosclerosis, diabetes, and cancer (60). The selection for a strong pro-inflammatory immune response, which is necessary to resist otherwise fatal infections in early life, is thus—as predicted by Williams' hypothesis—a double edge sword; the overproduction of inflammatory molecules may cause inflammatory diseases and even death later in life. Natural selection thus gives rise to mechanisms that both create and destroy the organism.

Surprising data from the last couple of years have even shown that this overproduction may be enhanced by various cultural "practices." Early experiences, which can affect adult health either by cumulative damage over time or by adversities that take place during sensitive periods (61), can take dramatic and often unexpected courses. Experience of maltreatment in childhood is, for example, a strong predictor of adult inflammation (62), and, more specifically, increases the risk for autoimmune disease (63). To control such malfunctions psychoneuroimmunologists thus have to treat culture no less than biology.

Also the adaptive immune system follows the logic laid down by Williams, but in a modified form. Newborn children come with immature adaptive immune systems and thus have to rely on maternally derived IgG and IgA for their first 6 months of life. However, this immunodeficiency of the young does not contradict Williams' prediction. Adaptive systems are designed by natural selection to mature over the life course and so their seeming failure in early life is part of their developmental program. The same goes for their deteriorating function with age, as evidenced by increasing tendencies to autoimmunity and immunodeficiencies, and as predicted by the antagonistic pleiotropy framework. For the adaptive immune system this malfunctioning is partly owing to a reconfiguration of T cell immunity, manifesting as the accumulation of senescent and dysfunctional cells (64), and a shift in subpopulation frequency as well as expressed repertoire of antibodies and T cell receptors (65).

8. Summing Up

Compelling evidence has demonstrated that early environments are important determinants of nervous, endocrine, and immune functions over the life course. As adaptive systems seem inherently disposed to degeneration, and since the prospects of controlling such evolutionary selected disintegration seem dim, a major aim of psychoneuroimmunological investigations should be to lay out early conditions that serve to increase the integrative processes and, of no less importance, to delay the disintegrative processes. Such investigations should acknowledge the importance of the experiential dimension, and should take a life cycle perspective in which the organism's timely unfolding is correlated to salient environmental contingencies. To develop, the organism needs to extract resources from the environment, and variation in the organism's local ecology will thus in large part determine the levels of available resources and thus the developmental course.

References

1. Ader R (1981) Psychoneuroimmunology. Academic, New York
2. Good RA (1981) Foreword: interactions of the body's major networks. In: Ader R (ed) Psychoneuroimmunology. Academic, New York, pp xvii–xix
3. Plaut SM, Friedman SB (1981) Psychosocial factors in infectious disease. In: Ader R (ed) Psychoneuroimmunology. Academic, New York., pp 3–30
4. Wittgenstein L (1960) The blue and brown books. Harper & Row, New York
5. Biondi M, Picardi A (1999) Psychological stress and neuroendocrine function in humans: the last two decades of research. Psychother Psychosom 68:114–150

6. Kull K (2001) Jakob von Uexküll: an introduction. Semiotica 134:1–59
7. Uexküll J (1982) The theory of meaning (original 1940). Semiotica 42:25–82
8. Ulvestad E (2007) Defending life. The nature of host-parasite relations. Springer, Dordrecht
9. Hoffmeyer J (2008) Biosemiotics. An examination into the signs of life and the life of signs. University of Scranton Press, Scranton
10. Hill K, Kaplan H (1999) Life history traits in humans: theory and empiricial studies. Annu Rev Anthropol 28:397–430
11. Craig AD (2009) How do you feel – now? The anterior insula and human awareness. Nat Rev Neurosci 10:59–70
12. Craig AD (2004) Human feelings: why are some more aware than others? Trends Cogn Sci 8:239–241
13. Frith C (2008) Making up the mind. How the brain creates our mental world. Blackwell, Oxford
14. Odling-Smee FJ, Laland KN, Feldman MW (2003) Niche construction. The neglected process in evolution. Princeton University Press, Princeton
15. Sterelny K (2007) Social intelligence, human intelligence and niche construction. Philos Trans R Soc Lond B Biol Sci 362:719–730
16. Laland KN, Odling-Smee J, Myles S (2010) How culture shaped the human genome: bringing genetics and the human sciences together. Nat Rev Genet 11:137–148
17. Beauregard M (2007) Mind does really matter: evidence from neuroimaging studies of emotional self-regulation, psychotherapy, and placebo effect. Prog Neurobiol 81:218–236
18. Getz L, Kirkengen AL, Ulvestad E (2011) The human biology – saturated with experience. J Nor Med Assoc 131:683–687
19. Henrich J, Heine SJ, Norenzayan A (2010) The weirdest people in the world? Behav Brain Sci 33:61–83
20. Gallagher S, Zahavi D (2008) The phenomenological mind. An introduction to philosophy of mind and cognitive science. Routledge, London
21. International human genome consortium (2001) Initial sequencing and analysis of the human genome. Nature 409:860–921
22. Kurth R, Bannert N (2010) Beneficial and detrimental effects of human endogenous retroviruses. Int J Cancer 126:306–314
23. Venner S, Feschotte C, Biémont C (2009) Dynamics of transposable elements: towards a community ecology of the genome. Trends Genet 25:317–323
24. Zhang Q, Raoof M, Chen Y et al (2010) Circulating mitochondrial DAMPs cause inflammatory responses to injury. Nature 464: 104–107
25. Sholtis SJ, Noonan JP (2010) Gene regulation and the origins of human biological uniqueness. Trends Genet 26:110–118
26. Dethlefsen L, McFall-Ngai M, Relman DA (2007) An ecological and evolutionary perspective on human-microbe mutualism and disease. Nature 449:811–818
27. Pennisi E (2011) Going viral: exploring the role of viruses in our bodies. Science 331:1513
28. Spor A, Koren O, Ley R (2011) Unravelling the effects of the environment and host genotype on the gut microbiome. Nat Rev Microbiol 9:279–290
29. Turnbaugh PJ, Hamady M, Yatsunenko T et al (2009) A core gut microbiome in obese and lean twins. Nature 457:480–484
30. Reyes A, Haynes M, Hanson N et al (2010) Viruses in the faecal microbiota of monozygotic twins and their mothers. Nature 466:334–338
31. Gonzalez A, Clemente JC, Shade A et al (2011) Our microbial selves: what ecology can teach us. EMBO Rep 12:775–784
32. Nicholson JK, Holmes E, Wilson ID (2005) Gut microorganisms, mammalian metabolism and personalized health care. Nat Rev Microbiol 3:431–438
33. Musso G, Gambino R, Cassader M (2011) Interactions between gut microbiota and host metabolism predisposing to obesity and diabetes. Annu Rev Med 62:361–380
34. Ivanov II, Littman DR (2011) Modulation of immune homeostasis by commensal bacteria. Curr Opin Microbiol 14:106–114
35. Lee YK, Mazmanian SK (2010) Has the microbiota played a critical role in the evolution of the adaptive immune system? Science 330:1768–1773
36. Heijtz RD, Wang S, Anuar F et al (2011) Normal gut microbiota modulates brain development and behavior. Proc Natl Acad Sci U S A 108:3047–3052
37. Boulanger LM (2009) Immune proteins in brain development and synaptic plasticity. Neuron 64:93–109
38. Van Der Zanden EP, Boeckxstaens GE, de Jonge WJ (2009) The vagus nerve as a modulator of intestinal inflammation. Neurogastroenterol Motil 21:6–17
39. Tracey KJ (2010) Understanding immunity requires more than immunology. Nat Immunol 1:561–564

40. Gareau MG, Silva MA, Perdue MH (2008) Pathophysiological mechanisms of stress-induced intestinal damage. Curr Mol Med 8: 274–281
41. Söderholm JD, Yang PC, Ceponis P et al (2002) Chronic stress induces mast cell-dependent bacterial adherence and initiates mucosal inflammation in rat intestine. Gastroenterology 123:1099–1108
42. Padgett DA, Glaser R (2003) How stress influences the immune response. Trends Immunol 24:444–448
43. Li J, Cowden LG, King JD et al (2007) Effects of chronic stress and interleukin-10 gene polymorphisms on antibody response to tetanus vaccine in family caregivers of patients with Alzheimer's disease. Psychosom Med 69: 551–559
44. McEwen BS, Gianaros PJ (2011) Stress- and allostasis-induced brain plasticity. Annu Rev Med 62:431–445
45. Hamburger V (1980) Embryology and the modern synthesis in evolutionary theory. In: Mayr E, Provine WB (eds) The evolutionary synthesis. Harvard University Press, Cambridge, pp 96–112
46. Mayr E (1961) Cause and effect in biology. Science 134:1501–1506
47. Reik W (2007) Stability and flexibility of epigenetic gene regulation in mammalian development. Nature 447:425–432
48. Fraga MF, Ballestar E, Paz MF et al (2005) Epigenetic differences arise during the lifetime of monozygotic twins. Proc Natl Acad Sci U S A 102:10604–10609
49. Rook GA (2010) 99th Dahlem conference on infection, inflammation and chronic inflammatory disorders: Darwinian medicine and the 'hygiene' or 'old friends' hypothesis. Clin Exp Immunol 160:70–79
50. Okada H, Kuhn C, Feillet H et al (2010) The 'hygiene hypothesis' for autoimmune and allergic diseases: an update. Clin Exp Immunol 160:1–9
51. Fitzsimmons CM, Dunne DW (2009) Survival of the fittest: allergology or parasitology? Trends Parasitol 25:447–451
52. Cairns J (1997) Matters of life and death. Perspectives on public health, molecular biology, cancer and the prospects for the human race. Princeton University Press, Princeton
53. Gluckman P, Hanson M (2005) The fetal matrix: evolution, development and disease. Cambridge University Press, Cambridge
54. Osmond C, Barker DJ (2000) Fetal, infant, and childhood growth are predictors of coronary heart disease, diabetes, and hypertension in adult men and women. Environ Health Perspect 108(suppl 3):545–553
55. World Health Organization (2008) The global burden of disease 2004 update. WHO Press, Geneva
56. Troen BR (2003) The biology of aging. Mt Sinai J Med 70:3–22
57. Williams GC (1957) Pleiotropy, natural selection, and the evolution of senescence. Evolution 11:398–411
58. De S (2011) Somatic mosaicism in healthy human tissues. Trends Genet 27:217–223
59. Pennington R, Gatenbee C, Kennedy B et al (2009) Group differences in proneness to inflammation. Infect Genet Evol 9:1371–1380
60. Licastro F, Candore G, Lio D et al (2005) Innate immunity and inflammation in ageing: a key for understanding age-related diseases. Immun Ageing 2:8
61. Shonkoff JP, Boyce WT, McEwen BS (2009) Neuroscience, molecular biology, and the childhood roots of health disparities: building a new framework for health promotion and disease prevention. JAMA 301:2252–2259
62. Danese A, Pariante CM, Caspi A et al (2007) Childhood maltreatment predicts adult inflammation in a life-course study. Proc Natl Acad Sci U S A 104:1319–1324
63. Dube SR, Fairweather D, Pearson WS et al (2009) Cumulative childhood stress and autoimmune diseases in adults. Psychosom Med 71: 243–250
64. Pawelec G, Akbar A, Caruso C et al (2004) Is immunosenescence infectious? Trends Immunol 25:406–410
65. Miller RA (1996) The aging immune system: primer and prospectus. Science 273:70–74

Chapter 3

Psychosocial Job Stress and Immunity: A Systematic Review

Akinori Nakata

Abstract

The purpose of this review was to provide current knowledge about the possible association between psychosocial job stress and immune parameters in blood, saliva, and urine. Using bibliographic databases (PubMed, PsychINFO, Web of Science, Medline) and the snowball method, 56 studies were found. In general, exposure to psychosocial job stress (high job demands, low job control, high job strain, job dissatisfaction, high effort–reward imbalance, overcommitment, burnout, unemployment, organizational downsizing, economic recession) had a measurable impact on immune parameters (reduced NK cell activity, NK and T cell subsets, CD4+/CD8+ ratio, and increased inflammatory markers). The evidence supports that psychosocial job stresses are related to disrupted immune responses but further research is needed to demonstrate cause–effect relationships.

Key words: Psychosocial job stress, Immune system, Psychoneuroimmunology, Systematic review, Work environment

1. Background

A poor psychosocial work environment has been linked with a broad array of adverse health outcomes. Studies have demonstrated that prolonged exposure to psychosocial job stress increases the risk for coronary heart disease (1–3), hypertension (4), immune-related disorders (5), musculoskeletal disorders (6), depression (7, 8), poor mental health (9), and stress-related disorders (10), as well as adverse health behaviors such as alcohol dependence, substance misuse, physical inactivity, poor sleep, and obesity (11–14). To elucidate the mechanisms responsible for these effects, researchers have explored the relationship between psychosocial job stress and the immune system, the body's chief defense against numerous diseases.

Qing Yan (ed.), *Psychoneuroimmunology: Methods and Protocols*, Methods in Molecular Biology, vol. 934,
DOI 10.1007/978-1-62703-071-7_3, © Springer Science+Business Media, LLC 2012

Psychoneuroimmunology (PNI) studies have shown that exposure to psychological stress is associated with a variety of immune indicators (15, 16). Stress is known to activate the sympathetic nervous system leading to changes in peripheral adrenaline and noradrenaline secretions, while a variety of endocrine factors such as cortisol, prolactin, and growth hormone are altered through the hypothalamic-pituitary function. The immune system receives signals from the central nervous system and endocrine system to respond and adapt to the stimuli, i.e., stress. If stress is manageable, it may promote adaptation. However, if stress is persistent and difficult to manage, it can lead over time to wear and tear on the body and brain, consequently causing multiple physiological dysfunctions, i.e., allostatic load (17). Psychosocial job stresses are often related to the latter, which may lead to irreversible or incurable health conditions if stress cannot be managed (18, 19).

This chapter contains a systematic literature review specifically focused on psychosocial job stress and the immune response. First, the types of psychosocial job stressors studied in this area are listed. Second, the immunological indicators generally selected for studies of the relationship between psychosocial job stress and immunity and the primary functions and roles of these parameters are explained. Third, evidence will be provided about how psychosocial job stress may alter immune responses.

2. Method

A systematic review of all English articles using PubMed, PsychINFO, Web of Science, and Medline was conducted to identify all observational studies assessing the association between psychosocial job stress and the immune system. References from relevant reviews and articles ("snowball method") were also scrutinized. The search terms included: *job stress*, *occupational stress*, *work stress*, *job strain*, *job control*, *job demands*, *workload*, *job satisfaction*, *effort–reward imbalance*, *overcommitment*, *unemployment*, *burnout*, *overwork*, *social support at work*, *supervisor support*, *and coworker support* in combination with the selected immunological markers: *lymphocyte*, *natural killer (NK) cell*, *helper T cell*, *cytotoxic T cell*, *CD4*, *CD3*, *CD8*, *CD25*, *CD27*, *CD28*, *CD29*, *CD45RA*, *CD45RO*, *immunoglobulin (Ig)*, *IgA*, *IgG*, *IgM*, *IgD*, *IgE*, *cytokine*, *interleukin*, *inflammation*, *C-reactive protein (CRP)*, *complement component* as well as more general immunological terms: *immune system*, *immune function*, and *immunity*. Studies were included in our review if they were studies of workers and had immunological outcomes using blood, saliva, or urine. Overall, 56 studies were identified for the period ending August 2011 and the sample sizes of these studies ranged from 25 to 1,563.

3. Results

A list of psychosocial job stress measures frequently used in PNI research is presented in Table 1. As shown in this table, a number of subjective and objective measures have been used to define job stress. Some measures derive from theory-based models and measure subjective feelings about the job. Job stress may be also be defined objectively by work environment changes such as unemployment, organizational downsizing, and economic recession. Most studies are based on subjective feelings (how employees perceive job stress) as a measure of stress.

Table 2 shows the examples of immune (-related) indicators frequently investigated in job stress research. As shown in this table, functional and quantitative aspects of immune markers are measured. NK cell activity (NKCA) and lymphocyte transformation tests are typical functional parameters while measurement of lymphocyte subsets, immunoglobulins, and cytokine concentrations are classified as quantitative parameters.

Tables 3, 4, and 5 as well as Tables 6, 7, and 8 present the summary of the studies reviewed. Tables 3, 4, and 5 present the possible associations between psychosocial job stressors and cellular immune markers while Tables 6, 7, and 8 summarize the relationships between psychosocial job stressors, humoral immune markers, and cytokine concentrations. If a study found a statistically significant relationship, the association was indicated in Tables 3, 4, 5, 6, 7, and 8 as a positive (↑) or negative (↓) association. If the study measured immune parameters but found no significant associations, it was stated as non-significant (NS). There were 46 cross-sectional and 10 prospective studies of which 49 studies used blood, six used saliva, and one used urine samples. There were 27 studies from Europe (Norway, Sweden, Finland, Netherland, Germany, Switzerland, Belgium, Italy, and UK), 19 studies from Asia (Japan, Korea, Malaysia, Singapore, and China), four studies from the Middle East (Israel), three studies from Oceania (Australia and New Zealand), and three studies from the US.

4. Discussion

4.1. Job Strain and Immunity

The job demands-control (JDC) model (hereafter referred to as the job strain model) is one of the most influential job stress models in occupational stress research. Because it is spare, practical, and testable, it has been widely adopted in occupational health studies. According to Karasek, a limited number of job-related psychosocial risk factors (job control/decision latitude and job demands) can be combined in a simple theoretical framework (job strain)

Table 1
List of psychosocial job stress measures frequently used in job stress research

	Type of job stresses
Subjective stress measures	Job demands (*job strain model*) Job control (*job strain model*) Job strain (*job demands/job control*) Effort (*effort–reward imbalance model*) Reward (*effort–reward imbalance model*) Overcommitment (*effort–reward imbalance model*) Social support at work (*job strain model*) Supervisor support (*job strain model*) Coworker support (*job strain model*) Workload (*NIOSH generic job stress model*, etc.) Variance in workload (*NIOSH generic job stress model*) Job dissatisfaction Role conflict (*NIOSH generic job stress model*) Role ambiguity (*NIOSH generic job stress model*) Mental/cognitive demands (*NIOSH generic job stress model*) Interpersonal conflict Skill underutilization (*NIOSH generic job stress model*) Burnout (*Maslach, Shirom*)
Objective stress measures	Unemployment Job insecurity Organizational downsizing/restructuring Economic recession Overtime/overwork

that can be an important determinant of worker health (20). Job control refers to employees' control over their tasks and how those tasks are executed, while job demands are psychological stressors (e.g., time pressure, conflicting demands, reaction time required, work amount, degree of concentration required, etc.) in the work environment. The job strain model postulates that job stress becomes highest when job demands are high and job control is low. A number of studies have demonstrated that job strain predicts coronary heart disease (3), stroke (21), type 2 diabetes (22), musculoskeletal pain (23), depression (7), sickness absence (24), and poor psychological well-being (25).

The job strain model is the most prevalent model used in studies of the psychosocial work environment and immunity and there are 12 studies reported to date (19, 26–36). One of the first studies that examined this relationship was from Sweden. In a sample of 49 workers with different occupations (air traffic controllers, waiters, physicians, etc.), Theorell et al. (1990) examined how job strain and workplace social support affected serum IgG levels and found

Table 2
Examples of immune (-related) indicators frequently used in job stress research

Indicators	Major roles/functions
Functional parameters	
Natural killer cell activity (NKCA)	NK cells are large granular cells possessing killer activity against certain tumor cells and virus-infected cells without prior sensitization. Reduced NKCA often indicates poor resistance to tumor cells and virus infected cells, leading to a higher cancer incidence and infection
Lymphocyte transformation test (mitogen stimulation)	A functional test of the ability of lymphocytes to respond to chemical substances called mitogens that encourage a cell to commence cell division triggering mitosis. There are several commonly used mitogens, i.e., phytohemagglutinin A (PHA), concanavalin A (ConA), and pokeweed mitogen (PWM); PPD (tuberculin), Candida antigen, and streptokinase-streptodornase. Lower value often indicates poor response to pathogens/antigens and reduced cellular immune function
CD4+/CD8+ ratio	An indicator for the status of the cellular immune system. The value depends on a balance of CD4+ and CD8+ T cells. The normal (non-clinical) range is between 0.60 and 220. Lower values are often found in HIV-infected patients and those with compromised immune system
Quantitative parameters	
Natural killer (NK) cells	Kill certain tumor and virus-infected cells. Lower counts may reflect poor resistance to tumor cells and virus-infected cells
B cells	Antibody (immunoglobulin, gammaglobulin) production. An extreme decrease of B cells is considered to be associated with suppression in production of immunoglobulins
T cells	Directly attack foreign antigens and regulate the immune system. An excessive increase of T cells is known to be associated with systemic inflammation, whereas a persistent decrease of T cells is related to immunodeficiency and psychological disorders such as depression
Cytotoxic T cells (CD8+)	Lysis of virus-infected cells, tumor cells, or allografted cells. Lower counts may reflect poor resistance to virus-infected cells and tumor cells
Helper T cells (CD4+)	Facilitate B cell proliferation and differentiation, immunoglobulin synthesis, assist cytotoxic T cells attacking antigens. An excessive increase in counts is associated with inflammation while a decrease of counts is found in HIV-infected patients
Memory T cells (CD4+ CD45RO+)	Subset of helper T cells that respond to previously encountered antigens. This cell can reproduce to mount a faster and stronger immune response than the first time the immune system responded to the antigens. Higher counts indicate inflammation while lower counts are often found in people exposed to hazardous chemical factors
Naive T cells (CD4+ CD45RA+)	Subset of helper T cells that have not yet encountered antigens. This cell responds to the newly encountered antigens and will turn into a reservoir of memory T cells

(continued)

Table 2 (continued)

Indicators	Major roles/functions
Immunoglobulin G, A, M (IgG, IgA, IgM)	Neutralize bacteria, viruses, and other environmental pathogens. Higher values may indicate primary infection or reactivation/reinfection to antigens
Interleukin (IL)-1	Proinflammatory cytokine primarily secreted by monocytes and macrophages. It stimulates B cells to produce antibody, NK cells to destroy foreign cells, resting T cells to produce more cytokines, and central nervous system to exert sickness behavior
Interleukin (IL)-4	Stimulates proliferation and differentiation of B cells into antibody-secreting cells
Interleukin (IL)-6	IL-6 is the major initiator of acute phase response by hepatocytes and a primary determinant of hepatic CRP production. It has both pro- and anti-inflammatory actions
Interleukin (IL)-10	Anti-inflammatory cytokine produced by T cells and inhibits the synthesis of IL-1 by macrophages and down-regulates expression of major histocompatibility antigens
Interferon (IFN)-γ	IFN-γ is primarily secreted by NK cells and T cells and has an ability to inhibit viral replication
Tumor necrosis factor (TNF)-α and -β	There are two types of tumor necrosis factors: TNF-α and TNF-β. TNF-β is cytotoxic against some tumors that can cause lysis and destruction of the cells. TNF-α stimulates the production of IL-6
Salivary IgA (s-IgA)	S-IgA is one of the antibodies that form a front line of defense in mucosal immunity and it is thought to be indicative of the functional status of the entire mucosal immune system. S-IgA deficiency represents a reduced level of protection for the body, and an increased risk of infection
C-reactive protein (CRP)	CRP is produced by the liver and the level of CRP rises when there is inflammation throughout the body. CRP rises up to 50,000-fold in acute inflammation, such as viral and bacterial infections. It has also been used as a very rough proxy for cardiovascular disease risk

that job strain was associated with an increase of serum IgG level but workplace social support attenuated its effect when job strain was at peak (33). This research group also examined the relationship between job strain and IgG and IgA in human service organizations, but failed to find significant associations between job strain and IgG or IgA (30). Studies from Japan and the Netherlands reported the relationship between job strain and lymphocyte subset counts (26–29). Among shift workers in the Netherlands, high job demands and high job control were related to decreases of CD4+ T cells and CD4+/CD8+ ratio (27). Three studies from Japan consistently reported that job strain was inversely related to counts of NK cells and CD4+ T cell subsets (26, 28, 29). More recent studies have focused on the relationship of job strain with inflammatory markers such as CRP, interleukin (IL)-6, tumor

Table 3
Association between psychosocial job stressors and cellular immune markers (functional markers)

First author	Country	Year	Sample (M/F)	Study design	Occupation	Exposure	NKCA	CD4+/ CD8+	LAA	LTT	Confounders
Arnetz	Sweden	1987	–/25W	L	Unemployed	Unemployment stress				↓	NM/NC
Arnetz	Sweden	1991	78M/246W	L	Blue-collar workers	Unemployment stress				↓	NM/NC
Endresen	Norway	1991	–/94W	CS	Bank employees	Job stress (communication, leadership, relocation, and workload)		NS		NS	NM/NC
Marriot	New Zealand	1994	45	CS	Meat factory workers	Unemployment stress		↓			NM/NC
Meijman	Netherlands	1995	24M/–	CS	Cargo handlers (shift workers)	High job demands		↓			NM/NC
Nakano	Japan	1998	45 (56) M/–	CS, CC	Taxi drivers vs. age-matched controls	Severe economic recession				↓	A
Nakamura	Japan	1999	42M/–	CS	Office workers	Burnout syndrome: Low personal accomplishments (LPA), high depreso-nalization (HD), high emotional exhaustion (HEE)	↓				A, Sm, Al, BMI

(continued)

Table 3 (continued)

First author	Country	Year	Sample (M/F)	Study design	Occupation	Exposure	NKCA	CD4+/CD8+	LAA	LTT	Confounders
Lerman	Israel	1999	68M/111W	CS	Mixed population (69 postg raduate students, 48 laboratory technicians, 46 research associates, 16 other occupations)	Burnout syndrome: High total burnout (HTB), high emotional exhaustion (HEE), high chronic fatigue (HCF), high cognitive weariness (HCW)					S, A, Edu
Morikawa	Japan	2005	–/61W	CS	Nurses	High quantitative workload High conflict with physicians	↓				A
Di Donato	Italy	2006	40M/44W	CS	University and museum employees	Occupational stress	↓				NM/NC
Cohen	USA	2007	96M/104W	L	Unemployed	Unemployment stress (4 months)	↓				A, S, R, Ed, Sm, Med
Kawaguchi	Japan	2007	–/128W	CS	Nurses	High quantitative workload High variance in workload	↓				A, WkEx, WkSch, Sm
Okamoto	Japan	2008	59M/15W	CS	Emergency physicians	Overwork (long work hours)	↓				NM/NC
Boscolo	Italy	2009	88M/–	CS	University employees	High workload High job insecurity	↓				A, Sm, Al

Bosch	Germany	2009	478M/59W	CS	Factory workers	High effort Low reward High ERI High overcommitment Low job control High job demands		↓		A, S, Ms, Ed, Sm, Ex, Al, BMI, PC, Dp
Nakata	Japan	2010	165M/141W	CS	White-collar workers (trading and pharmaceutical companies)	Low job satisfaction	↓			A, Sm, Al, Ex, Edu, Sl, BMI, Med, Dep, Conf
Lee	Korea	2010	–/38W	L	Nurses	High objective stress High subjective stress	NS			A, Sm
Nakata	Japan	2011	165M/141W	CS	White-collar workers (trading and pharmaceutical companies)	Overtime (hours of overtime per month)	NS			S, A, Al, Ex, Edu, Sl, BMI, Med, Dp, Conf, Com, Occup, Jobsat
Nakata	Japan	2011	190M/157W	CS	White-collar workers (trading and pharmaceutical companies)	High effort Low reward High ERI High overcommitment	↓			A, Sm, Al, Ex, Edu, Sl, BMI, Med, Dp, Conf, Com, Occup, Caf

M men; *F* women; *CS* cross-sectional; *CC* case–control; *L* longitudinal; *ERI* effort reward imbalance; *NKCA* natural killer cell activity; *LTT* lymphocyte transformation test; *LAA* leukocyte adhesiveness/aggregation test; *A* age; *S* sex; *R* race; *Ed* educational level; *Ms* marital status; *Sm* smoking; *Al* alcohol consumption; *Ex* physical exercise; *Sl* sleep, *Anx* anxiety; *BMI* body mass index; *Med* medication usage; *Conf* interpersonal conflict at work; *BL* blood lead concentration; *HRT* hormone replacement therapy; *WkEx* work experience; *WkSch* work schedule; *PC* physical condition; *Occup* occupation; *Caf* caffeine intake; *Com* commuting time; *Jobsat* job satisfaction; *IC* income, *NM/NC* not mentioned or not controlled for
↓ = decrease; ↑ = increase; NS = no significant change

Table 4
Association between psychosocial job stressors and cellular immune markers (NK, T and, B cells)

First author	Country	Year	Sample (M/F)	Study design	Occupation	Exposure	T cells	NK cells	B cells	Confounders
Endresen	Norway	1991	–/94W	CS	Bank employees	Job stress (communication, leadership, relocation, and workload)	NS			NM/NC
Marriot	New Zealand	1994	45	CS	Meat factory workers	Unemployment stress	NS	NS	NS	NM/NC
Kawakami	Japan	1997	76M/–	CS	Blue-collar workers (chemical company)	Low job control High job strain				A, Sm, BL
Nakamura	Japan	1999	42M/–	CS	Office workers	Burnout syndrome: Low personal accomplish-ments (LPA), high depresona-lization (HD), high emotional exhaustion (HEE)		↓		A, Sm, Al, BMI
De Gucht	Belgium	1999	17M/43W	CS	Nurses	High nursing stress	NS	NS		NM/NC
Nakata	Japan	2000	116M/–	CS	White-collar workers (power plant operators)	High job strain Low social support at work		↓		A, Sm
Bargellini	Italy	2000	39M/32W	CS	Physicians	Burnout: Low personal accomplishments (LPA), high depresonalization (HD), high emotional exhaustion (HEE)	↓			S, Sm, Occup, WkEx

Nakata	Japan	2002	231M/–	CS	White-collar workers (power plant operators)	Low job control			A, Sm, Al, Ex
Miyazaki	Japan	2003	98M/–	CS	Private company	Low social support		↓		A, Sm
Sakami	Japan	2004	71M/–	CS	Non-smoking firefighters	High quantitative workload	NS			A
Morikawa	Japan	2005	–/61W	CS	Nurses	High quantitative workload High conflict with physicians		NS		A
Miyazaki	Japan	2005	241M (142M)/–	CS	White-collar workers (manufacturing company)	High job demands combined with low social support at work	NS	NS		A, Al, Sm, Ex
Mommersteeg	Netherlands	2006	44M/50W 49 Cases/38 controls	CC	Participants recruited via websites	Burnout	NS	NS	NS	S, A, BMI matched (Med excluded)
Okamoto	Japan	2008	59M/15W	CS	Emergency physicians	Overwork (long work hours)		NS		NM/NC
Nakata	Japan	2010	165M/141W	CS	White-collar workers (trading and pharmaceutical companies)	Low job satisfaction		↓		A, Sm, Al, Ex, Edu, Sl, BMI, Med, Dep, Conf
Amati	Italy	2010	26M/75W	L	Nurses	Low job satisfaction	NS	↑	NS	NM/NC
Lee	Korea	2010	–/38W	L	Nurses	High objective stress High subjective stress	NS	NS	NS	A, Sm

(continued)

Table 4 (continued)

First author	Country	Year	Sample (M/F)	Study design	Occupation	Exposure	T cells	NK cells	B cells	Confounders
Bellingrath	Germany	2010	21M/34W	CS	School teachers	High ERI High over-commitment				A, Med, Dep, Sm
Nakata	Japan	2011	165M/141W	CS	White-collar workers (trading and pharmaceutical companies)	Overtime (hours of overtime per month)	NS	↓	NS	S, A, Al, Ex, Edu, Sl, BMI, Med, Dp, Conf, Com, Occup, Jobsat
Nakata	Japan	2011	190M/157W	CS	White-collar workers (trading and pharmaceutical companies)	High effort Low reward High ERI imbalance High overcommitment	NS	↓	NS	A, Sm, Al, Ex, Edu, Sl, BMI, Med, Dp, Conf, Com, Occup, Caf

M men; *F* women; *CS* cross-sectional; *CC* case–control; *L* longitudinal; *ERI* effort reward imbalance; *NKCA* natural killer cell activity; *LTT* lymphocyte transformation test; *LAA* leukocyte adhesiveness/aggregation test; *A* age; *S* sex; *R* race; *Ed* educational level; *Ms* marital status; *Sm* smoking; *Al* alcohol consumption; *Ex* physical exercise; *Sl* sleep; *Anx* anxiety; *BMI* body mass index; *Med* medication usage; *Conf* interpersonal conflict at work; *BL* blood lead concentration; *HRT* hormone replacement therapy; *WkEx* work experience; *WkSch* work schedule; *PC* physical condition; *Occup* occupation; *Caf* caffeine intake; *Com* commuting time; *Jobsat* job satisfaction; *IC* income; *NM/NC* not mentioned or not controlled for

↓ = decrease; ↑ = increase; NS = no significant change

Table 5
Association between psychosocial job stressors and cellular immune markers (CD4, CD25, CD27, and CD28 subsets)

First author	Country	Year	Sample (M/F)	Study design	Occupation	Exposure	Naïve CD4+ T cells	Memory CD4+ T cells	CD3+ CD25+ cells	CD4+ CD25+ cells	CD27+ CD28+ cells	CD27+ CD28- cells	CD27- CD28- cells	Confounders
Kawakami	Japan	1997	76M/–	CS	Blue-collar workers (chemical company)	Low job control High job strain		↓						A, Sm, BL
De Gucht	Belgium	1999	17M/43W	CS	Nurses	High nursing stress			NS	↑				NM/NC
Nakata	Japan	2000	116M/–	CS	White-collar workers (power plant operators)	High job strain Low social support at work	↓							A, Sm
Nakata	Japan	2002	231M/–	CS	White-collar workers (power plant operators)	Low job control		↓						A, Sm, Al, Ex
Bosch	Germany	2009	478M/59W	CS	Factory workers	High effort Low reward High ERI imbalance High overcommitment Low job control High job demands					NS	↑	↑	A, S, Ms, Ed, Sm, Ex, Al, BMI, PC, Dp

M men; *F* women; *CS* cross-sectional; *CC* case–control, *L* longitudinal; *ERI* effort reward imbalance; *NKCA* natural killer cell activity; *LTT* lymphocyte transformation test; *LAA* leukocyte adhesiveness/aggregation test; *A* age; *S* sex; *R* race; *Ed* educational level; *Ms* marital status; *Sm* smoking; *Al* alcohol consumption; *Ex* physical exercise; *Sl* sleep; *Anx* anxiety; *BMI* body mass index; *Med* medication usage; *Conf* interpersonal conflict at work; *BL* blood lead concentration; *HRT* hormone replacement therapy; *WkEx* work experience; *WkSch* work schedule; *PC* physical condition; *Occup* occupation; *Caf* caffeine intake; *Com* commuting time; *Jobsat* job satisfaction; *IC* income; *NM/NC* not mentioned or not controlled for
↓ = decrease, ↑ = increase, NS = no significant change

Table 6
Association between psychosocial job stressors and immunoglobulins and complement components

First author	Country	Year	Sample (M/F)	Study design	Occupation	Exposure	IgG	IgM	IgA	s-IgA	Antibody titers	C3	C4	Confounders
Ursin	Norway	1984	38M/40W	CS	School teachers (W) Merchant navy students (M)	High job stress	NS	↓	NS			↓	NS	A, S, WkEx
Endresen	Norway	1987	–/34W	CS	Nurses	High psychological job stress Low job satisfaction	NS	↓	↑			↑		NM/NC
Theorell	Sweden	1990	39M/10W	CS	Various occupations (air traffic controllers, waiters, physicians, etc.)	Job strain	↑							NM/NC
Endresen	Norway	1991	–/94W	CS	Bank employees	Job stress (communication, leadership, relocation, and workload)	NS	NS	NS			NS	NS	NM/NC
Henningsen	USA	1992	–/40W	L	Nurses	Occupational stress				↑				NM/NC
Zeier	Switzerland	1996	158M/–	CS	Air traffic controllers	High work demands				↑				NM/NC
Ng	Singapore	1999	–/124W	CS	Nurses	High general stress				↓				NM/NC
Nakata	Japan	2000	116M/–	CS	White-collar workers (power plant operators)	High job strain	↑	↑	NS					A, Sm

Ohlson	Sweden	2001	8M/95W	CS	Human service organizations	High job strain	NS	NS		A, S, Ms, Ed, Sm, Al
Yang	Singapore	2002	–/132W	CS	Nurses	High professional stress		↓		Ms, WkEx
Herttig	Sweden	2002	–/31W	L	Nurses/medical secretaries	Downsizing Reorganization	↓			NM/NC
Clays	Belgium	2005	892M/–	CS	Various occupations (private companies, public administration, bank, insurance companies, hospitals)	Low social support			CV CP- HP-	A, Edu, Occup, Sm, BMI, Al, Med
Wright	Australia	2011	43M/55W	CS	Disability workers	Effort, ERI Overcommitment		↓		A
Masilaman	Malaysia	2011	52M/240W	CS	Teachers	High job strain Low social support		↓		NM/NC

M men; *F* women; *CS* cross-sectional; *CC* case–control; *L* longitudinal; *C3* complement component 3; *C4* complement component 4; *IL* interleukin; *IFN* interferon; *TNF* tumor necrosis factor; *TGF* transforming growth factor; *CRP* C-reactive protein; *hs* high sensitive; *ERI* effort reward imbalance; *A* age; *S* sex; *R* race; *Ed* educational level; *Ms* marital status; *Sm* smoking; *Al* alcohol consumption; *Ex* physical exercise; *Sl* sleep; *Anx* anxiety; *BMI* body mass index; *Med* medication usage; *Conf* interpersonal conflict at work; *BL* blood lead concentration; *HRT* hormone replacement therapy; *WkEx* work experience; *WkSch* work schedule; *PC* physical condition; *Occup* occupation; *Caf* caffeine intake; *Com* commuting time; *Jobsat* job satisfaction; *IC* income; *CV* cytomegalovirus; *CP Chlamydia pneumoniae*; *HP Helicobactor pylori*; *NM/NC* not mentioned or not controlled for

↓ = decrease, ↑ = increase, NS = no significant change

Table 7
Association between psychosocial job stressors and cytokines (IL-1β, IL-2, IL-4, IL-6, IL-10)

First author	Country	Year	Sample (M/F)	Study design	Occupation	Exposure	IL-1β	IL-2	IL-4	IL-6	IL-10	Urinary IL-8	Confounders
Nakano	Japan	1998	45 (56) M/–	CS, CC	Taxi drivers vs. age-matched controls	Severe economic recession		↓	↑				A
De Gucht	Belgium	1999	17M/43W	CS	Nurses	High nursing stress		NS					NM/NC
Theroell	Sweden	2000	102M/141W	CC	Case: Those who consulted caregiver Control: Age, sex matched controls	Low job satisfaction			↑W -M				A
Hemingway	UK	2003	168M/115W	CS	Civil servants	Low job control High job demands				NS			A, S
Sakami	Japan	2004	71M/–	CS	Non-smoking firefighters	High quantitative workload			NS				A
Miyazaki	Japan	2006	241M(142M)/–	CS	White-collar workers (manufacturing company)	High job demands combined with low social support at work			↑				A, Al, Sm, Ex
Mommersteeg	Netherlands	2006	44M/50W 49 Cases/38 controls	CC	Participants recruited via websites	Burnout					↑		S, A, BMI matched (Med excluded)
Fukuda	Japan	2008	–/118W	CS	Nurses	High nursing stress						↑	A

von Kanel	Germany	2008	55M/112W	CS	School teachers	Burnout syndrome: low personal accomplishments (LPA), high depresonalization (HD), high emotional exhaustion (HEE)			↓			S, A, AL, Sm, Sl, BP, Med, BMI, HR
Hintikka	Finland	2009	93M/132W 19 Cases/206 controls	CC, FU	General population without employment	Unemployment stress				↑		A, S, Ms, Ed, Sm, Ex, Al, BMI, PC, Dp
Amati	Italy	2010	26M/75W	L (12 mon)	Nurses	Low job satisfaction	↑			↑		NM/NC
Lee	Korea	2010	–/38W	L (8 mon)	Nurses	High objective stress High subjective stress	NS					A, Sm
Bellingrath	Germany	2010	21M/34W	CS	School teachers	High ERI High overcommitment		NS	NS	↑	↓	A, Med, Dep, Sm

M men; *F* women; *CS* cross-sectional; *CC* case–control; *L* longitudinal; *C3* complement component 3; *C4* complement component 4; *IL* interleukin; *IFN* interferon; *TNF* tumor necrosis factor; *TGF* transforming growth factor; *CRP* C-reactive protein; *hs* high sensitive; *ERI* effort reward imbalance; *A* age; *S* sex; *R* race; *Ed* educational level; *Ms* marital status; *Sm* smoking; *Al* alcohol consumption; *Ex* physical exercise; *Sl* sleep; *Anx* anxiety; *BMI* body mass index; *Med* medication usage; *Conf* interpersonal conflict at work; *BL* blood lead concentration; *HRT* hormone replacement therapy; *WkEx* work experience; *WkSch* work schedule; *PC* physical condition; *Occup* occupation; *Caf* caffeine intake; *Com* commuting time; *Jobsat* job satisfaction; *IC* income; *NM/NC* not mentioned or not controlled for

↓ = decrease, ↑ = increase, NS = no significant change

Table 8
Association between psychosocial job stressors and cytokines (IFN-γ, TNF-α, TGF-β) and inflammatory markers

First author	Country	Year	Sample (M/F)	Study design	Occupation	Exposure	IFN-γ	TNF-α	TGF-β	IFN-γ/L-4	TNF-α/IL-4	TNF-α/IL-10	CRP/hsCRP	Confounders
Hemingway	UK	2003	168M/115W	CS	Civil servants	Low job control High job demands							NS	A, S
Grossi	Sweden	2003	–/63W 20 Cases/43 controls	CC	White-collar employees (social insurance offices)	Burnout syndrome		↑	NS				NS	A, BMI, HRT, Dep, Sm
Schnorpfeil	Germany	2003	272M/52W	CC	Airplane manufacturing plant	High job demands Low job control Low social support at work		↑					↑	A, S, Sm
Sakami	Japan	2004	71M/–	CS	Non-smoking firefighters	High quantitative workload	NS			NS				A
Shirom	Israel	2005	933M/630W	CS	Apparently healthy employees	Burnout syndrome							M–/W↑	A, Sm, BMI, Ex, HDL, fasting glucose, BP, triglycerides, HRT, Dep, Anx
Shirom	Israel	2006	917M/622W	CS	Apparently healthy employees	Low job satisfaction							M↑/W-	A, BMI, Sm, Ex, HRT, Dep, Anx, HDL, fasting glucose, BP, triglycerides

Hamer	UK	2006	92M/– (non-smoking)	CS	Civil servants	High effort-reward imbalance					↑	A, BMI
Miyazaki	Japan	2006	241M (142M)/–	CS	White-collar workers (manufacturing company)	High job demands combined with low social support at work		↓				A, Al, Sm, Ex
Mommersteeg	Netherlands	2006	44M/50W 49 Cases/38 controls	CC	Participants recruited via websites	Burnout	NS					S, A, BMI matched (Med excluded)
Langelaan	Netherlands	2007	290M/–	CS	Managers	Burnout					NS	Sm, Ex
Sun	China	2007	634M/585W	CS	Various industries	High job strain					NS	A, S, Ed, M, AL, Sm, Ex
Shirom	Israel	2008	738M/383W	L (18 mon)	Apparently healthy employees	High workload Low perceived control Low social support at work					NS	A, S, Ed, Sm, Ex, BMI, Med, Dp, HRT (W)
von Kanel	Germany	2008	55M/112W	CS	School teachers	Burnout syndrome: Low personal accomplishments (LPA), high depresonalization (HD), high emotional exhaustion (HEE)	NS		↑	NS		S, A, AL, Sm, Sl, BP, Med, BMI, HR

(continued)

Table 8 (continued)

First author	Country	Year	Sample (M/F)	Study design	Occupation	Exposure	IFN-γ	TNF-α	TGF-β	IFN-γ/L-4	TNF-α/IL-4	TNF-α/IL-10	CRP/hsCRP	Confounders
Janicki-Deverts	USA	2008	1,093M/–	FU (5 years)	Various occupations (not reported)	Unemployment stress							↑	A, R, BMI, IC, Year 5 employment, Year 7 CRP
Hintikka	Finland	2009	93M/132W 19 Cases/206 controls	CC, FU	General population without employment	Unemployment stress							↑	A, S, Ms, Ed, Sm, Ex, Al, BMI, PC, Dp
Amati	Italy	2010	26M/75W	L (12 mon)	Nurses	Low job satisfaction	↑	NS						NM/NC
Lee	Korea	2010	–/38W	L (8 mon)	Nurses	High objective stress High subjective stress	NS	↓						A, Sm
Bellingrath	Germany	2010	21M/34W	CS	School teachers	High ERI High overcommitment		↑						A, Med, Dep, Sm

M men; *F* women; *CS* cross-sectional; *CC* case–control; *L* longitudinal; *C3* complement component 3; *C4* complement component 4; *IL* interleukin; *IFN* interferon; *TNF* tumor necrosis factor; *TGF* transforming growth factor; *CRP* C-reactive protein; *hs* high sensitive; *ERI* effort reward imbalance; *A* age; *S* sex; *R* race; *Ed* educational level; *Ms* marital status; *Sm* smoking; *Al* alcohol consumption; *Ex* physical exercise; *Sl* sleep; *Anx* anxiety; *BMI* body mass index; *Med* medication usage; *Conf* interpersonal conflict at work; *BL* blood lead concentration; *HRT* hormone replacement therapy; *WkEx* work experience; *WkSch* work schedule; *PC* physical condition; *Occup* occupation; *Caf* caffeine intake; *Com* commuting time; *Jobsat* job satisfaction; *IC* income; *NM/NC* not mentioned or not controlled for

↓ = decrease, ↑ = increase, NS = no significant change

necrosis factor (TNF)-α, and white blood cell (WBC) counts, as well as allostatic load indicators (19, 31, 32, 34, 35). Four out of five studies (19, 31, 32, 34) found that job strain was not related to these inflammatory markers. However, one study demonstrated that high job demands and low social support at work were significantly related to an increase of CRP while low job control was associated with elevated TNF-α (35). Hence, lymphocyte subsets appear to be a more sensitive immune marker to job strain than inflammatory markers.

4.2. Effort–Reward Imbalance and Immunity

In parallel to the job strain model which exclusively focused on the job task profile, Siegrist formulated the effort–reward imbalance (ERI) model (37, 38), which is known to hold a significant predictive power for adverse health outcomes (39, 40). This model postulates that job strain is not merely a product of employee efforts but results from an imbalance between the efforts spent and the rewards (money, career opportunities, esteem, respect, and job security) received. The model also considers a personal characteristic referred to as overcommitment. Overcommitment refers to a set of attitudes, behaviors, and emotions reflecting excessive endeavor in combination with a strong desire for approval and esteem. Reviews of the ERI model concluded that employees reporting overcommitment and exerting a high level of effort, but receiving a low level of rewards, may experience an increased risk of psychological and physical health disorders (39, 40).

To date, several studies have used the ERI model in relation to immune parameters (41–45). In a sample of 537 German factory workers (89% men), Bosch et al. examined the link between ERI measures and CD4+/CD8+ ratio and late-differentiated (CD27–CD28–) CD8+ cytotoxic T cells (41). They found that reduced rewards were associated with a significantly lower CD4+/CD8+ ratio, and decreased rewards and heightened ERI were related to increased relative proportion and counts of late-differentiated cytotoxic T cells, suggesting that exposure to such chronic stress may promote immunosenescence (aging of the immune system). A study of German school teachers (34 women and 21 men) examined whether high ERI and overcommitment modulate the immune response after exposure to acute/stressful experimental tasks (an extemporaneous speech followed by mental arithmetic) (42). Authors hypothesized that those who perceived high job stress may maintain a poor immune status but their immune system can also be vulnerable when confronted with novel/acute stressors. The results revealed that the high ERI stress group at baseline had lowered CD4+ T cells, NK cells, and IL-10, and elevated TNF-α and IL-6 compared to the low ERI stress group, but immune responses to the subsequent acute experimental task were somewhat different for the high and low stress groups. Both high and low stress groups showed an increment of CD4+ T and NK cells but an increase of these cells in response to acute stress in the high stress group was dampened compared to the response of the low stress group. In addition, those under low stress had an increased secretion of anti-inflammatory (IL-10) cytokine and a decreased secretion of pro-inflammatory (IL-2) cytokine after exposure to acute stress but those with high stress showed an opposite reaction, i.e., a decrease of IL-10 and an increase of IL-2, after exposure to acute stressors. This means that the immune responses of those with low stress at baseline could flexibly respond to additional stress exposure but those under high stress may not have adaptable immune response. Another study with a similar experimental protocol demonstrated that the ERI score was significantly and positively associated with high-sensitivity (hs) CRP after exposure to acute mental stress in a sample of 92 healthy working men (43). More recently, a study of white-collar employees reported that the counts of NK cells were inversely associated with effort and ERI and positively associated with reward scores but not with overcommitment in men; the reward score was positively associated with NKCC and inversely associated with B cells (44). A study of disability workers (at adult training and support services and community residential units) in Australia reported on the relationship between ERI and salivary IgA (s-IgA) and found that reward was positively associated with s-IgA while the ERI ratio was inversely related to s-IgA, suggesting the impairment of the oral mucosal host defense system (45).

All in all, ERI, especially reward seems to be a significant indicator of reduced immune function but prospective studies are necessary to allow causal conclusions.

4.3. Social Support at Work and Immunity

Social networks and support have been associated with a broad range of physical and mental outcomes, including cardiovascular disorders (46), hypertension (47), depression (48), sleep disorders (11), and all-cause mortality (49). According to Kahn and Antonucci, social support is characterized by affective support (i.e., loving, liking, and respect), confirmation (i.e., confirming the moral and factual "rightness" of actions and statements), and direct help (e.g., aid in work, giving information or money) (50). These various aspects of social support are usually highly interrelated. Studies reported during the 1990s suggested that emotional and tangible social support is related to a better immune function (51). Among the clinical population, higher social support has been reported to be protective against stress-induced immunosuppression. For example, among ovarian cancer patients, social support was significantly correlated with NKCA even after adjusting for cancer stage (52). Similarly, among breast cancer patients, the perception of higher quality emotional support from a spouse or intimate other and perceived social support from the physician was associated with higher NKCA (53). Moreover, in several studies, social support was found to be a significant predictor of CD4+ T cell counts among human immunodeficiency virus (HIV) positive patients (54–56). A review of 81 studies on the relationship between social support and physiological processes concluded that social support is reliably related to beneficial effects in the cardiovascular, neuroendocrine, and immune systems (57).

Although social support has been identified as a significant candidate for alleviating stress-induced immunosuppression, not many studies have explicitly focused on the effects of workplace social support on immune outcomes. In the job stress research field, social support at work is often measured with regard to the source of support, i.e., support from supervisors or support from colleagues, although in many cases the sources of support are combined into one variable. Using search engines, 11 studies were identified that examined the relationship between social support at work and immunity (26, 28, 29, 33, 34, 36, 41, 58–61). Among these reports, seven studies (28, 33, 36, 41, 58–60) found significant beneficial effects of workplace social support on immune indicators such as increased CD4+/CD8+ ratio (41), NK cells (59), CD8+ T cells (28), IL-4 (60), and reduced late-differentiated (CD27−CD28−) CD8+ cytotoxic T cells (41), IL-6 (58), IgG (33), and s-IgA (36). It is important to note that these findings are consistent with the biological significance of the link between social support and immunity.

4.4. Job Satisfaction and Immunity

Job satisfaction, defined as the degree of pleasure a worker derives from his/her job, is one of the most widely studied constructs in occupational health psychology (62). Job satisfaction can be considered to be a global feeling about the job or as a related constellation of attitudes about various aspects or facets of the job. The former is often called global or general job satisfaction and the latter is called facet job satisfaction (63). It is often used as a summary measure of worker well-being because it captures not only micro-level daily interactions on the job but also macro-level factors related to selection into a job (64). Given its popularity, there is a considerable amount of literature that links job satisfaction with various health measures including mental and physical health status (65), health behaviors (66, 67), and sickness absences (68–71). A comprehensive meta-analysis based on 485 studies of job satisfaction and health reported that workers with low levels of satisfaction were more likely to experience anxiety, burnout, depression, cardiovascular disease, musculoskeletal disorders, and other physical illnesses, indicating that reduced job satisfaction is an important predictor of physical and psychological health (65). Some previous reports revealed that job satisfaction was positively associated with well-being over time (72, 73). Therefore, job satisfaction could be a key psychosocial determinant of worker health and well-being.

The connection between job satisfaction and health is widely acknowledged as mentioned earlier, but such findings are mostly based on subjective health outcomes derived from questionnaires or through self-report, and have not often been investigated through objective outcomes, especially immune measures. To date, only a handful of studies have attempted to examine the effects of job satisfaction on immunity (31, 58, 74–76). For example, a study of Norwegian female nurses ($n = 34$) found that a sum of facet-specific job satisfaction consisting of comfort, challenge, financial rewards, relations with coworkers, and resource adequacy and promotions, was significantly associated with decreased circulating IgA and complement component C3 but not with IgG or IgM (74). A large cohort study in Israel (917 men and 622 women) reported that facet-specific job satisfaction was inversely correlated with CRP in men ($B = -0.20, p < 0.05$) but not in women ($B = -0.10, p > 0.05$) (31). In contrast, global job satisfaction was inversely correlated with serum interleukin (IL)-6 in women but not in men in a sample of Swedish working people (141 women and 102 men) (75). A prospective study of job stress and immunity among nurses (75 women and 26 men) found that those who had undergone a decrease in job satisfaction over a 1-year period had increased levels of IL-1β, IL-6, and CD8+ CD57+ T cells, and a decreased level of interferon (IFN)-γ (58). More recently, Nakata et al. reported the relationship between job satisfaction and NKCA and lymphocyte subsets (T, B, and NK cells) among 306 healthy white-collar employees (76). Global job satisfaction, as measured by a 4-item scale, was significantly associated with NKCA and NK cell counts in women and positively related to NKCA but not NK cell counts in men; no significant association between job satisfaction and T or B cells was found in the study.

Taken altogether, these studies suggest that greater job satisfaction may have a positive impact on immune outcomes. However, the findings need to be interpreted cautiously because most studies were based on cross-sectional designs with a limited number of participants in some studies. An interesting question for future research is whether greater job satisfaction contributes to recovery/maintenance of NK cell immunity and host defense over time.

4.5. Unemployment, Job Insecurity, Economic Recession, Organizational Downsizing, and Immunity

As a result of globalization, increasing competition, and long-lasting global economic recession, people who are working under insecure and casual employment are increasing. Corresponding to such labor market status, unemployment, downsizing, restructuring, reorganization, and merging have become a common trend in modern work life. The loss of one's job as well as working under insecure conditions is highly stressful because, for most employed adults, work is a central part of one's life and identity and a major source of income (77). Studies of unemployment suggest that unemployment is not only related to future premature morbidity and mortality of unemployed individuals but is also known to be a threat of their families' health (78). Similarly, downsizing and restructuring are health risks not only for employees who lose their job, but also for those who remained in employment (79–81). As such, employees in insecure jobs are repeatedly found to have higher stress-related health problems because job insecurity involves both the threat of job loss and uncertainty regarding future employment (82, 83). Although a number of studies have found adverse effects of unemployment, job insecurity, and organizational restructuring on health (79–86), there are only a limited amount of studies that specifically focused on the relationship between unemployment, job insecurity, and the immune system (87–95).

One of the first studies that has dealt with unemployment and immunity was reported from Sweden (88). A study by Arnetz et al. evaluated the immunological impact of unemployment over a period of 12 months in women. In this study, two unemployment conditions (i.e., those who received traditional unemployment benefits only (Group A, $n=9$) and those who received the same benefits as Group A along with an opportunity to participate in a psychological program designed to counteract the negative psychosocial impact of unemployment and creating or finding new jobs (Group B, $n=8$)) were compared with a group of workers in stable jobs (Group C, $n=8$). At the 9- and 12-month follow-up periods (but not at 4- or 7-months), both unemployed groups had a significant decrease in their cellular immune response as measured by a lymphocyte transformation test, i.e., phytohemagglutinin A (PHA) and purified protein derivation of tuberculin (PPD), suggesting a functional decline of helper (CD4+) T cells. There were no significant differences between the groups regarding counts of lymphocyte subsets (CD4+, CD8+, NK, T, B, and total lymphocytes). The results indicate two important aspects of unemployment stress related to immunity. First, the effects of unemployment stress on cellular immune competence emerged after a period of time, even after a year, which indicates a long-lasting and time-lagged effect. Second, although it may largely depend on how psychological support was provided to the unemployed women in Group B, the effects of unemployment stress on immunity was not buffered by the psychological interventions used in this study. This research group later conducted a similar study of unemployment and immunity involving a larger sample of blue-collar workers ($n=354$, 75% women) with a longer follow-up period (2 years), and reported that unemployment was associated with a reduced response to PHA stimulation at the 12-month follow-up period but returned to baseline levels at the 20-month period (87). In the latter study, the authors have considered whether locus of control and mastery (which measures self-control attitude, social support, work involvement, coping, mood, mental well-being, sleep, and depression) could modulate the impact of unemployment stress and concluded that coping style is the key factor that could modulate immune outcome against unemployment stress.

Another study that uncovered the relationship between unemployment and immunity has been reported from the United States using a case–control follow-up study design of 100 unemployed persons and 100 matched employed healthy controls followed over a 4-month period (91). This study design is unique in that 25% of the unemployed people were followed until they became re-employed, to determine whether re-employed people may be released from the unemployment stress that was anticipated to suppress immune function. As expected, those who were persistently unemployed had significantly lower NKCA compared to matched employed workers throughout all measurement occasions (months 1, 2, 3, and 4). However, those who were re-employed regained their NKCA levels by 44–72% within 1 month after reemployment, which were comparable NKCA levels to matched employed workers. The results indicate that the termination of the major stressor is an important factor in recovering NKCA. It is important to note that the difference in NKCA between the unemployed and employed was neither due to smoking status (because smokers were excluded from the analysis) nor percentage of NK cells in the blood. Taken together, the results showed unemployment stress seems to reduce the function of T and NK cells but not the counts of lymphocyte subpopulations.

The effect of unemployment stress on the immune system has also been tested in the context of inflammatory processes. Janicki-Deverts et al. examined whether unemployment history predicts future CRP levels among young working males in the United States (Coronary Artery Risk Development in Young Adults (CARDIA) study) (89). After controlling for age, race, BMI, baseline CRP, unemployment status (at year 5), and average income across the study period, baseline unemployment status was associated with an increase of CRP levels between 5 and 8 years later. More recently, Hintikka et al. compared the levels of IL-6 and hs-CRP between the unemployed and other study participants who consisted of 131 currently with jobs, 14 in sick leave, 52 retired, 3 students, and 6 voluntarily not working (90). Unemployment was associated independently with an increase of IL-6 in a sex- and age-adjusted linear regression analysis but the increase was attenuated after controlling for sex, age, marital status, economic hardship, education, smoking, alcohol consumption, somatic diseases, depression, and BMI, while hs-CRP was not related to unemployment. The prospective association between unemployment and these markers was weak but additional cross-sectional analyses revealed that unemployment was associated with a fivefold greater odd for having an elevated inflammatory status. These findings may partly explain higher premature morbidity and mortality among involuntarily unemployed population.

With regard to job insecurity, Arnetz et al. examined the effects of different phases of unemployment, i.e., anticipation of job loss, actual job loss, and short- and long-term unemployment status with a lymphocyte transformation test using PHA (87). The study found that psychological stress was highest during the anticipatory phase although immunosuppression did not occur concurrently. Meanwhile, Boscolo et al. compared NKCA and lymphocyte subsets among workers with different levels of employment security and observed that young employees with a temporary/insecure employment status had a significantly reduced NKCA level compared to securely employed workers. However, no significant differences were found with regard to NK, T, and B cell subsets (93).

A study of Japanese taxi drivers evaluated the impact of the economic recession on the immune system using a case–control study design over 2 consecutive years (94). Immune responses to three different mitogens, PHA, concanavalin A (Con A), and Pokeweed mitogen (PWM) as well as levels of peripheral blood IL-2 and IL-4 levels were evaluated and compared between taxi drivers and age-matched controls in 1992 and 1993. In 1992, immune response to mitogens and cytokine levels were comparable between taxi drivers and controls (stably employed government researchers), however, in 1993, taxi drivers had significantly lower responses to mitogens as well as reduced IL-2 and increased IL-4 secretion. In 1992, there was no apparent economic recession, but in 1993 a major economic recession in Japan hit the taxi drivers drastically. The authors found that 76.4% of taxi drivers' income dropped from 1992 to 1993 whereas income in the control group increased from 1992 to 1993. The study also compared the immune responses of taxi drivers working under two different conditions: Those drivers who were permitted to work overtime (A-type) and those who were not permitted to work overtime (B-type). B-type taxi drivers exhibited a significantly lower response to all three mitogens and decreased IL-2 and increased IL-4 secretion than A-type taxi drivers. Because all taxi drivers' income was commission-based, a restriction of working time as in B-type condition, these drivers may find it difficult to attain a desirable income. In contrast, the A-type condition may have more flexibility in earning and control over time, which resulted in lower work-related stress levels in A-type drivers. In this case, it is notable that lower demands were associated with higher stress leading to immunosuppression suggesting that lower control over work demands resulted in increased stress levels.

There is one study which investigated the effects of organizational downsizing and reorganization on the immune response (95). Hertting and Theorell reported that after a reduction of 20% in personnel in the health care sector ($n=31$, 80% nurses) during 1995–1997, serum IgG was significantly decreased in 1998 compared to 1997. The authors concluded that as a result of a long-lasting adaptation process, a flattened circadian cortisol rhythm may have contributed to physiological dysfunction leading to an inhibited IgG level.

On balance, these studies revealed that the objective work environment as represented by unemployment, job insecurity, economic recession, and restructuring/downsizing is a potentially significant factor that lead to deterioration in the immune system, which may help explain premature morbidity and mortality in workers who had undergone such events.

4.6. Burnout and Immunity

Burnout is a chronic affective state characterized by persistent exhaustion, cynical work attitude, diminished competence, reduced energy, increased irritability, impaired sleep, and concentration problems that can occur irrespective of the type of profession (96). According to Maslach and Jackson, burnout consists of three main interrelated concepts, i.e., emotional exhaustion, depersonalization (cynicism), and reduced personal accomplishments, none of which overlap with any other concepts such as depression or anxiety, and which is conceptually distinct from a temporary state of fatigue (97). Burnout has been considered as an independent risk factor for mental disorders such as depression (98–100) as well as physical disorders, i.e., cardiovascular disease (101, 102), type 2 diabetes (103), and gastroenteritis (104). It is also considered as a strong risk factor of prolonged sickness absences (105–107) that may be connected with loss of productivity.

As burnout is a result of chronic work-related stress, occupational health researchers have explored the psychophysiological mechanisms of burnout. Several researchers have specifically focused on the immune responses to burnout and a total of eight studies have been reported to date (108–114). Bargellini et al. reported that physicians with low scores on personal accomplishment (which is one of three subcomponents of burnout) showed significant decreases in total lymphocytes, CD3+ T, CD4+ T, and CD8+ T cells as compared with physicians with higher scores (108). Nakamura et al. used the Maslach Burnout Inventory (96) among male office workers and found that depersonalization but not personal accomplishment or emotional exhaustion was inversely associated with NKCA (110). A study by Lerman et al. used a leukocyte adhesiveness/aggregation test as a non-specific marker of inflammation and reported that university employees with high burnout symptoms showed an increased leukocyte adhesiveness/aggregation (111). They also reported that subcomponents of burnout, i.e., emotional exhaustion, chronic fatigue, and cognitive weariness, were all significantly associated with leukocyte adhesiveness/aggregation. More recently, researchers have started to focus on the relationship between burnout and inflammatory cytokines/proteins because accumulating evidence suggests a direct relationship between burnout and arteriosclerotic diseases (115). In a large sample of healthy men and women, Toker et al. found that burnout was positively associated with hs-CRP in women but not in men (112). In contrast, no significant difference in CRP was found between burned-out employees and a control group among managers of a Dutch Telecom Company (114). In white-collar female employees in Sweden, those participants with high burnout exhibited higher plasma levels of TNF-α than counterparts with lower burnout scores but there were no significant differences in CRP and TNF-β levels between the two groups (113). Among school teachers in Germany, higher levels of total burnout symptoms were associated with a lower level of IL-4 and higher TNF-α/IL-4 ratio while lack of accomplishment was associated with diminished IL-4 and heightened TNF-α/IL-4 ratio (116). In more severe cases of burnout, Mommersteeg et al. reported that the burnout group had an increased production of anti-inflammatory cytokine IL-10 released by monocytes but not by T cells (109). The study did not find significant differences between the burnout group and healthy controls with regard to proinflammatory cytokines gamma interferon and TNF-α or counts of T, B, and NK cells.

In sum, burnout seems to be associated with immune parameters to some extent but further explorations are needed to find robust and sensitive immune markers for burnout.

4.7. Other Psycho-Social Job Stress and Immunity

Apart from job strain and ERI models, earlier studies have focused on certain type of jobs that were considered to be inherently stressful such as air traffic controllers (117), teachers (118), nurses (74, 119–122), and bank employees (123). Several studies focused on s-IgA (117, 119–121) and other studies focused on serum/plasma immunoglobulin G, A, and M (33, 74, 118). However, the associations between psychosocial job stress and the immunoglobulin markers were inconsistent between these studies. With regard to s-IgA, for example, Zeier et al. found that exposure to job stress caused increased s-IgA among air traffic controllers (117). In contrast, two studies in nurses reported a decrease of s-IgA due to a high nursing stress (120, 121), while in an 8-month longitudinal study, nurses with higher objective stress showed consistently higher s-IgA than their lower stress counterparts (124). The relationship between job stress and serum/plasma immunoglobulin levels seems also to be contradictory. Some studies reported that job stress increases IgG (28, 33), IgM (28), or IgA (74) levels, while other studies suggested that job stress reduces IgG (95) or IgM (74, 118) levels, or impact on IgG and IgA levels (30).

With regard to cellular immunity, eight studies have reported on the relationship between psychosocial job stressors and lymphocyte subsets and NKCA. Two studies from Italy reported that university employees with high levels of occupational stress, high anxiety levels, and job insecurity had reduced NKCA (93, 125). Among Japanese physicians, overwork was associated with decreased NKCA and CD4+ T cell counts (126). Similarly, two studies of Japanese nurses reported that high quantitative workload and frequent conflict with physicians were inversely associated with NKCA (127), while high quantitative workload and high variance in workload were inversely correlated with NK cell counts (61). A study which focused on overtime (amount of time beyond normal working hours) and cellular immunity reported that overtime was inversely associated with a decrease in NK cell counts in white-collar male and female workers (128). However, there are several studies that found an insignificant relationship between quantitative workload and cellular immune indicators. A study in an electric equipment manufacturing company reported that quantitative workload and mental demand was not independently related to counts of CD3+ T, CD4+ T, and CD8+ T cells among male employees (129). Similarly, no direct association between quantitative workload and T or NK cell counts were found in male white-collar workers (60). Inconsistent findings in these studies may be related to differences in intensity and length of stress exposures (acute vs. chronic), timing of blood sampling, differences in psychosocial job stress instruments used, and confounding factors considered.

Regarding urinary immune indicators, a study focused on nurses compared the level of urinary IL-8 between acute and chronic care (control group) departments and found that those in the acute care department exhibited higher stress and increased urinary IL-8 compared with the control group (130). Because urine sampling is non-invasive and painless, authors concluded that urinary IL-8 may be a convenient immune marker for stress assessment among nurses.

5. Future Directions and Conclusions

The relationship between psychosocial job stress and immunity has only been explored during the past few decades, and is therefore still in a developing phase within the discipline of PNI. In consideration of this fact, future studies should elaborate on the following methodological shortcomings. First, to strengthen the cause and effect relationship, prospective studies with multiple waves are needed. As listed in Tables 3, 4, 5, 6, 7, and 8, most investigations have been based on cross-sectional or case–control study designs. Although some studies used a prospective approach, they suffer from small sample sizes or high dropout rates, which make it difficult to generalize the results. Second, a number of confounding factors need to be taken into account in future studies. In earlier studies, confounders which modify dependent and independent variables, such as sociodemographic (age, sex, race, education, etc.) factors, health behaviors (smoking, sleep, alcohol consumption, exercise, caffeine, diet, etc.), physical/mental health status (comorbid disorders, body mass, etc.), and medication usage (antihypertensive or anti-depressive drugs, oral contraceptive use, etc.) are not always taken into account. It is also true that the immediate state before the blood sampling, i.e., how long participants slept the night before, timing (morning vs. night, beginning or end of the weekday) and condition (fasting vs. non-fasting blood sampling), menstrual cycle (women), and other exposures related to work (hazardous substances, radiation, etc.) need to be considered since they can have a direct impact on immune measurements. Third, it is essential to use well-established job stress measures with high validity and reliability; it is also important to use measures which cover various and broad aspects of working conditions. Stress measures should be carefully selected because some job stress measures may not be suitable for certain groups, occupations, and jobs. Fourth, immune indicators which measure both functional and quantitative aspects may be useful to measure systemic immune response to job stress. It is also desirable to find sensitive non-invasive (saliva or urine) measures that reflect job stress. These issues should be considered when one is designing a study regarding job stress and immunity.

In this review, we find that job stressors are associated with various immune parameters indicating disrupted immune functioning. The relationship between job stress and NK cell immunity was found to be robust but the relationships with other immune markers were less clear cut because of methodological issues raised above. A continued effort is needed to establish a cause and effect association between job stressors and immunity.

Acknowledgements

The findings and conclusions in this report are those of the authors and do not necessarily represent the views of the US National Institute for Occupational Safety and Health.

References

1. Siegrist J (2010) Effort-reward imbalance at work and cardiovascular diseases. Int J Occup Med Environ Health 23:279–285
2. Eller NH, Netterstrom B, Gyntelberg F et al (2009) Work-related psychosocial factors and the development of ischemic heart disease: a systematic review. Cardiol Rev 17:83–97
3. Kivimaki M, Virtanen M, Elovainio M, Kouvonen A, Vaananen A, Vahtera J (2006) Work stress in the etiology of coronary heart disease—a meta-analysis. Scand J Work Environ Health 32:431–442
4. Pickering T (1997) The effects of occupational stress on blood pressure in men and women. Acta Physiol Scand Suppl 640:125–128
5. Boscolo P, Youinou P, Theoharides TC, Cerulli G, Conti P (2008) Environmental and occupational stress and autoimmunity. Autoimmun Rev 7:340–343
6. van Rijn RM, Huisstede BM, Koes BW, Burdorf A (2010) Associations between work-related factors and specific disorders of the shoulder—a systematic review of the literature. Scand J Work Environ Health 36:189–201
7. Bonde JP (2008) Psychosocial factors at work and risk of depression: a systematic review of the epidemiological evidence. Occup Environ Med 65:438–445
8. Netterstrom B, Conrad N, Bech P et al (2008) The relation between work-related psychosocial factors and the development of depression. Epidemiol Rev 30:118–132
9. Stansfeld S, Candy B (2006) Psychosocial work environment and mental health—a meta-analytic review. Scand J Work Environ Health 32:443–462
10. Nieuwenhuijsen K, Bruinvels D, Frings-Dresen M (2010) Psychosocial work environment and stress-related disorders, a systematic review. Occup Med (Lond) 60:277–286
11. Nakata A, Haratani T, Takahashi M et al (2004) Job stress, social support, and prevalence of insomnia in a population of Japanese daytime workers. Soc Sci Med 59:1719–1730
12. Perdikaris P, Kletsiou E, Gymnopoulou E, Matziou V (2010) The relationship between workplace, job stress and nurses' tobacco use: a review of the literature. Int J Environ Res Public Health 7:2362–2375
13. Grunberg L, Moore S, Anderson-Connolly R, Greenberg E (1999) Work stress and self-reported alcohol use: the moderating role of escapist reasons for drinking. J Occup Health Psychol 4:29–36
14. Heraclides AM, Chandola T, Witte DR, Brunner EJ (2012) Work stress, obesity and the risk of type 2 diabetes: gender-specific bidirectional effect in the Whitehall II study. Obesity (Silver Spring) 20(2):428–433
15. Segerstrom SC, Miller GE (2004) Psychological stress and the human immune system: a meta-analytic study of 30 years of inquiry. Psychol Bull 130:601–630
16. Zorrilla EP, Luborsky L, McKay JR et al (2001) The relationship of depression and stressors to immunological assays: a meta-analytic review. Brain Behav Immun 15:199–226
17. McEwen BS, Gianaros PJ (2011) Stress- and allostasis-induced brain plasticity. Annu Rev Med 62:431–445
18. Bellingrath S, Weigl T, Kudielka BM (2009) Chronic work stress and exhaustion is associated with higher allostatic load in female school teachers. Stress 12:37–48
19. Sun J, Wang S, Zhang JQ, Li W (2007) Assessing the cumulative effects of stress: the association between job stress and allostatic load in a large sample if Chinese employees. Work Stress 21:333–347
20. Karasek RA (1979) Job demands, job decision latitude, and mental strain: implication for job design. Admin Sci Q 24:285–307
21. Tsutsumi A, Kayaba K, Ishikawa S (2011) Impact of occupational stress on stroke across occupational classes and genders. Soc Sci Med 72:1652–1658
22. Heraclides A, Chandola T, Witte DR, Brunner EJ (2009) Psychosocial stress at work doubles the risk of type 2 diabetes in middle-aged women: evidence from the Whitehall II study. Diabetes Care 32:2230–2235
23. Rugulies R, Krause N (2005) Job strain, iso-strain, and the incidence of low back and neck injuries. A 7.5-year prospective study of San Francisco transit operators. Soc Sci Med 61:27–39
24. Suominen S, Vahtera J, Korkeila K, Helenius H, Kivimaki M, Koskenvuo M (2007) Job strain, life events, and sickness absence: a longitudinal cohort study in a random population sample. J Occup Environ Med 49:990–996
25. Hausser JA, Mojzisch A, Nielsen M, Schulz-Hardt S (2010) Ten years on: a review of recent research on the job demand-control (-support) model and psychological well-being. Work Stress 24:1–35

26. Kawakami N, Tanigawa T, Araki S et al (1997) Effects of job strain on helper-inducer (CD4+CD29+) and suppressor-inducer (CD4+CD45RA+) T cells in Japanese blue-collar workers. Psychother Psychosom 66:192–198
27. Meijman TF, van Dormolen M, Herber RFM, Rogen H, Kuiper S (1995) Job strain, neuroendocrine activation, and immune status. In: Sauter SL, Murphy LR (eds) Organizational risk factors for job stress. American Psychological Association, Washington, DC, pp 113–126
28. Nakata A, Araki S, Tanigawa T et al (2000) Decrease of suppressor-inducer (CD4+ CD45RA) T lymphocytes and increase of serum immunoglobulin G due to perceived job stress in Japanese nuclear electric power plant workers. J Occup Environ Med 42:143–150
29. Nakata A, Tanigawa T, Fujioka Y, Kitamura F, Iso H, Shimamoto T (2002) Association of low job control with a decrease in memory (CD4+ CD45RO+) T lymphocytes in Japanese middle-aged male workers in an electric power plant. Ind Health 40:142–148
30. Ohlson CG, Soderfeldt M, Soderfeldt B, Jones I, Theorell T (2001) Stress markers in relation to job strain in human service organizations. Psychother Psychosom 70:268–275
31. Shirom A, Toker S, Berliner S, Shapir I, Melamed S (2006) Work-related vigor and job satisfaction relationships with inflammation biomarkers among employed adults. In: Fave A (ed) Dimensions of well-being: research and intervention. Franco Angeli, Milano, pp 254–274
32. Hemingway H, Shipley M, Mullen MJ et al (2003) Social and psychosocial influences on inflammatory markers and vascular function in civil servants (the Whitehall II study). Am J Cardiol 92:984–987
33. Theorell T, Orth-Gomer K, Eneroth P (1990) Slow-reacting immunoglobulin in relation to social support and changes in job strain: a preliminary note. Psychosom Med 52:511–516
34. Clays E, De Bacquer D, Delanghe J, Kittel F, Van Renterghem L, De Backer G (2005) Associations between dimensions of job stress and biomarkers of inflammation and infection. J Occup Environ Med 47:878–883
35. Schnorpfeil P, Noll A, Schulze R, Ehlert U, Frey K, Fischer JE (2003) Allostatic load and work conditions. Soc Sci Med 57:647–656
36. Masilamani R, Darus A, Su TA, Ali R, Mahmud AB, David K (2012) Salivary biomarkers of stress among teachers in an urban setting. Asia Pac J Public Health 24(2):278–287
37. Siegrist J, Starke D, Chandola T et al (2004) The measurement of effort-reward imbalance at work: European comparisons. Soc Sci Med 58:1483–1499
38. Siegrist J (1996) Adverse health effects of high-effort/low-reward conditions. J Occup Health Psychol 1:27–41
39. Tsutsumi A, Kawakami N (2004) A review of empirical studies on the model of effort-reward imbalance at work: reducing occupational stress by implementing a new theory. Soc Sci Med 59:2335–2359
40. van Vegchel N, de Jonge J, Bosma H, Schaufeli W (2005) Reviewing the effort-reward imbalance model: drawing up the balance of 45 empirical studies. Soc Sci Med 60:1117–1131
41. Bosch JA, Fischer JE, Fischer JC (2009) Psychologically adverse work conditions are associated with CD8+ T cell differentiation indicative of immunosenescence. Brain Behav Immun 23:527–534
42. Bellingrath S, Rohleder N, Kudielka BM (2010) Healthy working school teachers with high effort-reward-imbalance and overcommitment show increased pro-inflammatory immune activity and a dampened innate immune defence. Brain Behav Immun 24:1332–1339
43. Hamer M, Williams E, Vuonovirta R, Giacobazzi P, Gibson EL, Steptoe A (2006) The effects of effort-reward imbalance on inflammatory and cardiovascular responses to mental stress. Psychosom Med 68:408–413
44. Nakata A, Takahashi M, Irie M (2011) Effort-reward imbalance, overcommitment, and cellular immune measures among white-collar employees. Biol Psychol 88:270–279
45. Wright BJ (2011) Effort-reward imbalance is associated with salivary immunoglobulin a and cortisol secretion in disability workers. J Occup Environ Med 53:308–312
46. Barth J, Schneider S, von Kanel R (2010) Lack of social support in the etiology and the prognosis of coronary heart disease: a systematic review and meta-analysis. Psychosom Med 72:229–238
47. Bell CN, Thorpe RJ Jr, Laveist TA (2010) Race/ethnicity and hypertension: the role of social support. Am J Hypertens 23:534–540
48. Ikeda T, Nakata A, Takahashi M et al (2009) Correlates of depressive symptoms among workers in small- and medium-scale manufacturing enterprises in Japan. J Occup Health 51:26–37

49. Blazer DG (1982) Social support and mortality in an elderly community population. Am J Epidemiol 115:684–694
50. Kahn RL, Antonucci T (1980) Convoys over the life course: attachment, roles and social support. In: Baltes P (ed) Life span development and behavior, vol 3. Lexington Press, Boston
51. Uchino BN (2006) Social support and health: a review of physiological processes potentially underlying links to disease outcomes. J Behav Med 29:377–387
52. Lutgendorf SK, Sood AK, Anderson B et al (2005) Social support, psychological distress, and natural killer cell activity in ovarian cancer. J Clin Oncol 23:7105–7113
53. Levy SM, Herberman RB, Whiteside T, Sanzo K, Lee J, Kirkwood J (1990) Perceived social support and tumor estrogen/progesterone receptor status as predictors of natural killer cell activity in breast cancer patients. Psychosom Med 52:73–85
54. Theorell T, Blomkvist V, Jonsson H, Schulman S, Berntorp E, Stigendal L (1995) Social support and the development of immune function in human immunodeficiency virus infection. Psychosom Med 57:32–36
55. Persson L, Gullberg B, Hanson BS, Moestrup T, Ostergren PO (1994) HIV infection: social network, social support, and CD4 lymphocyte values in infected homosexual men in Malmo, Sweden. J Epidemiol Community Health 48:580–585
56. Ullrich PM, Lutgendorf SK, Stapleton JT (2003) Concealment of homosexual identity, social support and CD4 cell count among HIV-seropositive gay men. J Psychosom Res 54:205–212
57. Uchino BN, Cacioppo JT, Kiecolt-Glaser JK (1996) The relationship between social support and physiological processes: a review with emphasis on underlying mechanisms and implications for health. Psychol Bull 119:488–531
58. Amati M, Tomasetti M, Ciuccarelli M et al (2010) Relationship of job satisfaction, psychological distress and stress-related biological parameters among healthy nurses: a longitudinal study. J Occup Health 52:31–38
59. Miyazaki T, Ishikawa T, Iimori H et al (2003) Relationship between perceived social support and immune function. Stress Health 19:3–7
60. Miyazaki T, Ishikawa T, Nakata A et al (2005) Association between perceived social support and Th1 dominance. Biol Psychol 70:30–37
61. Kawaguchi Y, Toyomasu K, Yoshida N, Baba K, Uemoto M, Minota S (2007) Measuring job stress among hospital nurses: an attempt to identify biological markers. Fukuoka Igaku Zasshi 98:48–55
62. Spector PE (1997) Job satisfaction: application, assessment, causes, and consequences. Sage, Thousand Oaks, CA
63. van Saane N, Sluiter JK, Verbeek JH, Frings-Dresen MH (2003) Reliability and validity of instruments measuring job satisfaction—a systematic review. Occup Med (Lond) 53:191–200
64. de Castro AB, Gee GC, Takeuchi D (2008) Relationship between job dissatisfaction and physical and psychological health among Filipino immigrants. AAOHN J 56:33–40
65. Faragher EB, Cass M, Cooper CL (2005) The relationship between job satisfaction and health: a meta-analysis. Occup Environ Med 62:105–112
66. Hagihara A, Tarumi K, Nobutomo K (2000) Work stressors, drinking with colleagues after work, and job satisfaction among white-collar workers in Japan. Subst Use Misuse 35:737–756
67. Frone MR, Windle M (1997) Job dissatisfaction and substance use among employed high school students: the moderating influence of active and avoidant coping styles. Subst Use Misuse 32:571–585
68. Munch-Hansen T, Wieclaw J, Agerbo E, Westergaard-Nielsen N, Bonde JP (2008) Global measure of satisfaction with psychosocial work conditions versus measures of specific aspects of psychosocial work conditions in explaining sickness absence. BMC Public Health 8:270
69. Nakata A, Takahashi M, Irie M, Ray T, Swanson NG (2010) Job satisfaction, common cold, and sickness absence among white-collar employees: a cross-sectional survey. Ind Health 49:116–121
70. Roelen CA, Koopmans PC, Notenbomer A, Groothoff JW (2008) Job satisfaction and sickness absence: a questionnaire survey. Occup Med (Lond) 58:567–571
71. Andrea H, Beurskens AJ, Metsemakers JF, van Amelsvoort LG, van den Brandt PA, van Schayck CP (2003) Health problems and psychosocial work environment as predictors of long term sickness absence in employees who visited the occupational physician and/or general practitioner in relation to work: a prospective study. Occup Environ Med 60:295–300
72. Winefield AH, Tiggemann M, Goldney RD (1988) Psychological concomitants of satisfactory employment and unemployment in

young people. Soc Psychiatry Psychiatr Epidemiol 23:149–157

73. Barrios-Choplin B, McCarty R, Cryer B (1997) An inner quality approach to reducing stress and improving physical and emotional well-being at work. Stress Med 13:193–201
74. Endresen IM, Vaernes R, Ursin H, Tonder O (1987) Psychological stress-factors and concentration of immunoglobulins and complement components in Norwegian nurses. Work Stress 1:365–375
75. Theorell T, Hasselhorn HM, Vingard E, Andersson B, MUSIC-Norrtalje-Study-Group (2000) Interleukin 6 and cortisol in acute musculoskeletal disorders: results from a case-referent study in Sweden. Stress Med 16:27–35
76. Nakata A, Takahashi M, Irie M, Swanson NG (2010) Job satisfaction is associated with elevated natural killer cell immunity among healthy white-collar employees. Brain Behav Immun 24:1268–1275
77. Ensminger ME, Celentano DD (1988) Unemployment and psychiatric distress: social resources and coping. Soc Sci Med 27:239–247
78. Wilson SH, Walker GM (1993) Unemployment and health: a review. Public Health 107:153–162
79. Kivimaki M, Honkonen T, Wahlbeck K et al (2007) Organisational downsizing and increased use of psychotropic drugs among employees who remain in employment. J Epidemiol Community Health 61:154–158
80. Vahtera J, Kivimaki M, Pentti J (1997) Effect of organisational downsizing on health of employees. Lancet 350:1124–1128
81. Dragano N, Verde PE, Siegrist J (2005) Organisational downsizing and work stress: testing synergistic health effects in employed men and women. J Epidemiol Community Health 59:694–699
82. Virtanen P, Vahtera J, Kivimaki M, Pentti J, Ferrie J (2002) Employment security and health. J Epidemiol Community Health 56:569–574
83. Ferrie JE, Shipley MJ, Stansfeld SA, Marmot MG (2002) Effects of chronic job insecurity and change in job security on self reported health, minor psychiatric morbidity, physiological measures, and health related behaviours in British civil servants: the Whitehall II study. J Epidemiol Community Health 56:450–454
84. Laszlo KD, Pikhart H, Kopp MS et al (2010) Job insecurity and health: a study of 16 European countries. Soc Sci Med 70:867–874
85. Ferrie JE (2001) Is job insecurity harmful to health? J R Soc Med 94:71–76
86. Ferrie JE, Shipley MJ, Marmot MG, Stansfeld S, Smith GD (1995) Health effects of anticipation of job change and non-employment: longitudinal data from the Whitehall II study. BMJ 311:1264–1269
87. Arnetz BB, Brenner SO, Levi L et al (1991) Neuroendocrine and immunologic effects of unemployment and job insecurity. Psychother Psychosom 55:76–80
88. Arnetz BB, Wasserman J, Petrini B et al (1987) Immune function in unemployed women. Psychosom Med 49:3–12
89. Janicki-Deverts D, Cohen S, Matthews KA, Cullen MR (2008) History of unemployment predicts future elevations in C-reactive protein among male participants in the Coronary Artery Risk Development in Young Adults (CARDIA) study. Ann Behav Med 36:176–185
90. Hintikka J, Lehto SM, Niskanen L et al (2009) Unemployment and ill health: a connection through inflammation? BMC Public Health 9:410
91. Cohen F, Kemeny ME, Zegans LS, Johnson P, Kearney KA, Stites DP (2007) Immune function declines with unemployment and recovers after stressor termination. Psychosom Med 69:225–234
92. Marriott D, Kirkwood BJ, Stough C (1994) Immunological effects of unemployment. Lancet 344:269–270
93. Boscolo P, Di Donato A, Di Giampaolo L et al (2009) Blood natural killer activity is reduced in men with occupational stress and job insecurity working in a university. Int Arch Occup Environ Health 82:787–794
94. Nakano Y, Nakamura S, Hirata M et al (1998) Immune function and lifestyle of taxi drivers in Japan. Ind Health 36:32–39
95. Hertting A, Theorell T (2002) Physiological changes associated with downsizing of personnel and reorganisation in the health care sector. Psychother Psychosom 71:117–122
96. Maslach C, Schaufeli WB, Leiter MP (2001) Job burnout. Annu Rev Psychol 52:397–422
97. Maslach C, Jackson SE (1981) The measurement of experienced burnout. J Occup Behav 2:99–113
98. Middeldorp CM, Cath DC, Boomsma DI (2006) A twin-family study of the association between employment, burnout and anxious depression. J Affect Disord 90:163–169
99. Iacovides A, Fountoulakis KN, Kaprinis S, Kaprinis G (2003) The relationship between job stress, burnout and clinical depression. J Affect Disord 75:209–221

100. Ahola K, Honkonen T, Isometsa E et al (2005) The relationship between job-related burnout and depressive disorders—results from the Finnish Health 2000 study. J Affect Disord 88:55–62
101. Melamed S, Shirom A, Toker S, Berliner S, Shapira I (2006) Burnout and risk of cardiovascular disease: evidence, possible causal paths, and promising research directions. Psychol Bull 132:327–353
102. Honkonen T, Ahola K, Pertovaara M et al (2006) The association between burnout and physical illness in the general population—results from the Finnish Health 2000 study. J Psychosom Res 61:59–66
103. Melamed S, Shirom A, Toker S, Shapira I (2006) Burnout and risk of type 2 diabetes: a prospective study of apparently healthy employed persons. Psychosom Med 68:863–869
104. Mohren DC, Swaen GM, Kant IJ, van Amelsvoort LG, Borm PJ, Galama JM (2003) Common infections and the role of burnout in a Dutch working population. J Psychosom Res 55:201–208
105. Hallsten L, Voss M, Stark S, Josephson M (2011) Job burnout and job wornout as risk factors for long-term sickness absence. Work 38:181–192
106. Borritz M, Christensen KB, Bultmann U et al (2011) Impact of burnout and psychosocial work characteristics on future long-term sickness absence. Prospective results of the Danish PUMA Study among human service workers. J Occup Environ Med 52:964–970
107. Ahola K, Kivimaki M, Honkonen T et al (2008) Occupational burnout and medically certified sickness absence: a population-based study of Finnish employees. J Psychosom Res 64:185–193
108. Bargellini A, Barbieri A, Rovesti S, Vivoli R, Roncaglia R, Borella P (2000) Relation between immune variables and burnout in a sample of physicians. Occup Environ Med 57:453–457
109. Mommersteeg PM, Heijnen CJ, Kavelaars A, van Doornen LJ (2006) Immune and endocrine function in burnout syndrome. Psychosom Med 68:879–886
110. Nakamura H, Nagase H, Yoshida M, Ogino K (1999) Natural killer (NK) cell activity and NK cell subsets in workers with a tendency of burnout. J Psychosom Res 46:569–578
111. Lerman Y, Melamed S, Shragin Y et al (1999) Association between burnout at work and leukocyte adhesiveness/aggregation. Psychosom Med 61:828–833
112. Toker S, Shirom A, Shapira I, Berliner S, Melamed S (2005) The association between burnout, depression, anxiety, and inflammation biomarkers: C-reactive protein and fibrinogen in men and women. J Occup Health Psychol 10:344–362
113. Grossi G, Perski A, Evengard B, Blomkvist V, Orth-Gomer K (2003) Physiological correlates of burnout among women. J Psychosom Res 55:309–316
114. Langelaan S, Bakker AB, Schaufeli WB, van Rhenen W, van Doornen LJ (2007) Is burnout related to allostatic load? Int J Behav Med 14:213–221
115. Kitaoka-Higashiguchi K, Morikawa Y, Miura K et al (2009) Burnout and risk factors for arteriosclerotic disease: follow-up study. J Occup Health 51:123–131
116. von Kanel R, Bellingrath S, Kudielka BM (2008) Association between burnout and circulating levels of pro- and anti-inflammatory cytokines in schoolteachers. J Psychosom Res 65:51–59
117. Zeier H, Brauchli P, Joller-Jemelka HI (1996) Effects of work demands on immunoglobulin A and cortisol in air traffic controllers. Biol Psychol 42:413–423
118. Ursin H, Mykletun R, Tonder O et al (1984) Psychological stress-factors and concentrations of immunoglobulins and complement components in humans. Scand J Psychol 25:340–347
119. Henningsen GM, Hurrell JJ Jr, Baker F et al (1992) Measurement of salivary immunoglobulin A as an immunologic biomarker of job stress. Scand J Work Environ Health 18(suppl 2):133–136
120. Ng V, Koh D, Chan G, Ong HY, Chia SE, Ong CN (1999) Are salivary immunoglobulin A and lysozyme biomarkers of stress among nurses? J Occup Environ Med 41:920–927
121. Yang Y, Koh D, Ng V et al (2002) Self perceived work related stress and the relation with salivary IgA and lysozyme among emergency department nurses. Occup Environ Med 59:836–841
122. De Gucht V, Fischler B, Demanet C (1999) Immune dysfunction associated with chronic professional stress in nurses. Psychiatry Res 85:105–111
123. Endresen IM, Ellertsen B, Endresen C, Hjelmen AM, Matre R, Ursin H (1991) Stress at work and psychological and immunological parameters in a group of Norwegian female bank employees. Work Stress 5:217–227
124. Lee KM, Kang D, Yoon K et al (2010) A pilot study on the association between job stress

and repeated measures of immunological biomarkers in female nurses. Int Arch Occup Environ Health 83:779–789

125. Di Donato A, Di Giampaolo L, Reale M et al (2006) Effect of occupational stress and anxiety on natural killer lymphocyte activity of men and women employed in a university. Int J Immunopathol Pharmacol 19:79–84
126. Okamoto H, Tsunoda T, Teruya K et al (2008) An occupational health study of emergency physicians in Japan: health assessment by immune variables (CD4, CD8, CD56, and NK cell activity) at the beginning of work. J Occup Health 50:136–146
127. Morikawa Y, Kitaoka-Higashiguchi K, Tanimoto C et al (2005) A cross-sectional study on the relationship of job stress with natural killer cell activity and natural killer cell subsets among healthy nurses. J Occup Health 47:378–383
128. Nakata A, Takahashi M, Irie M (2012) Association of overtime work with cellular immune markers among healthy daytime white-collar employees. Scand J Work Environ Health 38:56–64
129. Sakami S, Maeda M, Maruoka T, Nakata A, Komaki G, Kawamura N (2004) Positive coping up- and down-regulates in vitro cytokine productions from T cells dependent on stress levels. Psychother Psychosom 73: 243–251
130. Fukuda H, Ichinose T, Kusama T, Sakurai R, Anndow K, Akiyoshi N (2008) Stress assessment in acute care department nurses by measuring interleukin-8. Int Nurs Rev 55:407–411

Chapter 4

Immune Cells Listen to What Stress Is Saying: Neuroendocrine Receptors Orchestrate Immune Function

Harlan P. Jones

Abstract

Over the past three decades, the field of psychoneuroimmunology research has blossomed into a major field of study, gaining interests of researchers across all traditionally accepted disciplines of scientific research. This chapter provides an overview of our current understanding in defining neuroimmune interactions with a primary focus of discussing the neuroendocrine receptor activity by immune cells. This chapter highlights the necessity of neuroimmune responses as it relates to a better understanding of the pathophysiological mechanisms of health and disease.

Key words: Neuroendocrine, Immune cells, Mechanisms, Central nervous system, Stress

1. Introduction

The immune system is recognized best for its role in protection against pathogens, which cause disease. As a first defense, the immune system elicits a robust non-specific response against evading pathogens by a collection of non-cellular and cellular responses termed the "innate" immune response. The second arm of the immune response is termed "adaptive or acquired" immunity. Adaptive immunity elicits a tailored and specific immune response against the ensuing pathogen and is unique in that it elicits memory to prior pathogenic exposures. Immune activation however, is not solely relegated to attack against foreign pathogens, but plays an integral role regulating homeostatic conditions related to immune surveillance against tumorogenesis and chronic inflammatory diseases (e.g., autoimmune disease, asthma, and rheumatoid arthritis). Thus, the immune system represents a complex network requiring tight regulatory control.

Qing Yan (ed.), *Psychoneuroimmunology: Methods and Protocols*, Methods in Molecular Biology, vol. 934,
DOI 10.1007/978-1-62703-071-7_4,

The central nervous system (CNS) coordinates the activation and release of neurotransmitter and hormonal factors that translate into physiological adaptations that protect the host from deleterious outcomes. Interactions between the neuroendocrine and immune systems are believed to be essential in defining the mechanisms regulating infectious and non-infectious disease states. The discipline of psychoneuroimmunology (PNI) serves as a platform in broadening our understanding of the collaborative roles of the immune and CNSs. Over the past four decades scientists have defined bi-directional pathways leading to novel concepts of behavioral and physiological health and disease on the basis of cellular and molecular interactions between the immune and CNS systems (1, 2). It is now accepted that the nervous system can receive input from the immune system via the release of cytokines and other immune mediators (3). Likewise, the immune system is also receptive to signals conveyed from neuroendocrine and neurotransmitter-mediated influences, suggesting a bi-directional interplay between the release of endocrine hormone factors, neurotransmitter activity, and cytokines, respectively (4, 5). The following sections discuss current knowledge relevant to influences of the nervous system mediators on immune function.

2. An Overview of the Classical Components of the Nervous System

The neuroendocrine, autonomic, and peripheral nervous systems represent the major pathways, linking immune and nervous system functioning. Within the CNS, the hypothalamic–pituitary–adrenal axis (HPA-axis) comprised of the paraventricular nucleus (PVN), the anterior pituitary gland and the adrenal glands mediate the release of corticotropin-releasing hormone (CRH) from the PVN, stimulating glucocorticoid release from the adrenal gland via activation of adrenocorticotropin hormone (ACTH). The actions of the CNS are largely characterized as immune suppressive (6, 7).

The autonomic nervous system (ANS), which consists of the peripheral sympathetic nervous system (SNS) innervates numerous sites of body and is commonly associated with the "Flight or Fight" response. Two neurotransmitters, epinephrine and norepinephrine, are synthesized from the amino acid, tyrosine and released from the synaptic end of SNS terminals (8, 9). Innervation of SNS is found in several tissues, including blood vessels, liver, kidney, intestines, lung, heart, and brain (10). In particular, Hadden et al. (11) discovered adrenergic receptors to be expressed by human peripheral blood lymphocytes. In the 1980s, Felten and Felten, provided a thorough landscape of the adrenergic innervation pathways within lymphoid tissues (12). Since, major immune organs such as lymph nodes, bone marrow, and spleen have been found to have SNS innervations and have been implicated in mediating cellular immune function (13). A second component of the ANS is the parasympathetic nervous system (PNS), which operates via vagus nerve innervation. The main neurotransmitter of the PNS is acetylcholine (Ach), which interacts with the G protein-coupled muscarinic acetylcholine receptors and the nicotinic ligand-gated ion channels. PNS innervation is believed to mediate immune function through projections within the postrema, connecting to the HPA and subsequently activating the SNS through the rostroventrolateral medulla. Through the efferent arc found in the dorsal motor nucleus, vagal activity is produced by the release of Ach at the vagal postsynaptic neurons. In terms of it its impact on immune function, vagal stimulation has been shown to evoke anti-inflammatory responses and in many ways counteracts the robust inflammatory response produced in response to initial infection or inflammatory insults (13, 14).

Through activation of these major nervous system pathways, we now know that immune responses in part receive distinct signals that instruct immune function. The discussions that follow address questions as to how neuronal factors of the nervous system convey instruction to the immune system and modify the phenotype of cellular immune constituents.

3. Neuroendocrine Receptor Expression by Immune Cells as Determinants of Cellular Immune Function

Neuroimmunomodulation is based on a number of intrinsic (e.g., genetic, organ, behavioral) and extrinsic factors (e.g., stressor, environmental exposures, and host–pathogen interactions) (15–18). Recently, attention has been placed on neuroimmune circuits produced through neuroendocrine and neuroendocrine receptor expression by immune cell populations. Immune cells such as macrophages/monocytes, dendritic cells, NK cells, neutrophils, T cells, and B cells express receptors for several neuroendocrine factors such as glucocorticoid, substance P, CRH, and catecholamines (norepinephrine and epinephrine) (19–23). Thus, it is postulated that the heterogeneity of receptor expression by immune cells are primary determinants of immune function.

3.1. Glucocorticoid Receptor-Mediated Responses

The glucocorticoid response has been shown to play an essential role in regulation of immune function and in turn impact health and disease. Most commonly is the known pharmacological benefit of its use in control of inflammatory responses. Insight into the role of glucocorticoids as regulators of immune function was demonstrated in early studies where overstimulation of the HPA was shown to be immunosuppressive, leading to susceptibility to infection (24, 25). Regulation of glucocorticoid responses on immune function is controlled by glucocorticoid receptors (GRs) expressed by immune cells. The glucocorticoid intracellular receptor system represents two receptors, the GR and the mineralocorticoid receptor (MR). Cortisol (Corticosterone in rodents) has the greatest affinity for the GR receptor, which is the dominant receptor expressed by immune cells (26, 27). Upon ligation, the inactivated GR found in the cytoplasm is translocated into the nucleus where it binds glucocorticoid response elements (GREs). Once in the nucleus, the GR homodimer regulates the transcription of key gene transcription factors including AP-1 and NFκB. NFκB in particular is a major factor involved in the regulation of cytokine responses (28, 29). GR regulation of NFκB acts as a repressor and in this manner is believed that downstream NFκB sequestration by GR-mediated IκB (second messenger) activity in the cytoplasm inhibits NFκB translocation into the nucleus and therefore alters cytokine gene expression (30). Other competing points of view have suggested that interactions between NFκB and GR are not exclusive for suppression of cytokine responses but rather may be dependent on the cell-type (31).

GRs are expressed on various cell types comprising the innate and adaptive arms of the immune system (32). In general, glucocorticoids suppress all aspects of an immune response including cellular trafficking (33), apoptosis (34, 35), maturation, and proliferation (36) among other specialized functions (e.g., adhesion, cytokine production, antigenic recognition, antigen presentation) (37). Such global suppression is mediated largely by glucocorticoid's inhibition of the production of pro-inflammatory cytokines IL-1β, IL-6, TNF-α, and chemotactic factors (38) as well as reductions in elastase, oxidative stress, and other inflammatory mediators (39). At the same time however, glucocorticoids promote the induction of the anti-inflammatory cytokines IL-10 and TGF-β (40, 70). This suggests a diversity of responses by GR-mediated responses that may indicate specialization of function based on the cellular phenotype. Macrophages/monocytes for example, which play a critical role in innate and activation of the adaptive arm of the immune response, are highly sensitive to GR-mediated responses (40, 41). Importantly, due to the identification of various inflammatory and anti-inflammatory phenotypes, recent evidence supports a role in GR-mediated responses in shaping immune function's response against pathogens (42, 43). Likewise, neutrophils, which play a key role in early innate immune responses against bacterial pathogens express GRs and are important targets in controlling neutrophilic inflammatory responses (44). In general, GR-mediated responses have been shown to decrease the up-regulation of neutrophil-associated adhesion and chemotactic receptor expression (45, 46). Thus, limiting the transmigration of neutrophils to sites of inflammation. Moreover, GR-mediated responses on neutrophils have been shown to delay apoptosis resulting in a shift to the necrotic phenotype (47). These opposing outcomes resulting from GR activation in macrophage and neutrophils as well other innate immune cell populations remains unresolved and poses a complex picture under circumstances in understanding the induction and resolution of innate inflammatory responses.

Glucocorticoid responses also impact the development of acquired immunity. Dendritic cells, for example, which serve as professional antigen presenting cells and critical stimulators of antigen-specific T cell responses express GRs (48, 49). Conventionally, prior to maturation (during recognition and uptake of antigen), immature DCs respond positively to GR activity, resulting in their expansion and migration to lymph nodes necessary for their interaction with naïve T cells. Mature DCs on the other hand respond negatively to GR activation. Previous studies have demonstrated a down regulation in the expression of surface maturation co-stimulatory molecules including MHC II, CD80, and CD40, which are required for cognate ligation with naïve T cells co-receptors for their differentiation and activation (50). Emerging evidence, however, suggests a different perspective of GR-mediated responses on DCs. Recent studies suggest that GR activity does not solely suppress of DC maturation, but may dictate the functional phenotype. Roca et al., demonstrated that GC exposure of DC results in the production of anti-inflammatory cytokines such as IL-10 and suppression of IL-12 reminiscent of a tolerogenic phenotype (51). T cells and B cells also express GRs. In particular, GRs expressed on T cells have been shown to play a pivotal role during T cell development in thymus (52). Based on glucocorticoid levels in thymus, studies have demonstrated the extent of T cell survival (53, 54). In addition, GR expression by T cells is an important determinant of T cell differentiation. TCR signaling is modulated by GR activity (52). Importantly, T cell cytokine production as determinants of T cell differentiation is significantly influenced by GR responsiveness. Preferences in cytokine production are significantly affected by GR activity. IFN-γ production is suppressed through GR activity by the repression of Tbet/STAT signaling pathways (55, 56). In fact, preferences in a loss of Th1-differentiation due to GR activity has been thought to explain the polarization of Th2 and Th17 responses associated with certain disease immunopathological diseases (e.g., allergic and autoimmune) (57, 58). Further investigation demonstrating the diversity of GR-mediated molecular signaling that causes preferences in T cell cytokine production will greatly advance our understanding of T cell-mediated disease pathologies.

3.2. Sympathetic Neurotransmitter Receptor-Mediation of Immune Function

The SNS is mediated by two major neurotransmitters, epinephrine and norepinephrine, which are synthesized from the amino acid, tyrosine, and released from the synaptic end of SNS. Innervation of SNS is found in several tissues, including blood vessels, liver, kidney, intestines, lung, heart, and brain (12, 59). Major immune organs such as lymph node, bone marrow, and spleen also have SNS innervations (60). Expression of adrenergic receptor subtypes has been detected on several immune cell populations including NK cells, Th1 cells, macrophages, and dendritic cells (61–65). Thus, it is believed that immune cells derive their functional properties in part by catecholaminergic neurotransmitter responses. The adrenergic receptors, which mediate the functional effects of these neurotransmitters are included in the GPCR (G protein-coupled receptor) family, and, therefore, their biological effect is mediated by coupling with different G-protein-associated signaling. Adrenergic receptors are subdivided into nine isotypes; three alpha-1 types ($\alpha 1_A$, $\alpha 1_B$ and $\alpha 1_C$), three alpha-2 types ($\alpha 2_A$, $\alpha 2_B$ and $\alpha 2_C$), and three beta-types (β1, β2 and β3).

Among all of the adrenergic receptors, β2 expression by T cells has received most attention. In particular, β2 adrenergic receptor expression and binding to epinephrine and norepinephrine results in decreased IFN-γ production by Th1 type helper T cells whereas no effects are discerned in Th2 type cells, because of the absence of receptor expression (66). In support, Panine-Bordignon et al. showed β2 agonists prevents Th1 development by selective inhibition of IL-12 by antigen presenting cells, while promoting Th2 cell phenotype (67). Because IL-12 is typically a cytokine expressed by dendritic cells and macrophages, it is of interests to investigate adrenergic-mediated responses in regulation of APC-T cell interactions. Norepinephrine is rapidly oxidized and turned into epinephrine. In this regard, our recent published studies demonstrated that preferences in β2 adrenergic receptor activation by DC result in a preferential Th17 phenotype (68). Further studies, which examine adrenergic receptor-specific responses to elicit distinct cellular immune function, will be important in fully defining the role of adrenergic responses in the setting of inflammatory disease.

3.3. Parasympathetic-Receptor-Mediated Immune Responses

The PNS is critical in maintaining physiological homeostasis to all major organs of the hosts including heart, lung, and gut. This is also true for controlling immune responses. While the sympathetic arm of the ANS is typically excitatory in nature, the primary role of the vagal system is thought to counterbalance SNS output as well as limit the activation of the CNS in the midst of ongoing inflammatory signals. For example, during acute infection, the HPA axis responds to elevations in inflammatory cytokines such as IL-1β and IL-6 provoking sickness-like behaviors. Importantly, through vagal stimulation the HPA is signaled allowing for an appropriate response to the infection (69). Likewise the efferent arm of the vagus is an essential deactivator of inflammatory responses (14). As mentioned above Ach is a key PNS neurotransmitter that can relay instruction directly to immune cells by Ach receptors (14). In particular, the alpha-7 (α7) nicotinic receptor is expressed on various immune cell populations such as macrophages (70). Studies have shown that α7 signaling results in the reduction in pro-inflammatory cytokine production (TNF-α, IL-β, IL-6) (70–72). In a similar manner as to CRs, Ach-mediated suppression of pro-inflammatory cytokine production has been found to be a result of repression of NFκB phosphorylation (72) as well as α7-mediated inhibition of the STAT3 pathways in immune cells (73). Although, studies have implicated Ach-mediated suppression of pro-inflammatory responses, equally relevant is the potential for the existence of feedback mechanisms in which α7 activation support the induction of anti-inflammatory cytokine expression such as IL-10 and TGF-β. Such studies would be helpful in targeting such pathways to attenuate conditions in certain chronic inflammatory conditions by promoting anti-inflammatory cellular phenotype.

3.4. Peripheral Corticotrophin-Releasing Hormone: An Emerging Neuronal Pathway Affecting Cellular Immune Function

Corticotrophin-releasing hormone (CRH), also known as corticotropin-releasing factor (CRF), is a neuroendocrine factor composed of 41-amino acids (74). CRH was originally known as a stress-induced factor produced in PVN of the hypothalamus that triggers production of adrenocorticotropic hormone (ACTH) in pituitary, and consequently, induces production of glucocorticoids. Two receptor isotypes (CRHR1 and CRHR2) have been reported to mediate its biological effects, which belong to the GPCR superfamily (75). In addition to its production and location in the CNS, CRH and its receptors have been identified in several other sites such as placenta, fetal membranes, and spleen (76–78). Recent evidences in our own research have demonstrated CRH and CRH receptors expressed by immune cells to play a pivotal role as determinants of disease outcome (79). In particular, several immune cell types such as mast cells, peripheral blood monocytes, macrophage, and lymphocytes including Th2 cells have been identified as a potential target of CRH (80, 81). Interestingly, CRH-mediated enhancement of immunological responses corresponding with specific receptor expression has been reported. Agelaki et al. showed that CRH stimulation induces pro-inflammatory cytokine production in the macrophage cell line RAW264.7. In this study, they also showed that LPS-induced systemic shock was suppressed by administration of CRHR1 antagonist (82). These findings implicate that free CRH released from the location of its production has direct effects on immune responses separate from HPA axis. In support, several ectopic production of CRH from extra hypothalamic tissues such as placenta and T cells has been reported (81, 83). In addition, Kalantaridou et al., also showed that embryonic trophoblast and maternal decidual cells produce CRH (76). This peripheral CRH plays crucial roles in implantation, as well as in the anti-rejection process that protects the fetus from the maternal immune system, primarily through apoptotic effects on activated T cells. Thus, peripheral CRH may have an influence on several biological activities associated with immune responses and therefore provide a potential mechanism for homeostatic maintenance against stress-induced immune disorders. In this regard, recent studies utilizing CRH receptor-specific antagonists have demonstrated quality of inflammatory responses based on preferences in CRH-receptor activity (84–86). Our unpublished results also highlight the significance of CRH receptor expression in manipulation macrophage and dendritic cell functions. Together, these and other studies point to alternative roles for a CNS-derived neuroendocrine factor in orchestrating immune function.

4. Conclusion

Much of what we understand regarding the relationships between nervous and immune system functioning stem from early studies describing the effects of adverse stress and disease susceptibility (87, 88). For example, under conditions of acute stress, immune responses were characterized as hyper-responsive. On the contrary, instances of chronic stress were typically deemed immunosuppressive. Consequently, the specificity of immune function was characterized based on preferences in neuroendocrine output. Interests in these effects became the emphasis in defining determinants of disease. To date, susceptibility to viral infection, bacterial infections, and cancer has been associated with neuroendocrine-mediated suppression of immune function. In contrast, the propensity of inflammatory responses associated with asthma, rheumatoid arthritis, and colitis has been linked to elevations in the SNS pathways. This dichotomy between neuro-immune responses poses much complexity and specificity in neuro-immune functioning.

Neuroendocrine control of immunity at the level of individual immune cell types raises interesting questions of neural and immune circuits that protect the host from deleterious outcomes. Knowledge of newly identified neuroendocrine receptor expression by innate and adaptive immune cells and consequently its downstream function will provide a new understanding of the bi-directional pathways which exist between the nervous and immune systems. An increased understanding will ultimately provide potential avenues for therapies.

References

1. Steinman L (2004) Elaborate interactions between the immune and nervous systems. Nat Immunol 5:575–581
2. Dantzer R et al (1998) Cytokines and sickness behavior. Ann N Y Acad Sci 840:586–590
3. Dantzer R et al (2000) Neural and humoral pathways of communication from the immune system to the brain: parallel or convergent? Auton Neurosci 85:60–65
4. Watkins LR et al (1995) Cytokine-to-brain communication: a review and analysis of alternative mechanisms. Life Sci 57:1101–1126
5. Hopkins SJ, Rothwell NJ (1995) Cytokines and the nervous system I. Expression and recognition. Trends Neurosci 18:83–88
6. Barnes PJ (1998) Anti-inflammatory actions of glucocorticoids: molecular mechanisms. Clin Sci 94:557–572

7. Kunicka JE et al (1993) Immunosuppression by glucocorticoids: inhibition of production of multiple lymphokines by in vivo administration of dexamethasone. Cell Immunol 149:39–49
8. Elenkov IJ et al (2000) The sympathetic nerve—an integrative interface between two supersystems: the brain and the immune system. Pharmacol Rev 52:595–638
9. Nance DM, Sanders VM (2001) Autonomic innervation and regulation of the immune system (1987–2007). Pharmacol Rev 53:487–525
10. Horin T et al (1995) The autonomic nervous system as a communication channel between the brain and the immune system. Neuroimmunomodulation 2:203–215
11. Hadden JW et al (1970) Lymphocyte blast transformation. I. Demonstration of adrenergic receptors in human peripheral lymphocytes. Cell Immunol 1:583–595
12. Felten DL, Felten SY (1988) Sympathetic noradrenergic innervation of immune organs. Brain Behav Immun 2:293–300
13. Elenkov IJ, Wilder RL, Chrousos GP, Vizi ES (2000) The sympathetic nerve—an integrative interface between two supersystems: the brain and the immune system. Pharmacol Rev 52: 595–638
14. Westerloo DJ (2010) The vagal immune reflex: a blessing from above. Wien Med Wochenschr 160:112–117
15. Steinman L et al (2003) The intricate interplay among body weight, stress, and the immune response to friend or foe. J Clin Invest 111:183–185
16. Wilder RL et al (1982) Strain and sex variation in the susceptibility to streptococcal cell wall-induced polyarthritis in the rat. Arthritis Rheum 25:1064–1072
17. Rozlog LA et al (1999) Stress and immunity: implications of viral disease and wound healing. J Periodontol 70:786–792
18. Glaser R, Liecolt-Glaser JK (1998) Stress-associated immune modulation: relevance to viral infections and chronic fatique syndrome. Am J Med 105:35S–42S
19. Argon A, Stanisz AM (1992) Are lymphocytes a target for substance P modulation in arthritis? Semin Arthritis Rheum 21:252–258
20. Webster EL et al (1990) Corticotropin-releasing factor receptors in mouse spleen: identification of receptor-bearing cells as resident macrophages. Endocrinology 27:440–452
21. Nance DM, Sanders VM (2007) Autonomic innervation and regulation of the immune system. Pharmacol Rev 53:487–525
22. Kohm AP, Sanders VM (2008) Norepinephrine and beta 2-adrenergic receptor stimulation regulate CD4+ T and B lymphocyte function in vitro and in vivo. Acta Biophys Sin (Shanghai) 40:595–600
23. Tompson EB (2008) Stepping stones in the path of glucocorticoid-driven apoptosis of lymphoid cells. Steroids 73:1025–1029
24. Elmquist JK, Scammell TE, Saper CB (1997) Mechanisms of CNS response to systemic immune challenge: the febrile response. Trends Neurosci 20:565–570
25. Mulla A, Buckingham JC (1999) Regulation of the hypothalamo-pituitary-adrenal axis by cytokines. Baillieres Best Pract Res Clin Endocrinol Metab 13:503–521
26. Dharbhar FS, McEwen BS, Spencer RL (1993) Stress response, adrenal steroid receptor levels and corticosteroid-binding globulin levels—a comparison between Spraque-Dawley, Fischer 344 and Lewis rats. Brain Res 616:89–98
27. Smith CC et al (1994) Differential mineral corticoid (type 1) and glucocorticoid (type 2) receptor expression in Lewis and Fischer rats. Neuroimmunomodulation 1:66–73
28. McKay L, Cidlowshki JA (1999) Molecular control of immune/inflammatory responses: interactions between nuclear factor-kB and steroid receptor-signaling pathways. Endocr Rev 20:435–459
29. Van der Burg B et al (1997) Nuclear factor-k B repression in antiinflammation an immunosuppression by glucocorticoids. Trends Endocrinol Metab 8:152–157
30. Brogan IJ et al (1999) Interaction of glucocorticoid receptor isoforms with transcription factors AP-1 and NF-kB: lack of effect of glucocorticoid receptor B. Mol Cell Endocrinol 157:95–104
31. Pearce D, Yamamoto K (1993) Mineralocorticoid and glucocorticoid receptor activities distinguished by nonreceptor factors at a composite response element. Science 259:1161–1165
32. Plaut M (1987) Lymphocyte hormone receptors. Annu Rev Immunol 5:621–669
33. Pitzalis C, Piitone N, Perretti M (2002) Regulation of leukocyte-endothelial interactions by glucocorticoids. Ann N Y Acad Sci 966:108–118
34. Tamada K et al (1998) IL-4-producing NK1.1+ T cells are resistance to glucocorticoid-induced apoptosis: implications for the Th1/Th2 balance. J Immunol 161:1239–1247
35. Planey S, Litwack G (2000) Glucocorticoid-induced apoptosis in lymphocyte. Biochem Biophys Res Commun 279:307–312
36. Alamai WY, Melemedjian OK (2002) Molecular mechanisms of glucocorticoid antiproliferative

effects: antagonism of transcription factor activity by glucocorticoid receptor. J Leukoc Biol 71:9–15

37. Steer JH et al (1998) Altered leucocytes trafficking and suppressed tumour necrosis factor a release from peripheral blood monocytes after intraarticular glucocorticoid treatment. Ann Rheum Dis 57:732–737
38. Wingett D, Forcier K, Nielson CP (1996) Glucocorticoid mediated inhibition of RANTES expression in human T lymphocytes. FEBS Lett 398:308–311
39. Barnes PJ (2010) Mechanisms and resistance in glucocorticoid control of inflammation. J Steroid Biochem Mol Biol 120:76–85
40. Liberman AC et al (2007) Glucocorticoids in the regulation of transcription factors that control cytokine synthesis. Cytokine Growth Factor Rev 18:45–56
41. Russo-Marie F (1992) Macrophages and the glucocorticoids. J Neuroimmunol 40:281–286
42. Tait AS, Butts CL, Sternberg EM (2008) The role of glucocorticoids and progestins in inflammatory, autoimmune, and infectious disease. J Leukoc Biol 84:924–931
43. Schif-Zuck S et al (2011) Saturated-efferocytosis generates proresolving CD11b low macrophages: modulation by resolvins and glucocorticoids. Eur J Immunol 41:336–379
44. Goulding NK et al (1998) Novel pathways for glucocorticoid effects on neutrophils in chronic inflammation. Inflamm Res 47:S158–S165
45. Strausbaugh HJ, Rosen SD (1998) A potential role for annexin 1 as a physiologic mediator of glucocorticoid-induced L-selectin shedding from myeloid cells. J Immunol 166:294–300
46. Kontula K et al (1983) Binding of progestins to the glucocorticoid receptor. Correlation to their glucocorticoid-like effects on in vitro functions of human mononuclear leukocytes. Biochem Pharmacol 32:1511–1518
47. McColl A et al (2007) Effects of glucocorticoids on apoptosis and clearance of apoptotic cells. ScientificWorldJournal 17:1165–1181
48. Ashwell JD, Lu FWM, Ms V (2000) Glucocorticoids in T cell development and function. Annu Rev Immunol 18:309–345
49. Zen M et al (2011) The kaleidoscope of glucocorticoid effects on immune system. Autoimmun Rev 10:305–310
50. Moser M et al (1995) Glucocorticoids downregulate dendritic cell function in vitro and in vivo. Eur J Immunol 10:2818–2824
51. Roca L et al (2007) Dexamethasone modulates interleukin-12 production by inducing monocyte chemoattractant protein-1 in human dendritic cells. Immunol Cell Biol 8:610–616
52. Vacchio MS, Lee JJ, Ashwell JD (1999) Thymus-derived glucocorticoids set the thresholds for thymocyte selection by inhibiting TCR-mediated thymocyte activation. J Immunol 163:1327–1333
53. Palinkas L et al (2008) Developmental shift in TcR-mediated rescue of thymocytes from glucocorticoid-induced apoptosis. Immunobiology 213:39–50
54. Purton JF et al (2004) Expression of the glucocorticoid receptor from the 1A promoter correlates with T lymphocyte sensitivity to glucocorticoid-induced cell death. J Immunol 173:3816–3824
55. Takeda T et al (2008) Crosstalk between the interleukin-6 (IL-6)-JAK-STAT and the glucocorticoid-nuclear receptor pathway: synergistic activation of IL-6 response element by IL-6 and glucocorticoid. J Endocrinol 159: 323–330
56. Adcock IM (2001) Glucocorticoid-regulated transcription factors. Pulm Pharmacol Ther 14:211–219
57. Van Oosten MJ et al (2010) Polymorphisms n the glucocorticoid receptor gene that modulate glucocorticoid sensitivity are associated with rheumatoid arthritis. Arthritis Res Ther 12:R159
58. Vazquez-Tello A et al (2010) Induction of glucocorticoid receptor-beta expression in epithelial cells of asthmatic airways by T-helper type 17 cytokines. Clin Exp Allergy 40(9):1312–1322
59. Belinger DL et al (2008) Sympathetic modulation of immunity: relevance to disease. Cell Immunol 2:27–56
60. Nance DM, Sanders VM (2007) Autonomic innervation and regulation of the immune system (1987–2007). Brain Behav Immun 21: 736–745
61. Madden KS, Sanders VM, Felten DL (1995) Catecholamine influences and sympathetic neural modulation of immune responsiveness. Annu Rev Pharmacol Toxicol 35:417–448
62. Logan RW, Ariona A, Sarkar DK (2011) Role of sympathetic nervous system in the entrainment of circadian natural-killer cell function. Brain Behav Immun 25:101–109
63. Woods JA (2000) Exercised and neuroendocrine modulation of macrophage function. Int J Sports Med 21:S24–S30
64. Maestroni GJ (2006) Sympathetic nervous system influence on the innate immune response. Ann N Y Acad Sci 1069:195–207
65. Shahabi S et al (2006) Sympathetic nervous system plays an important role in the relationship between immune mediated diseases. Med Hypotheses 67:900–903

66. Sanders VM et al (1997) Differential expression of the beta-2-adrenergic receptor by Th1 and Th2 clones: implications for cytokine production and B cell help. J Immunol 158:4200–4210
67. Panine-Bordignon P et al (1997) Beta2-agonists prevent Th1 development by selective inhibition of interleukin 12. J Clin Invest 100:1513–1519
68. Kim BJ, Jones HP (2010) Epinephrine-primed murine bone marrow-derived dendritic cells facilitate production of IL-17A and IL-4 but not IFN-g by CD4+ T cells. Brain Behav Immun 24:1126–1136
69. Borovikova LV et al (2000) Vagus nerve stimulation attenuates the systemic inflammatory response to endotoxin. Nature 405:458–462
70. Sato KZ et al (1999) Diversity of mRNA expression for muscarinic acetylcholine receptor subtypes and neuronal nicotinic acetylcholine receptor subunits in human mononuclear leukocytes and leukemic cell lines. Neurosci Lett 266:17–20
71. Borovikova LV et al (2000) Role of vagus nerve signaling in CNI-1493-mediated suppression of acute inflammation. Auton Neurosci 85:141–147
72. Yoshikawa H et al (2006) Nicotine inhibits the production of proinflammatory mediators in human monocytes by suppression of I-kappaB phosphorylation and nuclear factor-kappaB transcriptional activity through nicotinic acetylcholine receptor alpha7. Clin Exp Immunol 146:116–123
73. de Jonge WJ, van der Zanden EP (2005) Stimulation of the vagus nerve attenuates macrophage activation by activating the Jak2- STAT3 signaling pathway. Nat Immunol 6:844–851
74. Vale W et al (1981) Characterization of a 41-residue ovine hypothalamic peptide that stimulates secretion of corticotropin and beta-endorphin. Science 213:1394–1397
75. Chen R et al (1993) Expression cloning of a human corticotropin-releasing-factor receptor. Proc Natl Acad Sci U S A 90:8967–8971
76. Kalantaridou S et al (2007) Peripheral corticotropin-releasing hormone is produced in the immune and reproductive systems: actions, potential roles and clinical implications. Front Biosci 12:572–580
77. Tache Y, Kiank C, Stengel A (2009) A role for corticotropin-releasing factor in functional gastrointestinal disorders. Curr Gastroenterol Rep 11:270–277
78. Slominski A et al (2001) Cutaneous expression of corticotropin-releasing hormone (CRH), urocortin, and CRH receptors. FASEB J 15:1678–1693
79. Gonzales XF et al (2008) Stress-induced differences in primary and secondary resistance against bacterial sepsis corresponds with diverse corticotropin releasing hormone receptor expression by pulmonary CD11c+ MHC II+ and CD11c-MHC II+ APCs. Brain Behav Immun 22:552–564
80. Cao J et al (2005) Human mast cells express corticotropin-releasing hormone (CRH) receptors and CRH leads to selective secretion of vascular endothelial growth factor. J Immunol 174:7665–7675
81. Webster EL et al (1990) Corticotropin-releasing factor receptors in mouse spleen: identification of receptor-bearing cells as resident macrophages. Endocrinology 127: 440–452
82. Agelaki S et al (2002) Corticotropin-releasing hormone augments proinflammatory cytokine production from macrophages in vitro and in lipopolysaccharide-induced endotoxin shock in mice. Infect Immun 70:6068–6074
83. Wallon C, Soderholm JD (2009) Corticotropin-releasing hormone and mast cells in the regulation of mucosal barrier function in the human colon. Ann N Y Acad Sci 1165:206–210
84. Gao L et al (2007) Corticotropin-releasing hormone receptor type 1 and type 2 mediate differential effects on 15-hydroxy prostaglandin dehydrogenase expression in cultured human chorion trophoblasts. Endocrinology 148:3645–3654
85. Kokkotou E et al (2006) Corticotropin-releasing hormone receptor 2-deficient mice have reduced intestinal inflammatory responses. J Immunol 177:3355–3361
86. Moffatt JD, Lever R, Page CP (2006) Activation of corticotropin-releasing factor receptor-2 causes bronchorelaxation and inhibits pulmonary inflammation in mice. FASEB J 20:1877–1879
87. Watkins LR, Maier SF (2005) Immune regulation of central nervous system functions: from sickness responses to pathological pain. J Intern Med 257:139–155
88. Vedhara K et al (1999) Chronic stress in elderly carers of dementia patients and antibody response to influenza vaccination. Lancet 353: 627–631

Chapter 5

Physical Activity, Stress Reduction, and Mood: Insight into Immunological Mechanisms

Mark Hamer, Romano Endrighi, and Lydia Poole

Abstract

Psychosocial factors, such as chronic mental stress and mood, are recognized as an important predictor of longevity and wellbeing. In particular, depression is independently associated with cardiovascular disease and all-cause mortality, and is often comorbid with chronic diseases that can worsen their associated health outcomes. Regular exercise is thought to be associated with stress reduction and better mood, which may partly mediate associations between depression, stress, and health outcomes. The underlying mechanisms for the positive effects of exercise on wellbeing remain poorly understood. In this overview we examine epidemiological evidence for an association between physical activity and mental health. We then describe the exercise withdrawal paradigm as an experimental protocol to study mechanisms linking exercise, mood, and stress. In particular we will discuss the potential role of the inflammatory response as a central mechanism.

Key words: Exercise withdrawal, Mental stress, Mood, Physical activity, Inflammation, Psychophysiology, Wellbeing

1. Introduction

Mental illness is now recognized as a serious health risk, and accounts for approximately 14% of the global burden of disease. Depression, one of the most common mental disorders, ranks fourth among the leading causes of disability adjusted life years worldwide (1). Prospective studies have demonstrated that clinical and sub-clinical depression in initially healthy individuals relates to greater risk of future cardiovascular disease (CVD), diabetes, and mortality (2, 3). Depressive symptoms appear to be a risk factor for mortality following myocardial infarction (4) and in patients with coronary heart disease (5). In our recent meta-analysis of prospective cohort studies (6), depression also predicted a 29% increase in cancer incidence and an 8% reduction in cancer survival. In addition,

Qing Yan (ed.), *Psychoneuroimmunology: Methods and Protocols*, Methods in Molecular Biology, vol. 934, DOI 10.1007/978-1-62703-071-7_5, © Springer Science+Business Media, LLC 2012

observational data from 60 countries has demonstrated that depression produces the greatest decrement in health compared with other chronic diseases, and the comorbid state of depression incrementally worsens health compared with depression alone (7). Extensive epidemiological evidence has also demonstrated an association between chronic stress exposure and long-term health outcomes such as death and clinical CVD events. For example, chronic work stress, caregiver burden, hostility, loneliness, and poor social networks are all related to a greater risk of future CVD and mortality in initially healthy individuals (8–11). Conversely, evidence is beginning to emerge to show that positive psychosocial characteristics such as positive affect and wellbeing are associated with beneficial health outcomes (12). Psychosocial factors may therefore exert their effect on mental and physical health through similar behavioral and physiological mechanisms, but at present these mechanisms are not completely understood.

Depression and stress-related disorders have various modes of treatment, including pharmacotherapy, psychotherapy, and lifestyle or behavioral modification. However, evidence shows that pharmacotherapy is only effective in about one third of patients and some only have a partial response to treatment (13), prompting the need to identify other forms of treatment. Instead, more recently physical exercise has received a significant amount of attention with regards to stress reduction and improving mood. In this chapter we will present an overview of the evidence linking physical activity with stress reduction and mood, with particular attention on mechanisms. We will present evidence from several types of study design, including; (1) observational epidemiological cohort studies that follow large samples of the population over time; and (2) experimental studies that manipulate behaviors such as physical activity, or administer acute stressors in controlled laboratory settings.

2. Physical Activity, Stress, and Mood

The epidemiological cohort studies performed in this area are generally designed to assess the exposure variable (e.g., physical activity) at baseline and track various outcome measures (e.g., a measure of depressive symptoms) through follow-up so that changes over time can be examined. In a recent meta-analysis, we systematically retrieved 13 prospective cohort epidemiological studies (14–26) that examined the association between physical activity and risk of future depression. The total sample size consisted of 73,487 participants who were healthy and not clinically depressed at the baseline assessment. Three of the cohorts consisted of women only, three consisted of men only, and the remaining seven cohorts were of mixed gender. The follow-up period ranged from 2 to 25 years (mean average, 9.2 years). Physical activity was assessed through self-report measures and incident depression was measured from a variety of methods, including a physician diagnosis or the administration of different validated psychometric tools, such as the Centre for Epidemiologic Studies for Depression Scale. The pooled odds ratio (OR) of depression in the physically active compared with the sedentary was 0.78 (95% CI, 0.71–0.86, $P<0.001$), which suggests the active have a 22% reduced risk of developing depressive symptoms. There was significant heterogeneity, χ^2 (15)=47.06, $P<0.001$, although the results of Begg's asymmetry test suggested that publication bias was unlikely ($P>0.10$). Figure 1 displays the effect sizes from all of the included studies. Interestingly, the protective effects of physical activity appeared to be stronger in women (OR=0.69, 0.60–0.79, $P<0.001$) than in men (OR=0.81, 0.66–0.99, $P=0.045$), and this is noteworthy since women generally report more psychological distress and depression. The gender effect largely explained the high level of heterogeneity found in the overall results. It should be noted that wherever possible, odds ratios were extracted from

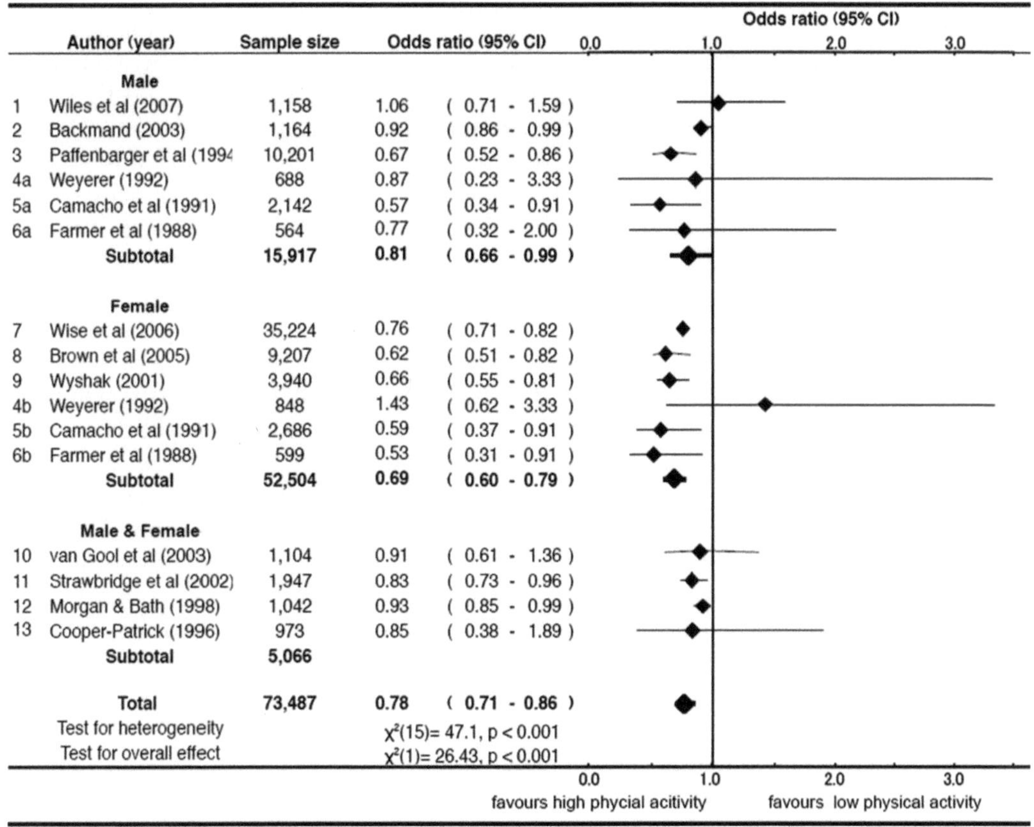

	Author (year)	Sample size	Odds ratio (95% CI)
	Male		
1	Wiles et al (2007)	1,158	1.06 (0.71 - 1.59)
2	Backmand (2003)	1,164	0.92 (0.86 - 0.99)
3	Paffenbarger et al (1994	10,201	0.67 (0.52 - 0.86)
4a	Weyerer (1992)	688	0.87 (0.23 - 3.33)
5a	Camacho et al (1991)	2,142	0.57 (0.34 - 0.91)
6a	Farmer et al (1988)	564	0.77 (0.32 - 2.00)
	Subtotal	**15,917**	**0.81 (0.66 - 0.99)**
	Female		
7	Wise et al (2006)	35,224	0.76 (0.71 - 0.82)
8	Brown et al (2005)	9,207	0.62 (0.51 - 0.82)
9	Wyshak (2001)	3,940	0.66 (0.55 - 0.81)
4b	Weyerer (1992)	848	1.43 (0.62 - 3.33)
5b	Camacho et al (1991)	2,686	0.59 (0.37 - 0.91)
6b	Farmer et al (1988)	599	0.53 (0.31 - 0.91)
	Subtotal	**52,504**	**0.69 (0.60 - 0.79)**
	Male & Female		
10	van Gool et al (2003)	1,104	0.91 (0.61 - 1.36)
11	Strawbridge et al (2002)	1,947	0.83 (0.73 - 0.96)
12	Morgan & Bath (1998)	1,042	0.93 (0.85 - 0.99)
13	Cooper-Patrick (1996)	973	0.85 (0.38 - 1.89)
	Subtotal	**5,066**	
	Total	**73,487**	**0.78 (0.71 - 0.86)**
	Test for heterogeneity		$\chi^2(15)= 47.1$, $p<0.001$
	Test for overall effect		$\chi^2(1)= 26.43$, $p<0.001$

Fig. 1. Forest plot that displays effect sizes from epidemiological studies on physical activity and risk of depressive symptoms.

multivariate models with the most complete adjustment for potential confounders, which importantly demonstrates that physical activity seems to be independently associated with risk of depression. The studies included in our analyses incorporated a number of potential confounders including social class, education, employment, marital status, smoking, and alcohol intake. Several studies also employed additional controls for chronic illnesses, physical disability, and stressful life events.

A major weakness of this area, however, is the reliance on self-reported physical activity. This is a limitation because mental health might cause reporting bias and some symptoms of mental illness might have conceptual overlap with physical activity behavior. For example, individuals with more depressive symptoms may under- or over-report the frequency of their physical activity or sedentary time. Furthermore, self-reported activity and sedentary time is somewhat arbitrary and imprecise as there is controversy at present as to how to differentiate between different exercise intensities e.g., light, moderate, vigorous (27). Physical activity can be assessed objectively using accelerometers, which are devices that measure body movements in terms of acceleration, which can then be used to estimate the intensity of physical activity over time. Most accelerometers are piezoelectric sensors that detect acceleration in one to three orthogonal planes (anteroposterior, mediolateral, and vertical). Very few studies have examined associations between objectively assessed physical activity and mental health, and those that have revealed inconsistent findings. For example, in a small cohort of elderly Japanese participants, physical activity was assessed objectively over 1 year, and inverse associations of activity with depression and stressful life events were observed (28, 29). In a small study of 32 non-psychiatric individuals, there was an inverse relationship between depressive symptoms and physical activity recorded over 5 days of accelerometry, with those performing the lowest levels of physical activity being at greatest risk of depressive symptoms (30). Similarly, in a sample of 73 students seeking help from a counseling service, depression was found to be negatively associated with daytime physical activity as assessed using 2-week accelerometry recordings (31). However, more recent evidence has not supported these findings, with results from 105 non-psychiatric participants showing no relationship between physical activity measured using accelerometers and depressed mood (32). The largest study to date by Janney et al. (33) used data from the NHANES 2003–2004 cohort of US non-institutionalized civilians, to investigate the use of mental health services and its association with physical activity as measured using accelerometers. Results showed that male users were significantly less active than non-users although no association was found for women. We have recently conducted several studies in this area. The first was a cross-sectional study in a representative sample of 921 English adults, which demonstrated

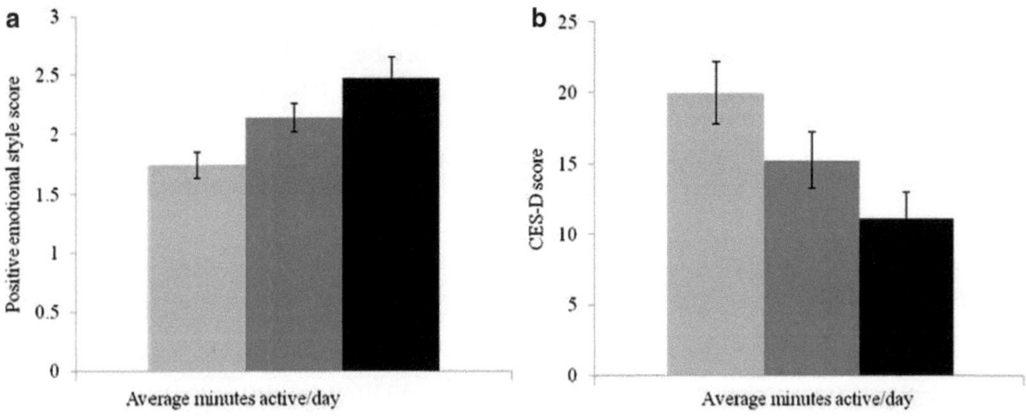

Fig. 2. The association between physical activity and (**a**) daily positive mood; (**b**) depressive mood measured from the Centre for Epidemiological Studies Depression (CES-D) scale. Physical activity groups are based on average daily activity recorded by accelerometry (*light bars*, ≤213.88 min/day; *grey bars*, 213.89–262.33 min/day; *black bars*, ≥262.34 min/day).

an association between objectively measured physical activity and self-rated health, although not with symptoms of psychological distress (34). In this study participants reporting very good health recorded, on average, 7 min/day (95% CI, 1–12 min/day, $P=0.019$) more moderate to vigorous activity compared with participants reporting fair–poor health. In a second study we examined the association between objectively measured habitual physical activity levels and daily mood in women (35). Participants wore an accelerometer device during waking hours for 1 week, and in addition recorded their daily moods. We observed robust associations between objectively assessed physical activity and more positive daily mood, which is displayed in Fig. 2 where physical activity groups reflect tertile of average daily minutes active recorded by accelerometry.

In addition to these discrepancies, it is not yet clear whether exercise intensity or duration is the key factor for determining mental health benefits. For example, epidemiological evidence using self-reported physical activity has suggested that the mental health benefits are positive regardless of the intensity of the activity (36). However, in a cohort of elderly Japanese participants, only the duration of objectively assessed moderate intensity activity was inversely associated with depressive symptoms (29). Evidence from randomized controlled trials also suggests greater effects on positive mood in participants undertaking moderate intensity exercise compared with vigorous (37), and in relation to symptoms of fatigue more favorable effects have been observed for light intensity activity (38). Taken together, the reason for the inconsistent findings might be attributable to different cut-off points adopted when interpreting data from accelerometers and thus the development of definitive guidelines tackling these issues are required. In addition, accelerometer devices are limited in that they cannot be worn for all activities such as swimming and contact sports, and defining "non-wear" time can therefore be problematic. In summary, self-report and objective measures both have their advantages and an optimal method is to combine both approaches. Taken together, however, the evidence suggests regular exercise is associated with higher positive and lower negative mood symptoms.

3. Physical Activity, Depressive Symptoms, and Inflammation

The immune system may play an important role in psychobiological processes that link psychosocial stress with CVD and other health outcomes (39, 40). In particular, there has been much interest in the association between depressive symptoms and inflammatory risk markers (41). Several studies have reported elevated concentrations of various inflammatory markers in differing populations reporting depressive symptoms, including the medically healthy (42, 43), elderly (44–46), and patients with acute coronary symptoms or existing CVD risk factors (39, 47, 48). Indeed, we recently hypothesized that inflammation may be one of the causal mechanisms by which depression manifests itself in acute coronary syndrome patients (49). Experimental work from our laboratory has also demonstrated a link between inflammation and mood. Using a vaccination model to induce a mild inflammatory challenge, greater increases in negative mood were observed after vaccine compared with placebo among 30 healthy male volunteers (50). In addition, negative changes in mood following vaccination were significantly correlated with increases in interleukin (IL)-6 production. Notably, no significant symptoms of nausea were reported, so it cannot be argued that negative mood arose because the participants were feeling ill.

A large amount of interest has also focused on the potential anti-inflammatory effects of exercise. It has been argued that the increases in circulating IL-6 that are observed after an acute bout of exercise promote an anti-inflammatory environment by increasing IL-1 receptor antagonist and IL-10 synthesis, while inhibiting pro-inflammatory markers such as tumor necrosis factor-alpha (TNF-α) (51). The cytokines released during exercise are thought to originate from exercising skeletal muscle, which work in a hormone-like fashion exerting specific endocrine effects on various organs and signaling pathways (52). Unlike IL-6 release during acute mental stress, which appears to be dependent on activation of the NFκB signaling pathway (53), intramuscular IL-6 expression is regulated by a network of signaling cascades that are likely to involve the CA^{2+}/NFAT and glycogen/p38 MAPK pathways. This might partly explain why exercise-induced IL-6 release is not acting as a strong pro-inflammatory agent. This hypothesis might also explain why a large number of observational studies have demonstrated an inverse association between regular physical activity and various pro-inflammatory markers in humans (54). Results from exercise trials have not always consistently found reductions in inflammatory markers following intervention although some of these findings are confounded by issues such as changes in fat mass that are an important source of inflammatory cytokine production (55). Indeed, increasing interest has focused on mechanisms by which exercise reduces visceral white adipose tissue inflammation, including reduced adipocyte size, increased blood flow, increased mitochondrial function and facilitated fatty acid oxidation, decreased cellular stress, and/or improved resistance to cell stress.

Given the described link between both mood and exercise with inflammatory pathways, it is feasible to hypothesize that better mental wellbeing experienced by regular exercisers might be partly explained by an underlying inflammatory mechanism. We conducted a study in a sample of 3,609 older adults from The English Longitudinal Study of Ageing, to examine if the association between persistent depressive symptoms and inflammatory markers over 2 years follow-up could be partly explained by physical activity behavior. Participants with recurrent elevated depressive symptomatology at both time points displayed significantly elevated levels of C-reactive protein (CRP) and fibrinogen at follow-up compared to non-depressed, and this relationship was partly explained through lower levels of physical activity in participants with depressive symptoms (56). The anti-inflammatory effects of exercise might also be relevant at a neurobiological level, since alterations in neurotransmitter function involving serotonin, norepinephrine, and dopamine are known to induce depression and are targets for currently available psychopharmacological treatments. Exercise is thought to alter serotonin metabolism, release endogenous opioids, and increase central noradrenergic neurotransmission which may all contribute to antidepressant and anxiolytic effects. The dopaminergic system is thought to play a key role in depression, and polymorphisms of the dopamine D2 receptor gene have also been implicated in physical activity behavior (57). Further research has focused on the hippocampus, where exercise-induced neurogenesis and growth factor expression have been proposed as potential mediators (58). An emerging theory is that exercise enhances several growth factors, such as brain derived neurotrophic factor (BDNF) and insulin like growth factor (IGF-1), which mediate the protective and therapeutic effects of exercise on depression. It has been shown that an acute bout of exercise increases peripheral levels of serum BDNF in an exercise intensity dependent fashion, but resting levels of BDNF does not seem to be affected by long-term exercise training (59) suggesting that other compensatory mechanisms might be at play. There is also evidence to suggest that the pro-inflammatory cytokines impair some of the growth factor signaling pathways in the brain (60), thus anti-inflammatory actions of exercise may again be important.

Another important aspect may be the interaction of the immune system with the hypothalamic pituitary adrenal (HPA) axis and autonomic nervous system. Following mental stress, the sensitivity of the immune system to dexamethasone inhibition (a synthetic version of the hormone cortisol that has potent anti-inflammatory properties) is reduced, as manifest by a reduction in this hormone's capacity to suppress the production of inflammatory cytokines (61). In endurance trained individuals, however, an acute bout of exercise has been shown to increase tissue sensitivity to glucocorticoids, which is thought to act as a mechanism to prevent an excessive muscle inflammatory reaction (62). HPA axis dysregulation and cortisol hyper-secretion has been implicated in mental health and some studies have shown lower stress-induced cortisol responses in physically trained individuals compared to the untrained (63, 64) suggesting that physical activity may act as a buffer against exaggerated or sustained stress responses. Nevertheless, we have failed to replicate these findings in our work that examined associations between objectively assessed physical activity levels and cortisol responses to acute mental stress (35). However, the association of the cortisol diurnal rhythm with physical activity behavior has not been investigated and further work is required in this area.

Previous research has indicated an intriguing link between efferent cholinergic activity of the vagus nerve (the parasympathetic arm of the autonomic nervous system) and inhibition of inflammatory processes (65). We have previously shown that physically fitter individuals maintained greater parasympathetic control during mental stress and also demonstrated lower inflammatory stress responses (66). The decline in parasympathetic control with aging is attenuated with regular exercise training (67), thus it is feasible that fitness-related improvements in parasympathetic activity could play a role in mediating the inhibition of stress-induced inflammatory processes.

In summary there is a link between physical activity and mood, and several physiological response systems have been implicated including the inflammatory, dopaminergic, and neuroendocrine systems. However, there is a lack of experimental and longitudinal evidence to show the long-term health consequences of the effect of physical activity on these biological pathways.

4. The Exercise Withdrawal Paradigm

Experimental trials of exercise training in patients and healthy volunteers have been effective in treating depressive symptoms with effect sizes ranging from 1.03 to 0.58, respectively (68). There appears to be substantial individual variation in responses, and the effect sizes vary depending on intervention duration, exercise type, bout duration, and intensity. Exercise training trials are costly and require a large amount of manpower in administering supervised exercise sessions. Additionally, one of the difficulties in interpreting data from short-term (often 8–12 weeks) exercise trials is that individual changes in fitness are usually modest, which suggests a short period of exercise training may not be sufficient to induce the type of chronic adaptations required to observe stress buffering effects. The exercise withdrawal paradigm therefore represents a useful, more practical alternative since mood disturbances can be elicited in habitual exercisers after 1–2 weeks withdrawal from their regular training activities, which provides a model to investigate the links between exercise, mood, and the underlying biology. We and others have hypothesized that mood disturbances caused by withdrawal from regular exercise might act as a mild inflammatory stimulus. However, recent studies have been unable to confirm this hypothesis. Several studies, including one of our own that have successfully induced an increased negative mood following several weeks of exercise withdrawal, did not find any changes in a range of inflammatory markers, such as IL-6, CRP, TNF-α, fibrinogen, and soluble intracellular adhesion molecule-1 (69, 70). Similarly, 1 week withdrawal from exercise in highly active men did not elicit any substantial changes in CRP, IL-6, TNF-α, and circulating leukocyte concentration (71). In the same study, no changes in inflammatory markers were observed among sedentary participants who undertook 30 min of brisk walking each day for 1 week. Healthy men that reduced their daily step count by 85% for 2 weeks developed impaired glucose tolerance, attenuation of postprandial lipid metabolism, and a 7% increase in intra-abdominal fat mass, although plasma cytokines and muscular expression of TNF was not altered (72). However, another study reported that reduced parasympathetic nervous activity as measured by heart rate variability was predictive of negative mood following exercise withdrawal (73). These findings are consistent with emerging data on underlying molecular mechanisms. For example, the expression of exercise-regulated muscle genes, such as the transcriptional co-activator PGC1α, that is thought to promote anti-inflammatory effects (74), is known to be rapidly induced after a single bout of acute exercise although quickly reverts back to basal levels. In contrast to the transient changes following acute exercise, greater levels of PGC1α are present in chronically trained exercised muscle than in untrained. Thus, there is a clear difference between short-term and long-term adaptations, which might explain why a short 2 week exercise withdrawal period in trained participants is insufficient to see changes. Furthermore, adherence to exercise withdrawal in regular, fit exercisers may be problematic because habitually active individuals are less likely to agree to stop their activity regime and perhaps compensate in some other ways to maintain a physically active lifestyle (e.g., taking up active commuting for the period of exercise withdrawal), which might influence the results.

In a further study we investigated the impact of exercise withdrawal on psychophysiological responses to mental stress because this method can sometimes detect differences that might not otherwise be seen under resting conditions. Indeed, although acute psychophysiological responses are not clinically meaningful in themselves, they represent the way in which individuals respond to daily stressors in their normal lives and if elicited regularly might have clinical relevance. Although the effects of cytokines are often thought to be transient, they may provoke a time-dependent sensitization so that the response to a later cytokine or stressor stimulus is enhanced, resulting in an increased vulnerability to depressed mood (75). We experimentally manipulated physical activity levels by asking a group of habitual exercisers to withdraw from their regular training for 2 weeks (76). The adherence to exercise withdrawal was mixed, as indicated by objective accelerometry physical activity records, but in participants with greater mood disturbances (assessed using the 28 item General Health Questionnaire) following 2 weeks withdrawal we observed significantly higher inflammatory responses to mental stress compared to those with low or no mood disturbance. These findings are presented in Fig. 3, which shows that participants in the highest tertile of mood disturbance demonstrated the greatest inflammatory responses to mental stress after statistical adjustments for age, gender, body mass index, and pre-intervention inflammatory stress response. In the same study, cortisol responses

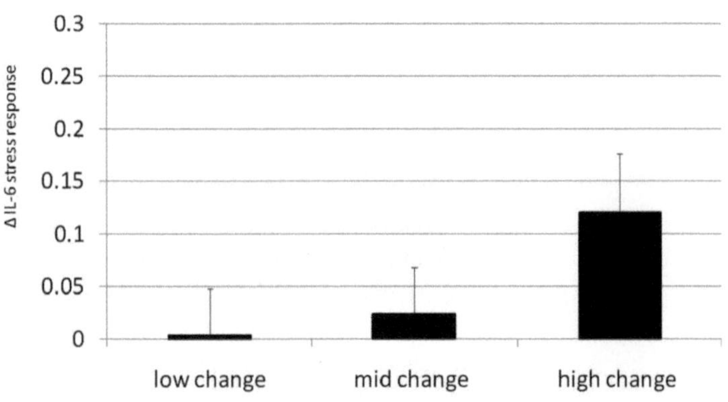

Fig. 3. The association between mood disturbance following 2 weeks exercise withdrawal and IL-6 responses to mental stress. Participants were 41 healthy men and women regularly engaged in exercise. Mood disturbance was assessed using the 28 item General Health questionnaire. Data are presented as mean ± SEM, adjusted for age, gender, body mass index, and pre-intervention inflammatory stress response.

to mental stress were higher in the exercise withdrawal phase compared to control period with a significant difference emerging at 20 min post-stress. These results, although preliminary, suggest that inflammatory and neuroendocrine factors may in part mediate the protective or buffering effect of physical activity on stress-related physiological activation.

To summarize, the exercise withdrawal paradigm offers a promising way in which to elucidate some of the causal pathways linking physical activity to stress and mood. Future work is needed to better understand the temporal relationship between exercise-induced mood disturbances and changes in inflammatory and neuroendocrine factors.

5. Summary

Regular physical activity is associated with better mental health and wellbeing. The methodologies used to investigate this area include observational population studies and smaller laboratory-based experimental work. In this article we have highlighted the exercise withdrawal paradigm as an experimental protocol to study mechanisms linking exercise, mood, and the underlying biology. We have presented some preliminary evidence to suggest that psychobiological responses to exercise, including adaptations to the immune system, HPA axis, and autonomic nervous system, might partly facilitate the links between physical activity and wellbeing.

Acknowledgements

The authors are supported by grant funding from the British Heart Foundation (UK).

References

1. Insel TR, Charney DS (2003) Research on major depression. JAMA 289:3167–3168
2. Kuper H, Marmot M, Hemingway H (2002) Systematic review of prospective cohort studies of psychosocial factors in the etiology and prognosis of coronary heart disease. Semin Vasc Med 2:267–314
3. Knol MJ, Twisk JW, Beekman AT, Heine RJ, Snoek FJ, Pouwer F (2006) Depression as a risk factor for the onset of type 2 diabetes mellitus. A meta-analysis. Diabetologia 49:837–845
4. van Melle JP, de Jonge P, Spijkerman TA, Tijssen JG, Ormel J, van Veldhuisen DJ, van den Brink RH, van den Berg MP (2004) Prognostic association of depression following myocardial infarction with mortality and cardiovascular events: a meta-analysis. Psychosom Med 66:814–822
5. Barth J, Schumacher M, Herrmann-Lingen C (2004) Depression as a risk factor for mortality in patients with coronary heart disease: a meta-analysis. Psychosom Med 66:802–813
6. Chida Y, Hamer H, Wardle J, Steptoe A (2008) Do psychosocial stress-related factors contribute to cancer incidence and survival? Nat Clin Pract Oncol 5:466–475

7. Moussavi S, Chatterji S, Verdes E, Tandon A, Patel V, Ustun B (2007) Depression, chronic diseases, and decrements in health: results from the World Health Surveys. Lancet 370: 851–858
8. Heffner KL, Waring ME, Roberts MB, Eaton CB, Gramling R (2011) Social isolation, C-reactive protein, and coronary heart disease mortality among community-dwelling adults. Soc Sci Med 72:1482–1488
9. Kivimäki M, Virtanen M, Elovainio M, Kouvonen A, Väänänen A, Vahtera J (2006) Work stress in the etiology of coronary heart disease–a meta-analysis. Scand J Work Environ Health 32:431–442
10. Chida Y, Steptoe A (2009) The association of anger and hostility with future coronary heart disease: a meta-analytic review of prospective evidence. J Am Coll Cardiol 53:936–946
11. Schulz R, Beach SR (1999) Caregiving as a risk factor for mortality: the Caregiver Health Effects Study. JAMA 282:2215–2219
12. Pressman SD, Cohen S (2005) Does positive affect influence health? Psychol Bull 131: 925–971
13. Trivedi MH, Rush AJ, Wisniewski SR, Nierenberg AA, Warden D, Ritz L, Norquist G, Howland RH, Lebowitz B, McGrath PJ, Shores-Wilson K, Biggs MM, Balasubramani GK, Fava M, STAR*D Study Team (2006) Evaluation of outcomes with citalopram for depression using measurement-based care in STAR*D: implications for clinical practice. Am J Psychiatry 163:28–40
14. Wiles NJ, Haase AM, Gallacher J, Lawlor DA, Lewis G (2007) Physical activity and common mental disorder: results from the Caerphilly study. Am J Epidemiol 165:946–954
15. Wise LA, Adams-Campbell LL, Palmer JR, Rosenberg L (2006) Leisure time physical activity in relation to depressive symptoms in the Black Women's Health Study. Ann Behav Med 32:68–76
16. Brown WJ, Ford JH, Burton NW, Marshall AL, Dobson AJ (2005) Prospective study of physical activity and depressive symptoms in middle-aged women. Am J Prev Med 29: 265–272
17. Backmand H, Kaprio J, Kujala U, Sarna S (2003) Influence of physical activity on depression and anxiety of former elite athletes. Int J Sports Med 24:609–619
18. van Gool CH, Kempen GI, Penninx BW, Deeg DJ, Beekman AT, van Eijk JT (2003) Relationship between changes in depressive symptoms and unhealthy lifestyles in late middle aged and older persons: results from the Longitudinal Aging Study Amsterdam. Age Ageing 32:81–87
19. Strawbridge WJ, Deleger S, Roberts RE, Kaplan GA (2002) Physical activity reduces the risk of subsequent depression for older adults. Am J Epidemiol 156:328–334
20. Wyshak G (2001) Women's college physical activity and self-reports of physician-diagnosed depression and of current symptoms of psychiatric distress. J Womens Health Gend Based Med 10:363–370
21. Morgan K, Bath PA (1998) Customary physical activity and psychological wellbeing: a longitudinal study. Age Ageing 27(suppl 3):35–40
22. Cooper-Patrick L, Ford DE, Mead LA, Chang PP, Klag MJ (1997) Exercise and depression in midlife: a prospective study. Am J Public Health 87:670–673
23. Paffenbarger RS Jr, Lee IM, Leung R (1994) Physical activity and personal characteristics associated with depression and suicide in American college men. Acta Psychiatr Scand Suppl 377:16–22
24. Weyerer S (1992) Physical inactivity and depression in the community. Evidence from the Upper Bavarian Field Study. Int J Sports Med 13:492–496
25. Camacho TC, Roberts RE, Lazarus NB, Kaplan GA, Cohen RD (1991) Physical activity and depression: evidence from the Alameda County Study. Am J Epidemiol 134:220–231
26. Farmer ME, Locke BZ, Moscicki EK, Dannenberg AL, Larson DB, Radloff LS (1988) Physical activity and depressive symptoms: the NHANES I Epidemiologic Follow-up Study. Am J Epidemiol 128:1340–1351
27. Pate RR, O'Neill JR, Lobelo F (2008) The evolving definition of "Sedentary". Exerc Sport Sci Rev 36:173–178
28. Yoshiuchi K, Inada S, Nakahara R, Akabayashi A, Park H, Park S, Shephard RJ (2010) Stressful life events and habitual physical activity in older adults: 1-year accelerometer data from the Nakanojo Study. Ment Health Phys Act 3:23–25
29. Yoshiuchi K, Nakahara R, Kumano H, Kuboki T, Togo F, Watanabe E, Yasunaga A (2006) Yearlong physical activity and depressive symptoms in older Japanese adults: cross-sectional data from the Nakanojo study. Am J Geriatr Psychiatry 14:621–624
30. Mendlowicz MV, Jean-Louis G, von Gizycki H, Zizi F, Nunes J (1999) Actigraphic predictors of depressed mood in a cohort of non-psychiatric adults. Aust N Z J Psychiatry 33:553–558

31. Barkley TJ, Tryon WW (1995) Psychomotor retardation found in college students seeking counseling. Behav Res Ther 33:977–984
32. Kawada T, Katsumata M, Suzuki H, Shimizu T (2007) Actigraphic predictors of the depressive state in students with no psychiatric disorders. J Affect Disord 98:117–120
33. Janney CA, Richardson CR, Holleman RG, Glasheen C, Strath SJ, Conroy MB, Kriska AM (2008) Gender, mental health service use and objectively measured physical activity: Data from the National Health and Nutrition Examination Survey (NHANES 2003–2004). Ment Health Phys Act 1:9–16
34. Hamer M, Stamatakis E (2010) Objectively assessed physical activity, fitness and subjective wellbeing. Ment Health Phys Act 3:67–71
35. Poole L, Steptoe A, Wawrzyniak AJ, Bostock S, Mitchell ES, Hamer M (2011) Associations of objectively measured physical activity with daily mood ratings and psychophysiological stress responses in women. Psychophysiology 48: 1165–1172
36. Asztalos M, De Bourdeaudhuij I, Cardon G (2010) The relationship between physical activity and mental health varies across activity intensity levels and dimensions of mental health among women and men. Public Health Nutr 13:1207–1214
37. Moses J, Steptoe A, Mathews A, Edwards S (1989) The effects of exercise training on mental well-being in the normal population: a controlled trial. J Psychosom Res 33:47–61
38. Puetz TW, Flowers SS, O'Connor PJ (2008) A randomized controlled trial of the effect of aerobic exercise training on feelings of energy and fatigue in sedentary young adults with persistent fatigue. Psychother Psychosom 77: 167–174
39. Vaccarino V, Johnson BD, Sheps DS, Reis SE, Kelsey SF, Bittner V, Rutledge T, Shaw LJ, Sopko G, Bairey Merz CN, National Heart, Lung, and Blood Institute (2007) Depression, inflammation, and incident cardiovascular disease in women with suspected coronary ischemia: the National Heart, Lung, and Blood Institute-sponsored WISE study. J Am Coll Cardiol 50:2044–2050
40. Hamer M, Molloy GJ, Stamatakis E (2008) Psychological distress as a risk factor for CVD events: pathophysiological and behavioral mechanisms. J Am Coll Cardiol 52: 2156–2162
41. Irwin MR, Miller AH (2007) Depressive disorders and immunity: 20 years of progress and discovery. Brain Behav Immun 21:374–383
42. Liukkonen T, Silvennoinen-Kassinen S, Jokelainen J, Räsänen P, Leinonen M, Meyer-Rochow VB, Timonen M (2006) The association between C-reactive protein levels and depression: results from the northern Finland 1966 birth cohort study. Biol Psychiatry 60:825–830
43. Panagiotakos DB, Pitsavos C, Chrysohoou C, Tsetsekou E, Papageorgiou C, Christodoulou G, Stefanadis C, ATTICA Study (2004) Inflammation, coagulation, and depressive symptomatology in cardiovascular disease-free people; the ATTICA study. Eur Heart J 25: 492–499
44. Kop WJ, Gottdiener JS, Tangen CM, Fried LP, McBurnie MA, Walston J, Newman A, Hirsch C, Tracy RP (2002) Inflammation and coagulation factors in persons >65 years of age with symptoms of depression but without evidence of myocardial ischemia. Am J Cardiol 89:419–424
45. Penninx BW, Kritchevsky SB, Yaffe K, Newman AB, Simonsick EM, Rubin S, Ferrucci L, Harris T, Pahor M (2003) Inflammatory markers and depressed mood in older persons: results from the Health, Aging and Body Composition study. Biol Psychiatry 54:566–572
46. Bremmer MA, Beekman AT, Deeg DJ, Penninx BW, Dik MG, Hack CE, Hoogendijk WJ (2008) Inflammatory markers in late-life depression: results from a population-based study. J Affect Disord 106:249–255
47. Empana JP, Sykes DH, Luc G, Juhan-Vague I, Arveiler D, Ferrieres J, PRIME Study Group (2005) Contributions of depressive mood and circulating inflammatory markers to coronary heart disease in healthy European men: the Prospective Epidemiological Study of Myocardial Infarction (PRIME). Circulation 111:2299–2305
48. Pizzi C, Manzoli L, Mancini S, Costa GM (2008) Analysis of potential predictors of depression among coronary heart disease risk factors including heart rate variability, markers of inflammation, and endothelial function. Eur Heart J 29:1110–1117
49. Poole L, Dickens C, Steptoe A (2011) The puzzle of depression and acute coronary syndrome: reviewing the role of acute inflammation. J Psychosom Res 71:61–68
50. Wright CE, Strike PC, Brydon L, Steptoe A (2005) Acute inflammation and negative mood: mediation by cytokine activation. Brain Behav Immun 19:345–350
51. Febbraio MA, Pedersen BK (2002) Muscle-derived interleukin-6: mechanisms for activa-

tion and possible biological roles. FASEB J 16:1335–1347

52. Pedersen BK (2011) Exercise-induced myokines and their role in chronic diseases. Brain Behav Immun 25:811–816
53. Bierhaus A, Wolf J, Andrassy M, Rohleder N, Humpert PM, Petrov D, Ferstl R, von Eynatten M, Wendt T, Rudofsky G, Joswig M, Morcos M, Schwaninger M, McEwen B, Kirschbaum C, Nawroth PP (2003) A mechanism converting psychosocial stress into mononuclear cell activation. Proc Natl Acad Sci U S A 100:1920–1925
54. Hamer M (2007) The relative influences of fitness and fatness on inflammatory factors. Prev Med 44:3–11
55. Hamer M, O'Donovan G (2010) Cardiorespiratory fitness and metabolic risk factors in obesity. Curr Opin Lipidol 21:1–7
56. Hamer M, Molloy GJ, de Oliveira C, Demakakos P (2009) Persistent depressive symptomatology and inflammation: to what extent do health behaviours and weight control mediate this relationship? Brain Behav Immun 23:413–418
57. Simonen RL, Rankinen T, Perusse L, Leon AS, Skinner JS, Wilmore JH, Rao DC, Bouchard C (2003) A dopamine D2 receptor gene polymorphism and physical activity in two family studies. Physiol Behav 78:751–757
58. Cotman CW, Berchtold NC, Christie LA (2007) Exercise builds brain health: key roles of growth factor cascades and inflammation. Trends Neurosci 30:464–472
59. Knaepen K, Goekint M, Heyman EM, Meeusen R (2010) Neuroplasticity—exercise-induced response of peripheral brain-derived neurotrophic factor: a systematic review of experimental studies in human subjects. Sports Med 40:765–801
60. Tong L, Balazs R, Soiampornkul R, Thangnipon W, Cotman CW (2008) Interleukin-1beta impairs brain derived neurotrophic factor-induced signal transduction. Neurobiol Aging 29:1380–1393
61. Rohleder N, Schommer NC, Hellhammer DH, Engel R, Kirschbaum C (2001) Sex differences in glucocorticoid sensitivity of proinflammatory cytokine production after psychosocial stress. Psychosom Med 63:966–972
62. Duclos M, Gouarne C, Bonnemaison D (2003) Acute and chronic effects of exercise on tissue sensitivity to glucocorticoids. J Appl Physiol 94:869–875
63. Rimmele U, Seiler R, Marti B, Wirtz PH, Ehlert U, Heinrichs M (2009) The level of physical activity affects adrenal and cardiovascular reactivity to psychosocial stress. Psychoneuroendocrinology 34:190–198
64. Traustadóttir T, Bosch PR, Matt KS (2005) The HPA axis response to stress in women: effects of aging and fitness. Psychoneuroendocrinology 30:392–402
65. Tracey KJ (2002) The inflammatory reflex. Nature 420:853–859
66. Hamer M, Steptoe A (2007) Association between physical fitness, parasympathetic control, and proinflammatory responses to mental stress. Psychosom Med 69:660–666
67. Carter JB, Banister EW, Blaber AP (2003) Effect of endurance exercise on autonomic control of heart rate. Sports Med 33:33–46
68. Rethorst CD, Wipfli BM, Landers DM (2009) The antidepressive effects of exercise: a meta-analysis of randomized trials. Sports Med 39:491–511
69. Poole L, Hamer M, Wawrzyniak AJ, Steptoe A (2011) The effects of exercise withdrawal on mood and inflammatory cytokine responses in humans. Stress 14:439–447
70. Kop WJ, Weinstein AA, Deuster PA, Whittaker KS, Tracy RP (2008) Inflammatory markers and negative mood symptoms following exercise withdrawal. Brain Behav Immun 22: 1190–1196
71. Lund AJ, Hurst TL, Tyrrell RM, Thompson D (2011) Markers of chronic inflammation with short-term changes in physical activity. Med Sci Sports Exerc 43:578–583
72. Krogh-Madsen R, Thyfault JP, Broholm C, Mortensen OH, Olsen RH, Mounier R, Plomgaard P, van Hall G, Booth FW, Pedersen BK (2010) A 2-wk reduction of ambulatory activity attenuates peripheral insulin sensitivity. J Appl Physiol 108:1034–1040
73. Weinstein AA, Deuster PA, Kop WJ (2007) Heart rate variability as a predictor of negative mood symptoms induced by exercise withdrawal. Med Sci Sports Exerc 39:735–741
74. Handschin C, Spiegelman BM (2008) The role of exercise and PGC1alpha in inflammation and chronic disease. Nature 454:463–469
75. Anisman H, Merali Z (2003) Cytokines, stress and depressive illness: brain-immune interactions. Ann Med 35:2–11
76. Endrighi R, Steptoe A, Hamer M (2011) Mood disturbance following exercise withdrawal is associated with greater inflammatory responses to stress. Psychosom Med 73:A110

Part II

Translation of Psychoneuroimmunology into Personalized Medicine: Potential Biomarkers and Clinical Implications

Chapter 6

Translational Implications of Inflammatory Biomarkers and Cytokine Networks in Psychoneuroimmunology

Qing Yan

Abstract

Developments in psychoneuroimmunology (PNI) need to be translated into personalized medicine to achieve better clinical outcomes. One of the most critical steps in this translational process is to identify systemic biomarkers for better diagnosis and treatment. Applications of systems biology approaches in PNI would enable the insights into the correlations among various systems and different levels for the identification of the basic elements of the psychophysiological framework. Among the potential PNI biomarkers, inflammatory markers deserve special attention as they play a pivotal role linking various health conditions and disorders. The elucidation of inflammatory markers, cytokine networks, and immune-brain-behavior interactions may help establish PNI profiles for the identification of potential targets for personalized interventions in at risk populations. The understanding of the general systemic pathways among different disorders may contribute to the transition from the disease-centered medicine to patient-centered medicine. Integrative strategies targeting these factors and pathways would be useful for the prevention and treatment of a spectrum of diseases that share the common links. Examples of the translational implications of potential PNI biomarkers and networks in diseases including depression, Alzheimer's disease, obesity, cardiovascular disease, stroke, and HIV are discussed in details.

Key words: Alzheimer's disease, Biomarkers, Cytokines, Depression, Inflammation, Obesity, Pathways, Personalized medicine, Psychoneuroimmunology, Systems biology

1. The Role of Psychoneuroimmunology Biomarkers in Personalized Medicine

Developments in psychoneuroimmunology (PNI) need to be translated into personalized medicine to achieve better clinical outcomes. One of the most critical steps in this translational process is to identify systemic biomarkers for better diagnosis and treatment. Biomarkers are objectively detected indicators of biomedical states (1). Biomarkers have great potentials for improving disease diagnosis, treatment selection, and prevention of side effects. Predictive and prognostic biomarkers for characterizing different subsets of patients have been used for outcome prediction and assessment in

Qing Yan (ed.), *Psychoneuroimmunology: Methods and Protocols*, Methods in Molecular Biology, vol. 934,
DOI 10.1007/978-1-62703-071-7_6, © Springer Science+Business Media, LLC 2012

a variety of diseases, such as cancer, cardiovascular diseases, respiratory diseases, rheumatoid arthritis, and neurological diseases (1).

Useful biomarkers should include the systems interactions and networks for the patient group profiling that are pathophysiologically similar (2). Discovery of biomarkers based on systems biology approaches may help understand multi-level factors and multi-directional interactions among psychological factors, the nervous system, the immune system, and the endocrine system ((2), also see Chapter 1). Insights into these interactions and the systems models would enable integrative prevention and therapeutic methods designed specifically for patient subgroups to reach the goals of personalized medicine.

These multi-level factors should include psychological and behavioral features such as emotional distress, and systemic physiological features such as immunological or neurological alterations (2). The connection of such factors with ultimate health conditions and disorders makes them appropriate candidate markers to be placed into the integrative frameworks for further personalized analysis (see Chapter 1). Although currently it is still hard to apply immune markers as biomarkers or diagnostic markers in the clinic, this rapidly developing field may make great contributions to the practice of personalized medicine. For instance, up to now the pathobiology of most psychiatric disorders is still unclear, with inaccurate diagnosis and empirical treatments that need improvement. The identification of biomarkers has been suggested to help achieve more precise diagnoses and better treatments in these disorders (3).

Among the potential PNI biomarkers, inflammatory markers deserve special attention as they play a pivotal role linking various health conditions and disorders including depression, obesity, cancer, and cardiovascular diseases (2). In fact, inflammation has been suggested as one of the best models for the translational purposes in personalized medicine (4). Patients with chronic diseases often have a high rate of inflammatory symptoms such as pain, sleep disorders, fatigue, as well as cognitive and mood changes. On the other hand, biobehavioral elements influence circulating inflammatory markers directly (5). The systemic profiling of inflammatory markers may have significant clinical implications for interventions to relieve those symptoms (6).

2. Applying Systems Biology Approaches in the Identification of Psychoneuro-immunology Biomarkers

Although genetic factors can be important biomarker candidates, these factors cannot function alone but are influenced by the gene-gene and gene-environment interactions. Gene-environment interactions have significant impacts on the identification of patient subgroups for personalized treatments in mood disorders (7).

Environmental factors such as epigenetic modifications and life experiences may affect the pathophysiological results of genetic susceptibility (see Chapter 2). These elements also include exposure types such as war trauma and time frames such as childhood abuse ((7), also see Chapter 1). Considering these complex factors, the integration of various types of information at different systems levels, including genetic variations, cellular pathways, and environmental factors are necessary for better diagnosis and treatments ((8), also see Chapter 1). Systems biology approaches would enable such integration.

Systems biology explores the interrelationships and networks among biomedical factors at various systems levels for the understanding and therapy of diseases (9). Systems biology combines mathematics and computational methods with empirical observations to be used for modeling multivariate networks for understanding complex systems ((9, 10), also see Chapter 20). Some strategies of systems biology that have been used to model molecular networks include ordinary differential equations (ODE) and general network models such as topological and statistical models (10). The cutting-edge technologies such as the high throughput methods may contribute to the finding of potential biomarkers by screening proteome mixtures at various disease states. A meaningful explanation of data from these methods requires investigation at multiple systems levels. A systems biology approach will make significant contributions to the interpretation of the behavior of these biomarker candidates (3).

For example, although singular factors are important in the pathogenesis of psychiatric disorders such as depression and anxiety, dysfunctional neural circuits and signaling pathways have been suggested to play significant roles (11). A combination of multiple genetic and environmental factors has been found to influence certain brain circuits in these disorders (12). Systemic profiling of the diseases need to be based on large datasets from analyses at various levels. These analyses should include gene expression and pathways at the molecular and cellular levels, multiple brain regions at the tissue/organ levels, and the transcriptome of a developmental series of brains within the time dimension (13). Thus systemic and multi-level analyses are needed for finding biomarkers and correlating genotypes with the disease phenotypes.

From the systems biology perspective, correlations among various systems need to be investigated for the identification of the basic elements of the psychophysiological framework. The brain and peripheral tissues including the cardiovascular and immune systems communicate in a bidirectional or even multi-directional approach, both "top-down and bottom-up" with autonomic and neuroendocrine pathways involved (14). Certain fronto-temporal cortical regions cooperate reciprocally with subcortical structures, responsible for affective, hormonal, immune, and stress responses, as well as the status of homeostasis (14). Inflammatory markers such as proinflammatory cytokines and signaling pathways can serve as crucial indices of these networks. Exploration of such structure-function connections between the mind and body may contribute to effective therapies for many chronic diseases.

In fact, systemic pathways have been found to be more useful as biomarkers than individual proteins for the transition from disease-centered medicine to preventive medicine (15). Many immune pathways can influence the brain and behavior. Interacting elements of the immune-brain interrelationships include the cytokines such as nuclear factor-κB (NF-κB) and neurotransmitters such as serotonin and dopamine (16). Such interactions are important in behavioral alterations such as anxiety, depression, anorexia, fatigue, sleep impairment, and cognitive dysfunctions (see Chapter 1). These immune-brain pathways can also affect environmental and vulnerability factors including stress, aging, and food intake (16). To discover personalized targets, it would be necessary to understand these immune-brain-behavior interrelationships. Potential preventive and treatment strategies can be designed by targeting these pathways of disorders among those at risk populations (2).

3. Cytokine Networks and Systemic Biomarkers

Cytokines enable the intercellular communication and transmit signals in the immune system. To this date more than 100 human cytokines have been identified (17). Cytokines form complex networks with multiple signaling pathways intersecting and influencing each other. They have synergistic or antagonistic functions. These molecules are involved in the bidirectional neural–immune interactions at various levels. Cytokine signals can be autocrine, i.e., the same cell generates the cytokine and also responds to it; or paracrine, i.e., the cytokine is generated by one cell and have effects on another (10). At the molecular level, cytokines and other molecules such as neurotransmitters and neuropeptides enable the communications among the nervous, endocrine, and immune systems. At the system level, neural–immune interactions have been associated with emotionality (10).

Cytokines may affect cognition through diverse mechanisms, such as by mediating bidirectional communications between the central nervous system (CNS) and the peripheral immune system, and involving in the hypothalamic-pituitary-adrenal (HPA) axis activation in stress and depression (18). Proinflammatory cytokines can communicate with a cytokine network in the brain and influence the brain functions associated with behaviors including neurotransmitter metabolism and neuroendocrine functions. These functions are involved in the modulation of mood, motivation, and alarm. Cytokine-mediated interactions between neurons and glial cells are associated with inflammatory mechanisms within the CNS in cognitive impairment (18). Such impacts may lead to behavioral changes and neuropsychiatric problems including anxiety, depression, anorexia, fatigue, cognitive dysfunction, and sleep disorders. For example, brain cytokines including interleukin-1β (IL-1β) and IL-6 have been related to various health conditions from food intake to anxiety-like behaviors (4). Investigation in such inflammation related pathways has been suggested a high priority in psychiatric diseases, because these pathways have played critical roles in diseases such as mood disorders and schizophrenia (19).

Specifically, many molecules and pathways are involved in such immune-brain interactions, such as NFκB, p38 mitogen activated protein kinase (MAPK), and various cytokine signaling networks. The relevant pathways also include those of indoleamine 2,3 dioxygenase (IDO) and kynurenine (KYN), the neurotransmitter pathways involving serotonin and dopamine, as well as neurocircuits (16). These immune-brain pathways interact with factors at various levels including chronic stress, aging, and obesity, and result in neuropsychiatric disorders. Animal studies have shown that proinflammatory pathways are involved in lower availability of tryptophan (TRP), with elevated activity of IDO and higher levels of KYN in the CNS (19). Changes in the KYN pathways have been found important in psychiatric disorders. For example, such changes may cause alterations of serotonin and other neurotransmitters and lead to depression (19).

In addition, the janus kinase/signal transducer and activator of transcription (JAK/STAT) pathway downstream of cytokine receptors and growth factor receptors are involved in sending signals from the cell surface to the nucleus (20). Cytokine signaling via this pathway is essential for long-term memory and cellular responses including cell survival, differentiation, and motility (21). The JAK2/STAT pathway can be activated in the pericontusional cortex and has been related to the neurological function recovery following traumatic brain injury (TBI) (20). Understanding of these pathways and networks may have profound clinical implications for better diagnosis and for the identification of systemic targets in preventive and translational medicine. The following sections will discuss the roles of the inflammatory markers and networks in various diseases in details.

4. Inflammatory Markers, Cytokine Networks, and Psychoneuro-immunology Profiles: Some Examples

4.1. Depression

Knowledge integration of the PNI of depression may help with the personalized treatment of depression and its medical comorbidities. To achieve this goal in the heterogeneous groups of patients, the differences in the immune profiles should be distinguished in addition to the profiles of symptoms and demographic elements (2). For example, depression has been closely related to both immune suppression and immune activation. The differentiation between the markers of immune suppression and immune activation would be needed for the discovery of individual differences (22).

Depressed patients often have altered cellular immunity such as reduced natural killer (NK) cell cytotoxicity. These patients have higher peripheral blood levels of immune activation markers including IL-6, IL-1, tumor necrosis factor-α (TNF-α), interferon (IFN)-α and γ, and C-reactive protein (CRP) (22–24). Elevations of peripheral blood chemokines and cellular adhesion molecules, as well as stress-induced NFκB have been found in patients with major depression (25). These molecules can be potential biomarkers of increased inflammation in depression. On the other hand, successful antidepressant treatments may help down-regulate the inflammatory markers back to normal in depressed patients (26). An association between inflammation and treatment resistance has also been observed.

Such connections of the immunological markers have indicated that immune malfunction may be a critical feature of depression and the medical comorbidities. For example, acute and chronic administrations of proinflammatory cytokines or cytokine inducers have been found to induce depressive symptoms (24). Chronic inflammation is also closely related to the pathophysiology of immune suppression in disorders including cancer and rheumatoid arthritis (23). Exploration of these immunoregulatory mechanisms from large samples of patients with depression may help elucidate the associations between immune suppression and immune activation (23). Investigations of such variations in immunologic disparity based on shared immune profiles may enable the understanding of individual differences and characterization of the subgroups in patients with depression and relevant diseases (23).

In addition, proinflammatory cytokines and relevant genetic polymorphisms are critical in depression-related disorders and behaviors. Polymorphisms in the IL-1β gene have been related to treatment response and changes in emotional processing (25). The endogenous opioid peptide beta-endorphin is involved in the modulation of proinflammatory cytokine production via the mu-opioid receptor-dependent pathways (27). Functional polymorphisms of the mu-opioid receptor gene (OPRM1, SNP: A118G) have been found to influence circulating cytokines and the health-related quality of life (QOL) (27). Exploration of such functional influences of genetic polymorphisms will be meaningful for personalized medicine.

To be useful as therapeutic targets, protein biomarkers need to be put back into the systemic pathways. Inflammatory and neurodegenerative pathways play essential roles in depression. For example, the stress-associated cytokines and oxidative brain damage have impacts on the IDO pathway. Such alterations reduce the generation of TRP and serotonin (5-HT) (24). Specifically, chronic exposure to innate immune cytokines such as IFN-α may lead to the altered activity of diurnal HPA axis and behavioral changes such as depression in medically ill individuals (28). IFN-α may affect CNS inflammatory pathways, neurotransmitter metabolism, and monoamine metabolism to form the pathway to depression. This protein may induce metabolic enzymes such as IDO and cytokine signaling pathways of p38 MAPK, and influence the production of 5-HT (26). Dopamine depletion and the basal ganglia may also be involved, because IFN-α can induce alterations in regional brain activity and behavior such as fatigue (26). Activation of neural circuits such as the dorsal anterior cingulate cortex related to anxiety and alarm may lead to cytokine-induced behavioral changes.

In another example, up-regulated production of IFN-γ in the periphery systems and brain activates a merger of TRP-KYN and guanine-tetrahydrobiopterin (BH4) metabolic pathways (29). Such changes may result in the inflammation cascade associated with aging and aging-associated medical and psychiatric disorders (AAMPD), including depression, anxiety, metabolic syndrome, diabetes, and vascular cognitive impairment. IFN-γ-inducible KYN/pteridines inflammation cascade is influenced by IFN-γ (+874) T/A genotypes encoding cytokine productions (29). IFN-γ-inducible cascade is also affected by environmental factors, such as vitamin B6 deficiency, and by pharmacological agents. The elucidation of these mechanisms and pathways may provide new strategies for anti-aging and anti-AAMPD interventions.

The proinflammatory cytokines have been related to the onset of the glucocorticoid resistance as well as the overdrive of the HPA axis. Such inflammatory and neurodegenerative pathways are involved in the brain damage in depression through reduced neurogenesis and elevated neurodegeneration (24). Stressors may affect the neurotransmitter systems such as GABAergic and monoamine functioning (30). Such changes can limit neurogenesis, cause the dysregulation of growth factors such as BDNF, and affect cellular viability via NFκB and MAP kinase pathways. These processes are also associated with the comorbidity among depression and neurological conditions, such as Parkinson's and Alzheimer's diseases, as well as cardiovascular-related pathology (30). The identification of these potential pathways and biomarkers will be helpful for discovering the therapeutic targets for depression.

These targets may include proinflammatory cytokines and their receptors, IDO pathways, and neurotrophic factors (24).

The above examples also indicate that the identification of the potential biomarkers of depression will facilitate the understanding of a spectrum of disorders. For instance, depression and behavioral changes are often observed among patients with the metabolic syndrome (MetS), with the possible involvement of chronic activation of innate immunity. Inflammation may provide the link between MetS and depressive symptoms such as neurovegetative, mood, and affective-cognitive properties (31). Those with MetS may have more depressive symptoms related to inflammatory biomarkers including CRP and IL-6. In addition, peripheral blood high-sensitive CRP (hsCRP) has been suggested to be used in the quantification of inflammation based on the association of inflammation with diseases such as cardiovascular disease. Guidelines for using such factors may be helpful for the identification of subgroups among depressed patients for immune-targeted therapies (25).

Another essential behavioral factor is sleep disorder. Blood concentrations of inflammatory factors have been correlated with the severity of depressive symptoms such as sleep disorders, cognitive dysfunction, and fatigue (25). Depressed patients with disordered sleep have shown nocturnal elevated levels of inflammatory markers IL-6 and soluble intercellular adhesion molecule (sICAM) (32).

Depression and inflammation are commonly seen in cancer patients. Psychological interventions have been found effective in relieving depression-related symptoms including pain and fatigue (33). A randomized clinical trial among breast cancer patients showed that such interventions also led to decreased levels of inflammation markers including white blood cell count and neutrophil count. The study suggested that the effects on inflammation could be mediated by relieving depressive symptoms (33).

Based on these understandings, cytokine antagonists have been suggested to have antidepressant features. For example, the TNF-α antagonist, etanercept has been found beneficial in relieving depressive symptoms and regulating rapid eye movement sleep in those with alcohol dependence (34). Anti-inflammatory cytokines such as IL-10 may inhibit the occurrence of depressive-like behavior after exposure to inflammatory stimuli (25).

In addition to targeting cytokines directly, another potential method for the treatment of depression is targeting inflammatory signaling pathways. For example, the inhibition of the p38 MAPK pathway was shown to reverse the process of behavioral changes in animal studies (25). Such strategy is also helpful for the treatment of other inflammatory disorders such as cardiovascular disease and pulmonary diseases including asthma. By focusing on targeting the systemic inflammation as the connection among various health conditions, these strategies may also be helpful for changing the emphasis from disease-focused medicine to human-centered medicine (4).

4.2. Alzheimer's Disease

Alzheimer's disease (AD) is a chronic neurodegenerative disease of the brain. The brain is involved in complex peripheral immune interactions, while inflammatory processes can profoundly influence brain functions. Activation of innate immune mechanisms causes increased levels of proinflammatory cytokines. Cytokines interact with cholinergic and dopaminergic pathways, and mediate inflammatory processes in neurodegenerative diseases such as AD and vascular dementia (18). Peripheral or central cytokine dysregulation could influence cognition such as impaired sleep regulation, micronutrient deficiency caused by appetite suppression, and many endocrine interactions. Peripheral cytokine dysregulation may also be associated with cognitive aging (18). Such understanding may provide a new framework for elucidating the roles of cytokines in neurodegenerative disorders such as AD. Anti-inflammatory cytokine signaling may mediate molecular adjuvant therapy of AD.

Inflammation plays an important role in the pathogenesis of AD. A study on the secretion pattern of monocytes in patients with AD and mild cognitive impairment (MCI) showed higher levels of cytokines including IL-1β, IL-6, and TNF-α, as well as a lower competence of these cells responding to inflammatory challenges (35). The study indicated that monocytes can be potential targets for understanding the progression from MCI to AD.

Specifically, the cytokine IL-1β is an important component in inflammatory pathways that may make neurons vulnerable to degeneration (36). This cytokine may damage neurons by disturbing the PI3-K/Akt pathway-mediated protection by BDNF, as well as the activations of Akt, MAPK/ERK, and CREB. The polymorphisms of the proinflammatory cytokine IL-1β also play a role in AD. AD has been related to the TT genotype of IL-1β +3953 SNP, and a potential association with the −511 TT genotype (37). The polymorphisms have been related to the pathogenic progress of the brain and the cognitive decline. In addition, increased levels of IL-18 were found in stimulated blood mononuclear cells from AD patients having the CC genotype at the position −607 (38). ICAM-1 can be found in astrocytes in CNS pathologies including multiple sclerosis and AD (39). ICAM-1 ligation may activate extracellular signal-regulated kinase (ERK) ERK1/ERK2 and p38 MAPKs, and induce mRNA expression of proinflammatory cytokines including IL-1α, IL-1β, IL-6, and TNF-α (39).

On the other hand, expression of the IL-4 gene was found to attenuate AD pathogenesis in mice models (40). Sustained expression of IL-4 led to decreased astro/microgliosis, amyloid-beta peptide (Abeta) oligomerization and deposition, and improved neurogenesis. Higher levels of IL-4 also improved spatial learning. Such findings have suggested that neuronal anti-inflammatory cytokine signaling can be used as a potential target for non-Abeta-mediated treatment of AD (40).

In addition, the elucidation of the multiple functions of IL-10 in the brain may enable a better understanding of neurodegenerative diseases and the development of novel interventions for major debilitating diseases of the CNS (41). IL-10 is synthesized in the CNS and is involved in limiting clinical symptoms of stroke, multiple sclerosis, Alzheimer's disease, meningitis, and the behavioral changes upon bacterial infections. Expression of IL-10 is increased in many diseases in the CNS to improve survival of neurons and all glial cells in the brain. This is done via inhibiting the pro-apoptotic cytokines and stimulating cell survival signals. Stimulation of IL-10 receptors is associated with the regulation of many signaling pathways such as Jak1/Stat3, PI 3-kinase, MAPK, suppressor of cytokine signaling (SOCS), and NFκB (41). Such changes may improve cell survival by blocking ligand- and mitochondrial-induced apoptotic pathways. IL-10 also leads to anergy in brain-infiltrating T cells via suppressing cell signaling by the co-stimulatory CD28-CD80/86 pathway (41). Therefore, IL-10 may have anti-inflammatory functions in the brain by limiting the production of proinflammatory cytokines, inhibiting cytokine receptor expression, and blocking receptor activation.

Using systems biology approaches, several processes have been found as molecular features of AD. These features include the reduction of mitochondrial metabolism, higher production of reactive oxygen species and misfolded proteins, altered synaptic protein machinery of transmission, tau hyperphosphorylation, and altered ubiquitination (42). However, up to now no single growth factor or cytokine has been confirmed as a biomarker for diagnosing AD or dementia such as MCI. On the other hand, several growth factors and/or cytokines/chemokines in cerebrospinal fluid (CSF) and blood can be combined to form a "patient profile signature" for the diagnosis of AD and MCI with high specificity (43). These potential biomarker profiles include growth factors such as epidermal growth factor (EGF), and cytokines/chemokines such as IL-11, CCL5 (RANTES), CCL15 (MIP1delta, macrophage inflammatory protein-1delta, MIP5), and CCL18 (MIP4, macrophage inflammatory protein-4 or PARC) (43).

4.3. Obesity

Obesity is featured with chronic low-grade inflammation, hyperleptinemia, and hypothalamic leptin resistance (44). Leptin is an adipocyte-derived hormone involved in the regulation of food intake and energy homeostasis. It can activate fatty acid oxidation, insulin release, and peripheral insulin action. Leptin receptor is a member of the class I cytokine receptor superfamily. Leptin deficiency or resistance can lead to obesity, diabetes, and infertility. Leptin signal transduction pathways are associated with peripheral lipid metabolism through AMP-activated protein kinase and hepatic stearoyl-CoA desaturase-1 pathways (45). Leptin functions are related to the regulation of phosphatidylinositol 3-kinase (PI3K), PTP-1B, and SOCS-3 (46). SOCS3 inhibits STAT3 pathway and suppresses the PI3K pathway of leptin signaling in the hypothalamus (47). These interactions have been associated with the development of central leptin resistance and obesity.

Inflammatory markers play a critical role in emotional distress and behavioral symptoms of obese individuals. Studies on the association between adiposity, inflammation, eating behavior, and emotional status among obese women found that body mass index (BMI) was positively related to inflammatory markers and adipokines such as leptin and adiponectin (48). These potential markers including IL-6 and hsCRP are also connected to the depression and anxiety aspects of neuroticism. On the other hand, gastric surgery could lead to significant weight loss, lower levels of inflammatory markers especially hsCRP, lower levels of anxiety, and progress in emotional status and eating behavior (48). These results suggested strong correlations between adiposity, inflammation, stress, and behavioral factors in obesity.

4.4. Cardiovascular Disease and Stroke

Studies have found that those with depressive mood had increased levels of inflammatory markers involved in coronary heart disease (CHD) incidence, including IL-6, CRP, and ICAM-1 (49). Such results confirmed the association between depressive mood and CHD events. The cytokine granulocyte colony-stimulating factor (G-CSF) binds to its receptor G-CSF-R and activates several signaling transduction pathways such as PI3K/Akt, Jak/Stat, and MAP kinase (50). Such activation stimulates survival, proliferation, differentiation, and mobilization of hematopoietic stem and progenitor cells. These mechanisms are involved in myocardial infarction, heart failure, and stroke (50).

Cytokines are crucial mediators of the inflammatory response in stroke. Both proinflammatory and anti-inflammatory cytokines are generated in the ischemic brain. Anti-inflammatory cytokines including IL-10 improve cell survival. However, proinflammatory cytokines including TNF-α can lead to cell death (51). Cytokines can interact with the JAK/STAT pathway, leading to changes associated with cell death or survival. Cerebral ischemia results in acute inflammation and primary brain damage. Activation of the innate immune system is involved in this inflammatory process, mediated by proinflammatory cytokines including IL-1β and IL-6. Generation of these cytokines is initiated by toll-like receptors (TLRs) involved signaling pathways (52). Negative feedback suppression of TLRs and proinflammatory cytokine signaling pathways is associated with ischemic tolerance in the brain with a protective mechanism.

Understanding of these mechanisms and pathways may contribute to the prevention and treatment of stroke and related diseases.

These approaches may include anti-neutrophil, anti-ICAM-1, and anti-proinflammatory cytokine strategies. Potential pathways that can be targeted include transcriptional regulators of inflammatory gene expression such as NF-κB and proteasome, and signaling pathways such as ICE-cascade and MAPK/MKK/ERK cascades that are related to inflammation and neuronal cell death (53).

4.5. HIV

It would be interesting to investigate the role of the HPA axis and the sympathetic nervous system (SNS) in biobehavioral effects on HIV-1 pathogenesis and disease progression. Studies have indicated that HPA and SNS effector molecules may increase HIV-1 replication in cellular models through the influences on viral infectivity, viral gene expression, and the innate immune response to infections (54). Regulation of leukocyte biology by neuroeffector molecules may be involved in the mediation of how psychosocial factors affect HIV-1 pathogenesis (54). Neural and endocrine parameters have been found as potential and useful biomarkers for evaluating the effects of behavioral interventions as novel strategies for inhibiting HIV-1 disease progression (54).

HIV-1 exposure may trigger proinflammatory genes associated with the JAK/STAT pathway in human brain microvascular endothelial cells (HBMEC) (55). HIV-1 gp120 protein can stimulate STAT1 and activate IL-6 and IL-8 secretion in HBMEC. The crosstalk between STAT1, mitogen activated protein kinase kinase (MEK), and PI3K pathways may cause the dysfunction of the blood–brain barrier (BBB). Suppression of STAT1 activation may be used for therapeutic strategies to inhibit neuroinflammation and BBB dysfunction in HIV/AIDS (55).

In addition, HIV-associated neurologic disorders (HAND) are serious problems among HIV-infected individuals. HIV encephalitis is often involved in the most severe form of HAND, with glial activation, cytokine-chemokine dysregulation, and neuronal damage and loss (56). HIV encephalitis has been associated with higher levels of the mitogen platelet-derived growth factor (PDGF) B chain in the brain, which can be modified by ERK1/2 and JNK signaling pathways and the downstream transcription factor early growth response 1 (56). Exposure of astrocytes to PDGF-B may cause the production of proinflammatory cytokines MCP-1 and IL-1β. Such understanding may help with the discovery of intervention strategies for HAND.

It is necessary to understand the effects of psychological interventions on HIV disease markers such as neuroendocrine hormone regulation and immune status. A meta-analysis found that behavioral interventions for HIV-positive persons have been efficacious in improving psychological status with beneficial effects on neuroendocrine and immune functions (57).

5. Conclusion and Future Perspectives

In summary, the elucidation of inflammatory markers, cytokine networks, and immune-brain-behavior interactions may help establish PNI profiles for the identification of potential targets for personalized interventions in at risk populations (16, 19). Levels of inflammation-related proteins in the blood can be measured for diagnosis and for monitoring treatment responsiveness by drugs affecting inflammation-related pathways, such as antidepressants and mood stabilizers. Although such investigations are still in their early stages, developments in this direction may lead to some breakthroughs to meet the challenges in the current biomedicine (4).

Because the same factors may be involved in different pathways and health conditions, targeting such factors may be potentially helpful for blocking various pathways in diseases. For instance, chronic exposure to cytokines including IFN-α has been found to influence regional brain activity, leading to the depletion of dopamine, and affecting the activity of the diurnal HPA axis (28). These alterations may result in depression. In addition, IFN-α may also influence metabolic enzymes such as IDO and cytokine signaling pathways such as p38 MAPK (38). Such changes may affect the synthesis and reuptake of serotonin, causing behavioral alterations including psychomotor slowing and fatigue (26). The common factors such as IFN-α can be used as the potential therapeutic targets.

In addition, the understanding of the general pathways among different disorders may contribute to the transition from the disease-centered medicine to human-centered medicine. This is because these common pathways may serve as the potential therapeutic targets, rather than the diseases (4). For instance, stressors may cause changes in the neurotransmitter systems such as GABAergic and monoamine functioning, leading to the dysregulation of growth factors such as BDNF, and influencing cellular viability such as via NFκB and MAP kinase pathways (30). These changes are important in many stress-related diseases such as depression, Parkinson's disease, Alzheimer's disease, and cardiovascular disease (30).

Integrative strategies targeting these pathways would be useful for the prevention and treatment of a spectrum of diseases that share the common links. For example, minocycline has anti-inflammatory effects, and can inhibit the activation of microglia and the generation of IL-1, p38 MAPK, as well as NF-κB (25). In another example, the drug etanercept targeting the TNF-α-related pathways has been found to have beneficial effects in many diseases including depression, alcohol addiction, and arthritis (19, 34). NF-κB plays a critical role in inflammation and its behavioral effects. A form of vitamin E called tocopherol has been found to inhibit NF-κB, the related neuroinflammatory, as well as behavioral changes (25). With the identification of potential biomarkers and systemic networks, it would be possible to establish PNI profiles for differentiating patient subgroups for more accurate diagnosis and optimal therapies toward personalized medicine.

References

1. Yan Q (2010) Translational bioinformatics and systems biology approaches for personalized medicine. Methods Mol Biol 662:167–178
2. Yan Q (2011) Translation of psychoneuroimmunology into personalized medicine: a systems biology perspective. Person Med 8:641–649
3. Reckow S, Gormanns P, Holsboer F et al (2008) Psychiatric disorders biomarker identification: from proteomics to systems biology. Pharmacopsychiatry 41(suppl 1):S70–S77
4. Yan Q (2011) Toward the integration of personalized and systems medicine: challenges, opportunities and approaches. Person Med 8:1–4
5. O'Connor M-F, Bower JE, Cho HJ et al (2009) To assess, to control, to exclude: effects of biobehavioral factors on circulating inflammatory markers. Brain Behav Immun 23:887–897
6. Dantzer R, Capuron L, Irwin MR (2008) Identification and treatment of symptoms associated with inflammation in medically ill patients. Psychoneuroendocrinology 33:18–29
7. Klengel T, Binder EB (2011) Using gene–environment interactions to target personalized treatment in mood disorder. Person Med 8:23–34
8. Yan Q (2008) The integration of personalized and systems medicine: bioinformatics support for pharmacogenomics and drug discovery. Methods Mol Biol 448:1–19
9. Yan Q (2010) Immunoinformatics and systems biology methods for personalized medicine. Methods Mol Biol 662:203–220
10. Goncharova LB, Tarakanov AO (2007) Molecular networks of brain and immunity. Brain Res Rev 55:155–166
11. Zhang Y, Filiou MD, Reckow S et al (2011) Proteomic and metabolomic profiling of a trait anxiety mouse model implicate affected pathways. Mol Cell Proteomics 10(12):M111.008110
12. Gormanns P, Mueller NS, Ditzen C et al (2011) Phenome-transcriptome correlation unravels anxiety and depression related pathways. J Psychiatr Res 45:973–979
13. Sequeira PA, Martin MV, Vawter MP (2012) The first decade and beyond of transcriptional profiling in schizophrenia. Neurobiol Dis 45(1):23–36
14. Taylor AG, Goehler LE, Galper DI et al (2010) Top-down and bottom-up mechanisms in mind-body medicine: development of an integrative framework for psychophysiological research. Explore (NY) 6:29–41
15. Yan Q (2011) Understanding and applying personalized therapeutics at systems level: role for translational bioinformatics. Curr Pharmacogenomics Person Med 9:137–147
16. Capuron L, Miller AH (2011) Immune system to brain signaling: neuropsychopharmacological implications. Pharmacol Ther 130:226–238
17. The systems biology database of cytokines. Available from http:// www.pharmtao.com/ cytokines. Accessed Jan 2012
18. Wilson CJ, Finch CE, Cohen HJ (2002) Cytokines and cognition—the case for a head-to-toe inflammatory paradigm. J Am Geriatr Soc 50:2041–2056
19. Dean B (2011) Understanding the role of inflammatory-related pathways in the pathophysiology and treatment of psychiatric disorders: evidence from human peripheral studies and CNS studies. Int J Neuropsychopharmacol 14: 997–1012
20. Zhao J-B, Zhang Y, Li G-Z et al (2011) Activation of JAK2/STAT pathway in cerebral cortex after experimental traumatic brain injury of rats. Neurosci Lett 498:147–152
21. Copf T, Goguel V, Lampin-Saint-Amaux A et al (2011) Cytokine signaling through the JAK/STAT pathway is required for long-term memory in Drosophila. Proc Natl Acad Sci U S A 108:8059–8064
22. Pike JL, Irwin MR (2006) Dissociation of inflammatory markers and natural killer cell activity in major depressive disorder. Brain Behav Immun 20:169–174
23. Blume J, Douglas SD, Evans DL (2011) Immune suppression and immune activation in depression. Brain Behav Immun 25:221–229
24. Catena-Dell'Osso M, Bellantuono C, Consoli G et al (2011) Inflammatory and neurodegenerative pathways in depression: a new avenue for antidepressant development? Curr Med Chem 18:245–255
25. Haroon E, Raison CL, Miller AH (2012) Psychoneuroimmunology meets neuropsychopharmacology: translational implications of the impact of inflammation on behavior. Neuropsychopharmacology 37(1):137–162

26. Miller AH (2009) Norman Cousins Lecture. Mechanisms of cytokine-induced behavioral changes: psychoneuroimmunology at the translational interface. Brain Behav Immun 23:149–158
27. Matsunaga M, Isowa T, Murakami H et al (2009) Association of polymorphism in the human mu-opioid receptor OPRM1 gene with proinflammatory cytokine levels and health perception. Brain Behav Immun 23:931–935
28. Raison CL, Borisov AS, Woolwine BJ et al (2010) Interferon-alpha effects on diurnal hypothalamic-pituitary-adrenal axis activity: relationship with proinflammatory cytokines and behavior. Mol Psychiatry 15:535–547
29. Oxenkrug GF (2011) Interferon-gamma-inducible kynurenines/pteridines inflammation cascade: implications for aging and aging-associated psychiatric and medical disorders. J Neural Transm 118:75–85
30. Anisman H, Merali Z, Hayley S (2008) Neurotransmitter, peptide and cytokine processes in relation to depressive disorder: comorbidity between depression and neurodegenerative disorders. Prog Neurobiol 85:1–74
31. Capuron L, Su S, Miller AH et al (2008) Depressive symptoms and metabolic syndrome: is inflammation the underlying link? Biol Psychiatry 64:896–900
32. Motivala SJ, Sarfatti A, Olmos L et al (2005) Inflammatory markers and sleep disturbance in major depression. Psychosom Med 67:187–194
33. Thornton LM, Andersen BL, Schuler TA et al (2009) A psychological intervention reduces inflammatory markers by alleviating depressive symptoms: secondary analysis of a randomized controlled trial. Psychosom Med 71:715–724
34. Irwin MR, Olmstead R, Valladares EM et al (2009) Tumor necrosis factor antagonism normalizes rapid eye movement sleep in alcohol dependence. Biol Psychiatry 66:191–195
35. Guerreiro RJ, Santana I, Brás JM et al (2007) Peripheral inflammatory cytokines as biomarkers in Alzheimer's disease and mild cognitive impairment. Neurodegener Dis 4:406–412
36. Tong L, Balazs R, Soiampornkul R et al (2008) Interleukin-1 beta impairs brain derived neurotrophic factor-induced signal transduction. Neurobiol Aging 29:1380–1393
37. Di Bona D, Plaia A, Vasto S et al (2008) Association between the interleukin-1beta polymorphisms and Alzheimer's disease: a systematic review and meta-analysis. Brain Res Rev 59:155–163
38. Bossù P, Ciaramella A, Salani F et al (2008) Interleukin-18 produced by peripheral blood cells is increased in Alzheimer's disease and correlates with cognitive impairment. Brain Behav Immun 22:487–492
39. Lee SJ, Drabik K, Van Wagoner NJ et al (2000) ICAM-1-induced expression of proinflammatory cytokines in astrocytes: involvement of extracellular signal-regulated kinase and p38 mitogen-activated protein kinase pathways. J Immunol 165:4658–4666
40. Kiyota T, Okuyama S, Swan RJ et al (2010) CNS expression of anti-inflammatory cytokine interleukin-4 attenuates Alzheimer's disease-like pathogenesis in APP+PS1 bigenic mice. FASEB J 24:3093–3102
41. Strle K, Zhou JH, Shen WH et al (2001) Interleukin-10 in the brain. Crit Rev Immunol 21:427–449
42. Juhász G, Földi I, Penke B (2011) Systems biology of Alzheimer's disease: how diverse molecular changes result in memory impairment in AD. Neurochem Int 58:739–750
43. Olson L, Humpel C (2010) Growth factors and cytokines/chemokines as surrogate biomarkers in cerebrospinal fluid and blood for diagnosing Alzheimer's disease and mild cognitive impairment. Exp Gerontol 45:41–46
44. Ahima RS (2006) Adipose tissue as an endocrine organ. Obesity (Silver Spring) 14(suppl 5):242S–249S
45. Zhang F, Chen Y, Heiman M et al (2005) Leptin: structure, function and biology. Vitam Horm 71:345–372
46. Ahima RS, Qi Y, Singhal NS (2006) Adipokines that link obesity and diabetes to the hypothalamus. Prog Brain Res 153:155–174
47. Metlakunta AS, Sahu M, Yasukawa H et al (2011) Neuronal suppressor of cytokine signaling-3 deficiency enhances hypothalamic leptin-dependent phosphatidylinositol 3-kinase signaling. Am J Physiol Regul Integr Comp Physiol 300:R1185–R1193
48. Capuron L, Poitou C, Machaux-Tholliez D et al (2011) Relationship between adiposity, emotional status and eating behaviour in obese women: role of inflammation. Psychol Med 41:1517–1528
49. Empana JP, Sykes DH, Luc G et al (2005) Contributions of depressive mood and circulating inflammatory markers to coronary heart disease in healthy European men: the Prospective Epidemiological Study of Myocardial Infarction (PRIME). Circulation 111:2299–2305
50. Klocke R, Kuhlmann MT, Scobioala S et al (2008) Granulocyte colony-stimulating factor (G-CSF) for cardio- and cerebrovascular regenerative applications. Curr Med Chem 15: 968–977

51. Planas AM, Gorina R, Chamorro A (2006) Signalling pathways mediating inflammatory responses in brain ischaemia. Biochem Soc Trans 34(pt 6):1267–1270
52. Karikó K, Weissman D, Welsh FA (2004) Inhibition of toll-like receptor and cytokine signaling–a unifying theme in ischemic tolerance. J Cereb Blood Flow Metab 24:1288–1304
53. Zhang W, Stanimirovic D (2002) Current and future therapeutic strategies to target inflammation in stroke. Curr Drug Targets Inflamm Allergy 1:151–166
54. Cole SW (2008) Psychosocial influences on HIV-1 disease progression: neural, endocrine, and virologic mechanisms. Psychosom Med 70:562–568
55. Yang B, Akhter S, Chaudhuri A et al (2009) HIV-1 gp120 induces cytokine expression, leukocyte adhesion, and transmigration across the blood–brain barrier: modulatory effects of STAT1 signaling. Microvasc Res 77:212–219
56. Bethel-Brown C, Yao H, Callen S et al (2011) HIV-1 Tat-mediated induction of platelet-derived growth factor in astrocytes: role of early growth response gene 1. J Immunol 186: 4119–4129
57. Carrico AW, Antoni MH (2008) Effects of psychological interventions on neuroendocrine hormone regulation and immune status in HIV-positive persons: a review of randomized controlled trials. Psychosom Med 70: 575–584

Chapter 7

Cytokines as Potential Biomarkers for Parkinson's Disease: A Multiplex Approach

Darcy Litteljohn and Shawn Hayley

Abstract

Cytokines, which are immunological messengers facilitating both intra- and inter-system communication, are considered central players in the neuroinflammatory cascades associated with the neurodegenerative process in Parkinson's disease (PD) and other neurological disorders. They have also been implicated in depression and other cognitive (e.g., memory impairment, dementia) and affective disturbances (e.g., anxiety) that show high co-morbidity with neurodegenerative diseases. As such, cytokines may hold great promise as serological biomarkers in PD, with potential applications ranging from early diagnosis and disease staging, to prognosis, drug discovery, and tracking the response to treatment. Subclassification or risk stratification in PD could be based (among other things) on reliably determined cytokine panel profiles or "signatures" of particular co-morbid disease states or at-risk groups (e.g., PD alone, PD with depression and/or dementia). Researchers and clinicians seeking to describe cytokine variations in health vs. disease will benefit greatly from technologies that allow a high degree of multiplexing and thus permit the simultaneous determination of a large roster of cytokines in single small-volume samples. The need for such highly paralleled assays is underscored by the fact that cytokines do not act in isolation but rather against a backdrop of complementary and antagonistic cytokine effects; ascribing valence to the actions of any one cytokine thus requires specific knowledge about the larger cytokine milieu. This chapter provides a technological overview of the major cytokine multiplex assay platforms before discussing the implications of such tools for biomarker discovery and related applications in PD and its depressive and cognitive co-morbidities.

Key words: Multiplex assays, Cytokine, Inflammation, Parkinson's disease, Co-morbidity, Biomarker, Psychoneuroimmunology

1. Introduction

Biomarkers are objective and reliably determined biological indicators of physiological and pathological processes. Once validated, biomarkers can be used as surrogate end-points (i.e., for clinical ones) to track biological responses to treatment, provided that they correlate well with disease progression (and clinical scales)

Qing Yan (ed.), *Psychoneuroimmunology: Methods and Protocols*, Methods in Molecular Biology, vol. 934,
DOI 10.1007/978-1-62703-071-7_7, © Springer Science+Business Media, LLC 2012

and predict the clinical endpoint(s) without being directly affected by the treatment (1). As it currently stands, several promising clinical, genetic, serological, and imaging biomarkers have been suggested for a number of complex neurological illnesses, including Alzheimer's disease (AD) and Parkinson's disease (PD). However, owing largely to a paucity of successful replication studies and the relative novelty of many of these markers, diagnosis and tracking of disease progression remain largely the purview of clinical acumen (2). This is problematic given that clinically derived diagnoses are sometimes fallible; indeed, early PD—a window of time during which disease-modulating therapies are likely to be most effective—is misdiagnosed by even experienced clinicians ~25% of the time (3).

In addition to their potential diagnostic value, biomarkers hold promise for disease staging, progression, prognosis, and tracking biological responses to treatment (i.e., markers of trait, state, rate, and fate) (4). Disease subclassification represents another worthwhile directive of biomarker research, particularly in the context of CNS spectrum disorders (e.g., autism, schizophrenia) and diseases of uncertain or suspected mixed etiology, such as PD and depression. Indeed, biomarker profiling can be applied to CNS diseases that show a high degree of co-morbidity in the hopes of delineating specific biological patterns or "signatures" that characterize a particular co-morbid state or a heightened vulnerability to co-morbidity (e.g., PD alone or co-morbid with depression or dementia). This information could, in turn, conceivably inform the development of more highly targeted and personalized adjuvant therapies that could be initiated at early, potentially pre-co-morbid disease stages.

While multiple mechanisms likely contribute to the pathogenesis of neurological diseases such as PD, AD, and cerebral stroke, neuroinflammation and oxidative stress are considered primary mediators of degenerative brain events. Microglia are the key CNS inflammatory cells and a large body of research has implicated activation of these cells, as well as the neuroinflammatory responses they mediate, in the neurodegenerative progression of PD and other neurological disorders (5). However, in practice, microglial cells are poor targets for biomarker identification as they lack disease specificity and only relatively expensive, time-consuming, and technically demanding brain imaging techniques (e.g., positron emission tomography) can resolve their activation state in vivo. While a multimodal, combinatorial approach to biomarker discovery is probably most prescient (e.g., drawing from clinical, genetic, serological, and imaging modalities), biological fluid parameters, including blood and cerebrospinal fluid (CSF) markers, are perhaps the most economically viable and efficient options. In the case of neurological disorders, CSF, given its close proximity to and unique relationship with the brain (CSF bathes the brain and spinal cord), should in theory hold great promise for biomarker discovery. Yet, blood-derived markers have the advantage of being rather easily and safely collected; this contrasts with the more invasive lumbar puncture procedures for removal of spinal fluid, which can themselves lead to blood contamination of CSF samples. Indeed, circulating proteins are far more abundant in plasma and serum than in CSF, although the relationship between brain and peripheral protein levels can be quite complex and potentially misleading.

Cytokines, which are soluble glycoprotein immune system messengers and include various chemokines (possess chemoattractant properties) and growth factors (regulate cell growth and differentiation), are at once both key mediators of microglial activation and primary effectors of these immunocompetent cells. In addition to local cytokines that are synthesized de novo within the brain (where they act in an autocrine or paracrine manner), peripherally derived cytokines too exert tremendous influence over brain processes, mainly by: (1) acting on peripheral immune cells (leukocytes); (2) gaining entry into the brain (extravasation, active transport mechanisms, release by infiltrating T cells); and (3) binding receptors of the blood brain barrier (BBB) to promote and perpetuate central inflammatory cascades (6). In this way, cytokines have been implicated in various oxidative (e.g., superoxide, pro-oxidant enzyme induction) and apoptotic pathways (e.g., caspases, heat shock proteins) to cellular toxicity and neurodegeneration (6). Indeed, evidence from clinical and animal studies has suggested an important role of cytokines in the development of PD and other neurodegenerative conditions, as well as some of the co-morbid neuropsychiatric symptoms (e.g., depression, anxiety) that often accompany and in some instances predate the primary degenerative disorder (5). The fact that cytokines are readily detectable in peripheral fluids such as blood, CSF, and saliva, together with their relevance and significance for brain pathology, makes these specialized immunotransmitters logical candidates for biomarker identification in PD and other neurodegenerative disorders of confirmed or suspected inflammatory origins.

Enzyme-linked immunosorbent assay (ELISA), which uses solid-phase detection chemistry to measure a particular target analyte in solution (capture antibody is coated onto the wells of a microtitre plate), has long been considered the gold standard of cytokine quantitation. While this fully quantitative and (at best) semi-automated method boasts high specificity, sensitivity, and throughput (assuming a 96-well plate format), only one cytokine can be measured per assay. Single-analyte testing, while certainly useful for some clinical and research applications, for instance confirmatory cytokine testing in clinical practice and trial monitoring, is severely limited as a tool for biomarker discovery, with the exception perhaps of candidate marker validation. However, even this can be costly and inefficient, especially when the sample is precious or volume is limited (e.g., stored clinical or rodent blood specimens) and/or when interrogating the levels of four or more cytokines (7).

Owing to their highly redundant and pleiotropic properties, cytokines are best considered not in isolation, but as a network of biologically active immunological mediators whose collective output can effectuate significant physiological and pathological change. Thus, the actions of any one cytokine must be considered in the context of the larger cytokine network to which it belongs and in whose activity it partakes. In this regard, highly multiplexed or paralleled assays that are capable of measuring the simultaneous concentrations of numerous cytokines in single, small-volume samples are needed to accurately characterize the inflammatory cytokine makeup of a particular disease-state (or normal physiological condition). This is especially important in the case of PD and other degenerative brain disorders where cytokines are considered primary mediators of disease pathogenesis and hence, constitute important targets for hypothesis-driven biomarker analysis and related applications such as drug discovery and personalized medicine.

1.1. PD and Co-morbid Depression: Role of Cytokines

PD has classically been conceptualized as a disorder primarily of motor functioning. Yet, symptoms tend to vary widely among PD patients, with a substantial number of individuals displaying neuropsychiatric and other co-morbid symptoms (e.g., autonomic problems, sleep disturbances) in addition to the core motor disturbances (bradykinesia, cogwheel rigidity, resting tremor). Of the co-morbid psychiatric symptoms, depression is particularly common, with 40–50% of PD patients showing clinically significant depression (8). While co-morbid depression, anxiety, and other psycho-emotional symptoms can have fairly obvious negative effects on quality of life among PD patients they may also come to affect the course of the primary neurodegenerative illness itself. In fact, PD patients with a high degree of depressive co-morbidity often perform more poorly on motor tasks and tests of executive cognitive functioning (9). Moreover, these individuals are clearly distinguishable from their non-depressed counterparts on functional brain imaging, displaying decreased metabolism within the frontal cortex-basal ganglia-thalamic loop (10) and impaired neuronal activity of motor regulatory elements of the basal ganglia (e.g., subthalamic nucleus) (11).

Depression in the context of neurological illness might be due to the distress attributable to the primary disease or its diagnosis, or alternatively might stem from common underlying pathobiological processes (10); the causes of such depression need not be mutually exclusive (see Fig. 1). According to the first perspective, depression may arise in the context of PD due to substantial psychosocial disease burden. In this respect, job loss, marital strain, and bleak outlook on the future owing to the progressive and

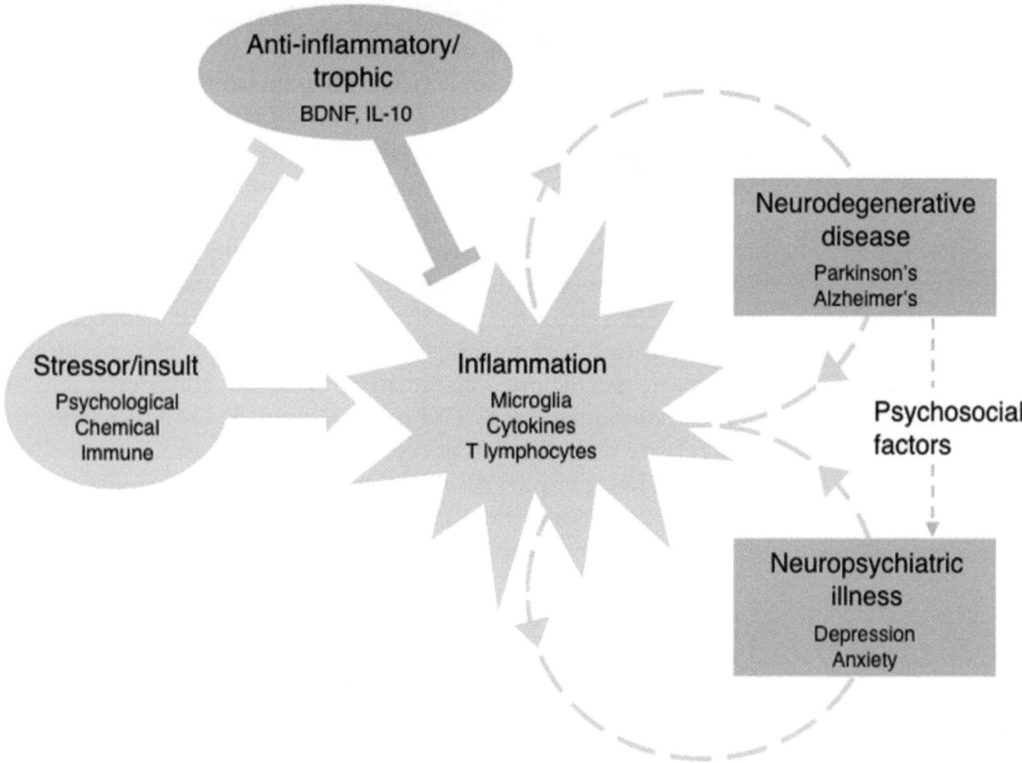

Fig. 1. Psychoneuroimmunological contributions to PD and its co-morbid depressive illness. *BDNF* brain-derived neurotrophic factor; *IL-10* interleukin-10.

debilitating nature of PD have all been correlated with risk of co-morbid depression among these individuals (12). Yet, depression and other neuropsychiatric symptoms may sometimes precede motor impairment and the clinical diagnosis of PD, making it unlikely that such pathology is uniformly secondary to psychological distress (8). In such cases, the depression might reflect early degenerative, neuroinflammatory, or other pathological processes that would likely result in disturbances of multi-neurotransmitter systems involving extra-nigrostriatal brain centers. Interestingly, depression along with olfactory (hyposmia) and sleep disturbances (insomnia, REM behavior sleep disorder) have garnered substantial attention as potential clinical biomarkers of early/prodromal PD or an increased susceptibility for developing the disorder (13); however, alone these markers clearly lack sufficient disease specificity. Yet, it is also important to note that some estimates suggest that the ~40–50% of PD patients with co-morbid anxiety/depression did not have such symptoms prior to PD motor onset and that the neuropsychiatric symptoms only emerged following substantial damage to brainstem or other monoaminergic regions (14). Whatever the case, common cytokine-associated immunobiological disturbances appear to be linked to both primary motor and co-morbid neuropsychiatric pathology.

In the case of PD, elevated levels of numerous pro-inflammatory cytokines, including IL-1β, IL-2, IL-6, TNF-α, and IFN-γ, were detected within the cortex, basal ganglia, and/or limbic regions on postmortem exam of PD brains (15). Animal studies using different toxin-based models of PD have similarly demonstrated enhanced regional brain accumulation of many of these cytokines (5). Moreover, several groups showed that animals could be made resistant or refractory to toxin-induced neuronal and behavioral pathology by knocking out, via genetic ablation or pharmacological blockade, specific pro-inflammatory cytokines considered relevant for human disease (e.g., TNF-α, IFN-γ, IL-6) (16, 17). However, the relative contribution of central (microglia, astrocytes, perhaps neuronal) vs. peripheral (T lymphocytes and other immune cells) cytokine production in PD and its toxin-based animal models is still a matter of debate. The fact that peripherally derived cytokines can gain access to and have significant effects within the CNS, especially in times of disease and/or with advancing age (facilitated by BBB breakdown), nonetheless suggests that the status of peripheral cytokine networks could potentially speak to the current or cumulative state of affairs in the degenerating brain (e.g., presence, type, location, extent of damage). In this regard, many of the same cytokines found increased in autopsied PD brain (e.g., TNF-α, IL-1β, IFN-γ) were also detected at elevated levels, both basally and upon stimulation with lipopolysaccharide (LPS), in the blood and CSF of PD patients (18). Moreover, severity of parkinsonism has been shown to correlate with the levels of at least some of these peripheral cytokines (18, 19).

Evidence from human, other primate, and rodent studies has likewise argued convincingly in favor of the view that cytokines contribute to the evolution of major depression and probably other affective pathologies. As in PD, blood (circulating and mitogen-provoked) and CSF levels of many pro-inflammatory cytokines, including TNF-α, IL-1α, IL-6, and IFN-γ, were found elevated along with other inflammatory factors (e.g., acute phase proteins) in depressed patients, especially those with relatively severe (melancholic) or treatment-resistant illness (6, 20, 21). As well, it was reported that the normal IL-6 circadian rhythm was disturbed among depressed patients (22), and that the usually strong positive correlation between plasma IL-6 and IL-10 concentrations was completely absent in these individuals (23). In the latter study, blood levels of IL-10 were actually diminished among depressed patients while IL-6 levels trended towards being increased, suggesting that the loss of a counter-balancing, immunoregulatory association between the two cytokines (IL-10 levels normally increase in response to pro-inflammatory IL-6 induction) may contribute to inflammation-related depression symptoms (23).

Positive correlations have also been observed between severity of depressive symptoms and the blood concentration of several cytokines, including IL-1β, IL-6, and TNF-α (6); and several reports have hinted at the ability of common antidepressant drugs (e.g., SSRIs) to normalize blood levels of at least some cytokines in depressed individuals (e.g., IL-1β, IL-6) (24). These reports are consistent with other studies linking antidepressants to the modulation of the T-helper type-1 (Th1)/Th2 cytokine balance, specifically the suppression of pro-inflammatory Th1-type cytokines (IFN-γ, IL-12) in favor of the more anti-inflammatory Th2-type cytokines (IL-10, IL-4) (25). However, ongoing controversy surrounding whether and which cytokine changes are normalized with successful antidepressant treatment, stirred by multiple conflicting studies (see ref. (24) for a recent meta-analysis), tends to suggest that cytokines might serve best as trait markers of certain sub-types of this highly heterogeneous disease.

In addition, cancer and hepatitis C patients receiving IFN-α immunotherapy were found to develop prominent neuropsychiatric symptoms, including a depressive-like syndrome that was amenable to antidepressant treatment (26). Correspondingly, rodents treated with IFN-α displayed marked signs of anhedonia, impaired hippocampal neurogenesis, and a reduction of cortical neuronal fiber density (27, 28). Moreover, we have shown that systemic IFN-α administration provoked neurochemical changes implicated in depression (altered 5-HT and NE activity) within several stressor-sensitive brain regions (29). Similarly, numerous other pro-inflammatory cytokines, including TNF-α, IFN-γ, and members of the interleukin family of cytokines (IL-1β, IL-6 and IL-2), have also been linked to depressive-like neural and behavioral pathology in rodents (6, 30). Exposure to cytokines or cytokine-inducing immune agents (e.g., LPS, polyinosinic:polycytidylic acid (poly I:C)) might have especially marked CNS consequences when encountered in the context of concomitant xenobiotic, physical, or psychological stressor challenge, each of which can contribute to a breakdown of the BBB, thus facilitating the entry of peripheral immune factors into the brain. For instance, we found that the impact of IFN-α upon neurotransmitter and glucocorticoid activity was greatly augmented when the cytokine was administered on the backdrop of a psychosocial stressor (disruption of social order) (29), as would be expected in human immunotherapy patients experiencing considerable distress.

Multiple lines of evidence have thus helped shape and promote the emerging belief that inflammatory processes critically involving the actions of many pro- and anti-inflammatory cytokines may be a critical common pathway to neurological illness and co-morbid depression. It stands to reason, then, that cytokines may be ideal candidate biomarkers for neurodegenerative disorders such as PD and AD, particularly in the context of early screening among neurological patients for the presence or risk of co-morbid psychiatric pathology. We believe that dysregulation of peripheral cytokine markers (and potentially other inflammation-related factors) may reflect brain pathology because: (1) cytokine-associated inflammatory processes are causally related to neurodegeneration; (2) cytokine cascades are mounted in direct response to ongoing pathology; and (3) cytokines partake in CNS-based crosstalk across the BBB.

Yet, it should be underscored from the outset that cytokines, as orchestrators of the inflammatory immune system and facilitators of myriad psycho-neuro-endocrine-immune interactions, are by their very nature disease ***nonspecific***. While specificity can be promoted (and in theory perhaps achieved) by combining individual cytokine markers into multianalyte disease profiles or signatures, there is bound to be some degree of residual overlap between disease-states. It is our position therefore that cytokines, and hence the multiplexed cytokine panels discussed in this chapter, may be best suited as adjunctive tools or "add-ons" to clinical diagnostics and potentially other biomarker modalities. In this way, cytokine multiplexing could conceivably help to improve the accuracy of early and differential PD diagnosis, and to refine co-morbid disease risk stratification in PD and other neurological disorders.

2. Cytokine Multiplex Assays

The last couple of decades have seen the development of several promising cytokine multiplex technologies, spurred on largely by the limitations of traditional ELISA and other conventional quantitative methods (e.g., radioimmunoassay) for handling the ever-expanding multiplex requirements of present-day research and clinical applications. While the focus of this chapter will be restricted primarily to protein-level cytokine multiplex assays, it should be mentioned that nucleic acid-based multiplexing tools have also been developed and applied with some success to drug discovery and the elucidation of cytokine-associated disease mechanisms (31, 32). In this regard, while proteins are certainly the key molecular players in cellular biological processes, changes in cytokine transcription and translation, as well as post-translational protein modifications (e.g., glycosylation, phosphorylation, acetylation), can have important consequences for both cytokine expression and function. Thus, an integrated strategy combining analytical molecular and proteomic approaches will be best suited to detecting both gross and nuanced changes in cytokine network expression among healthy vs. diseased populations. Similarly, while a discussion of global comparative proteomic methods (e.g., mass spectrometry, ultra-high-density protein microarray chip technology) is outside the scope of this chapter, their importance to biomarker discovery in PD and other complex brain diseases should not be understated (see ref. (33) for a good review).

Drawing from traditional sandwich ELISA principles, virtually all current cytokine multiplex assays feature solid-phase capture and label-based detection chemistries in either of two basic formats: cytometric bead-based arrays or planar solid-platform-based arrays. As shown in Fig. 2, anti-cytokine capture antibodies are immobilized in parallel assays onto solid supports, which take the form either of rigid two-dimensional platforms/membranes or three-dimensional polystyrene (and more recently magnetic) microspheres. Following incubation with biological samples, captured analyte (cytokines or other biomolecular targets) is detected by labeled reporter antibodies. The method of detection differs between assay platforms and ranges from fluorescent and chemiluminescent techniques to electrogenerated chemiluminescence (or electrochemiluminescence, ECL). Differences in dynamic range, sensitivity, degree of multiplexing, and cost (equipment and consumables) exist among the different multiplex platforms, and between these newer technologies and conventional ELISA. These and other issues will be discussed in the sections that follow.

2.1. Bead-Based Arrays: Technological Overview

The defining characteristic of bead-based arrays, otherwise known as liquid, suspension or flow cytometric arrays, is the use of multiple different populations of antibody-conjugated microspheres

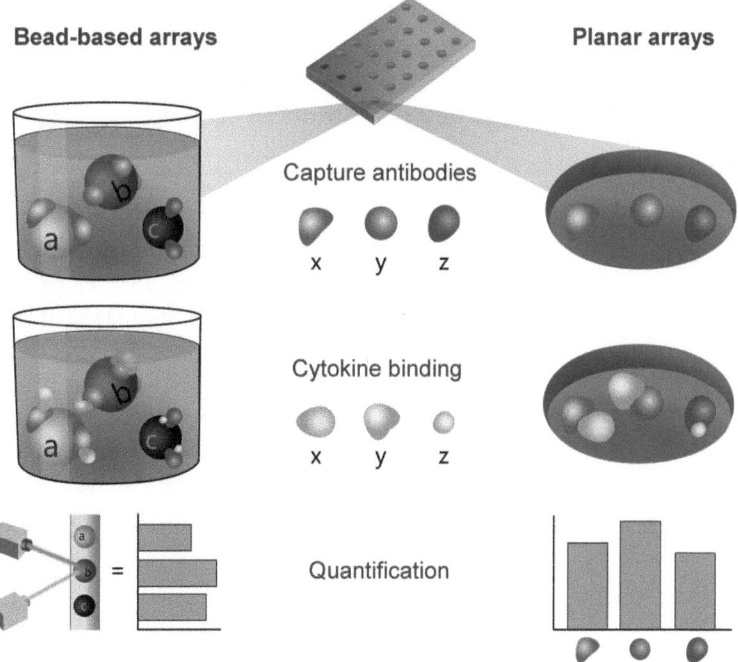

Fig. 2. Overview of bead-based and planar multiplex technologies.

for building multiplex immunoassays. The polystyrene beads, usually no larger than 10 μm in diameter, are size and/or color-coded (with one or more internal fluorophore), rendering them distinguishable via light scatter or internal fluorescence-intensity ratio upon flow cytometric analysis. Fluorophore-conjugated reporter antibodies, with an emission spectrum distinct from the encoding fluorophores, provide the analyte-dependent immunoassay signal, which is also read out using flow cytometry. Finally, experimentally derived calibration curves are used to relate signal response of the distinct microsphere sets (typically 50–100 beads within each bead population) to the concentration of target analytes in sample. While the bead-based approaches to multiplexing pose several distinct disadvantages (e.g., increased vulnerability to cross-reactivity between antibodies and other proteins in solution) (34), analyte quantification is usually performed with high sensitivity (pg/mL), wide dynamic range (at least 3 logs), and good precision. Bead-based multiplex platforms are also readily automated by a wide range of liquid handling systems.

The Luminex 100/200 system (Luminex Corp.) uses proprietary xMAP (multianalyte profiling) technology and a flow cytometry-based Luminex analyzer to detect up to 100 different analytes in a single microplate well containing 25 μL sample (50 μL if running duplicates). Up to 100 distinct sets of microspheres (~5.6 μm MicroPlex polystyrene beads) are internally dyed with different ratios of red and infrared fluorophores, which have coincidental excitation spectra but distinct emission bands (35). Each bead population is conjugated to a different cytokine-specific capture antibody and thus bears a unique immunoassay. The suspended beads, following incubation with sample or standards and streptavidin-phycoerythrin-(PE)-conjugated detection antibodies in porous 96-well filter plates, are aspirated (by vacuum) into the Luminex analyzer's flow chamber. Passing rapidly and individually through the flow cell, a red classification laser (635 nm) identifies the particular cytokine bound (based on the microsphere's spectral address) and a second green reporter laser (532 nm) quantifies the immunoassay response signal. Standard calibration curve generation and data analysis are facilitated by specialized multiplex curve-fitting software packages supporting the four or five parameter logistic nonlinear regression models (e.g., MasterPlex QT).

Numerous mouse and human multiplex cytokine kits (with ~10–20 cytokines on each panel) are commercially available (e.g., Millipore, Bio-Rad, Invitrogen, Panomics), although Luminex's open-architecture xMAP technology allows researchers to customize multiplex immunoassay panels (with in theory up to 100 different analytes, but in practice typically <30 due to potential issues of antibody cross-reactivity). We typically utilize custom designed kits comprising both pro-inflammatory (IFN-α, TNF-α, IL-1β, IL-6, IL-8, IL-12) and anti-inflammatory (IL-4, IL-10, TGF-β) cytokines.

High-throughput 96-well microplates allow ~40 samples to be run in duplicate; the remaining wells contain standards and various quality controls. To control for nonspecific antibody binding and thus increase the signal-to-noise ratio, we generally use two separate positive controls at two different concentrations. As well, a negative control serves as a background measure that is subtracted from all sample wells. Using this procedure we have recently published several papers demonstrating time-dependent brain and blood cytokine variations in response to various PD- and/or depression-relevant xenobiotic (paraquat), psychogenic (social housing manipulations, chronic stress), and immunogenic insults (LPS, poly I:C) (30, 36, 37).

The Luminex 100/200 system has probably become the foremost bead-based multiplexing system used in research and clinical settings; however, two xMAP technology-based platforms recently introduced by Luminex Corp., namely the FLEXMAP 3D and MAGPIX systems, hold the promise of substantial improvements in multiplexing capability and cost efficiency, respectively. Two major differences separate the FLEXMAP 3D system from its Luminex 100/200 predecessor. Firstly, polystyrene microspheres are impregnated with different ratios of three (as opposed to two) internal fluorophores, enabling the discrimination of up to 500 discrete bead populations and consequently, the multiplexing of up to 500 different assays (in theory). Secondly, instrumentation innovations, including dual sample fluidics paths and 384-well plate compatibility, provide for higher throughput and faster readout times. The FLEXMAP 3D system also boasts a wider dynamic range compared to the Luminex 100/200 (4.5 logs vs. 3.5 logs) and is highly amenable to automation.

While the strength of the FLEXMAP 3D system thus lies in the capacity for high-density and high-throughput screening, the newer MAGPIX system offers an (relatively) affordable means of performing fully quantitative, low-to-medium density (up to 50 analytes), and high-throughput (~40 samples) applications. According to company literature, even when running single-plex tests the MAGPIX system provides cost-savings over traditional ELISA because it circumvents the need for filter plates; yet, capital equipment costs should certainly not be overlooked (38). Further strengths of this instrument are its compact size (W × D × H: 16.5 cm × 60 cm × 43 cm) and portability. Like the Luminex 100/200 and FLEXMAP 3D systems, the MAGPIX platform is built on established xMAP technology; however, the slightly larger (6.4 μm) polystyrene MagPlex beads used in the MAGPIX system are embedded with superparamagnetic ferrite (iron oxide) nanoparticles. These microspheres behave magnetically only upon application of an extrinsic magnetic field (domains become temporarily aligned) and have the distinct advantage of being readily amenable to high-throughput automation. Indeed, since magnetic beads can be immobilized with magnets during washing steps, the requirement for vacuum/suction-driven filter plate washers (i.e., using a physical barrier to entrap beads while permitting solution to pass through) and the potentially serious complications associated with this method, such as filter plate leaking and clogging, can be abrogated (39, 40).

Similar to the older-generation MicroPlex spheres, spectral coding of MagPlex beads is accomplished by impregnating different microsphere sets with specific combinations of fluorescent dyes; this permits the multiplexing of up to 50 analytes in a single sample. Further setting the MAGPIX system apart is its use of light-emitting diodes (LEDs) instead of lasers to excite the classification and reporter fluorophores, and its reliance on CCD fluorescence imaging and detection (an externally applied magnetic field temporarily immobilizes the beads), as opposed to flow cytometric quantification methods. While few studies have been published using the new MAGPIX system, assay reproducibility and performance (e.g., sensitivity, linear dynamic range, standard recovery) using multiplex kits from at least two different suppliers (Bio-Rad and Millipore) appear to be comparable to the established Luminex 100/200 system (41). MagPlex bead compatibility has also been established for both the Luminex 100/200 and FLEXMAP 3D platforms, allowing for up to 80-plex or 500-plex assays, respectively.

Similar to the approach taken by Luminex with its xMAP technology, both eBioscience's FlowCytomix array and the BD (Beckton Dickinson) Cytometric Bead Array (CBA) use antibody-coated microbeads (4.4 μm and 5.5 μm, and 7.5 μm, respectively) to capture multiple target analytes in solution. Distinct bead populations are identified on flow cytometry either by internal fluorescence-intensity ratio (CBA) or the combination of a monofluorescent signal and bead size (FlowCytomix); in both cases, PE fluorescence intensity generates the assay response signal. Since the various fluorophores used in the FlowCytomix and CBA systems are readily excitable at 488 nm, any flow cytometer equipped with a standard blue laser can be used for assay readout; this represents a potentially substantial cost-savings advantage over the Luminex systems. However, the degree of multiplexing supported by the FlowCytomix and CBA platforms is somewhat limited compared to the xMAP technology-based arrays, ranging from around 20 different analytes per sample in the FlowCytomix array to upwards of 30 in the CBA system.

2.2. Planar Arrays: Technological Overview

Like the multiplex bead-based assays, planar membrane-based approaches to multiplexing borrow heavily from traditional sandwich ELISA principles. Cytokine-specific capture antibodies are arrayed onto any one of several types of solid support, most commonly the individual wells of polystyrene microtitre plates. While assay identification in bead-based arrays relies upon the physical (size) and/or optical encoding (internal fluorescent intensity) of antibody-conjugated bead sets, planar multiplexes instead use a positional coding scheme, wherein the location of spotted antibody in a two-dimensional array (e.g., within a microwell) defines a particular immunoassay. Following incubation with biological samples or standards, labeled detection antibodies form immunosandwiches with bound analyte and surface-immobilized capture antibody. Typically, assay reaction signals are read out using a streptavidin/horseradish peroxidase (HRP)-based chemiluminescence system, although at least one commercial platform features ECL imaging and detection. The sensitivity (pg/mL) and dynamic range (3–4 logs) of these assays is generally comparable to if not better than traditional ELISA.

The technologically similar Multiplex ELISA from Quansys Bioscience, alternately called Q-Plex array technology, and the SearchLight Chemiluminescent Protein Array kits from Aushon Bioscience use standard 96-well microplates as the solid support structure for multiple ELISA assays in parallel. The Q-Plex also supports a 384-well platform. Multiplexing in these high-throughput sandwich ELISA systems is achieved by spotting up to 16 (SearchLight) or 25 (Q-Plex) different capture antibodies onto the bottom of each microwell in a spatially discrete manner. The precise *x*, *y* coordinates of a spot within a given well thus defines a distinct capture antibody population/immunoassay across all wells in a plate. After incubation with biological specimens and standards, bound analyte is visualized with streptavidin-HRP and chemiluminescent detection. High-resolution fluorescence scanning (with a CCD imaging system) captures an image of the plate, from which the concentration of target analytes in the multiple samples is determined using any number of array software programs. Analogously, Research & Diagnostics Systems' Mosaic ELISA permits the simultaneous determination of up to eight different analytes in as little as 13–50 μL of sample. As with the Q-plex and SearchLight technologies, good throughput is achieved by running duplicate samples in 96-well microtitre plates. However, the Mosaic platform does not at present support customization, as kit selection is limited to two pre-spotted panels of 6 (human growth factor panel) or 8 capture antibodies (human cytokine panel).

An alternative to multiplexing with chemiluminescent detection, Aushon Biosystems' SearchLight Infrared (IR) Array kits use DyLight 800 labeled streptavidin conjugates, which feature near-IR fluorescence and narrow emission profiles, for detecting up to 24 different cytokines (human or mouse) in single small-volume samples. The core principles of this assay are the same as for the SearchLight chemiluminescent array (e.g., multiplex sandwich ELISA, capture antibodies spotted in defined arrays into the wells of a 96-well plate), but the near-IR fluorometric analysis requires an Odyssey or Aerius IR Imaging System (LI-COR) and appropriate array analysis software. Also featuring fluorescence detection, the FAST Quant system from Whatman, part of GE Healthcare, uses nitrocellulose-coated glass FAST slides as the solid-phase substrate for multiplexed assays in lieu of the familiar 96-well microtiter plates. In this method, 8–10 different capture antibodies are arrayed in triplicate onto 16 nitrocellulose pads per slide. Since triplicate values are obtained for each analyte in sample/standard (and due to the solid-phase nature of the assay), there is no need to run duplicate samples; this helps to both conserve sample and promote assay throughput (42). Indeed, as each FAST Quant kit contains four slides, and more than one kit can be run using the same standards (albeit at the same time), the FAST Quant system is readily amenable to high-throughput. A fluorescence scanner is required to image Cy5 signal intensity (these kits use a streptavidin–Cy5 detection system) and data analysis is performed with specialized protein array software (e.g., MicroVigene).

Using pre-arrayed FAST slides, Whatman has only recently started offering the FAST Quant 40 Human kit, a higher-density array capable of simultaneously quantifying 40 cytokines in human samples. In this configuration, the 40 immunoassays are actually divided into two sub-arrays of immobilized capture antibodies (18-plex and 22-plex, respectively). Each sub-array is printed eight times per slide, corresponding to the 16 nitrocellulose pads, and requires its own standards. Thus, while assay selection, customizability, and throughput are diminished (the kit of four slides can run 24 samples), the FAST Quant 40 Human assay represents a significant upgrade in plex level over the older 8–10-plex kits.

Meso Scale Diagnostics' (MSD, a division of Meso Scale Discovery) MULTI-SPOT assay systems use oxidative-reduction ECL detection technology for multiplexing up to ten analytes per well (containing ~25 μL of sample) of a specialized 96-well carbon electrode microplate. Up to ten different capture antibody populations are directly adsorbed in array format on high-binding capacity carbon electrodes embedded in the bottom of 4-, 7-, or 10-spot MULTI-SPOT plates. The desired plex level determines which of the three basic MULTI-SPOT plate geometries is used; a 1-spot MICRO-ARRAY plate is also offered for single-plex applications. Following incubation with analytes in sample, detection antibodies labeled with proprietary electrochemiluminescent SULFO-TAG NHS ester reagent (ruthenium (II) tris-bipyridine; $Ru(bpy)_3^{2+}$) complete the sandwich immunocomplex and provide the analyte-dependent luminescence signal when electrochemically stimulated in the presence of the ECL coreactant, tripropylamine (TPA).

Briefly, upon application of a voltage to the plate electrodes using any one of several SECTOR imaging systems, both ruthenium (label/luminophore) and TPA (ECL coreactant in read buffer) are oxidized at the electrodes' surface. TPA^{+} rapidly and spontaneously loses a proton to form the highly reactive neutral TPA^{+} intermediate, which reduces the ruthenium-bipyridine moiety to form a divalent excited state ruthenium complex ($Ru(bpy)_3^{2+*}$). On relaxation back to the ground state a photon at ~620 nm is emitted (43). Multiple oxidative-reduction cycles involving ruthenium SULFO-TAG labels and TPA (which is consumed in the reaction) amplifies the luminescent signal and in so doing enhances assay sensitivity. In the SECTOR reader, an ultra-low noise CCD camera images the luminescent intensity of the ECL labels, enabling quantitation of analytes with appropriate data analysis tools. MSD's ECL-based approach to multiplexing offers several distinct advantages, including ultra high sensitivity (lower limit of detection <1 pg/mL for most cytokines), minimal nonspecific background signals (which contributes to high sensitivity), a broad linear dynamic range (up to 5 logs), and compatibility with complex biological matrices such as vaginal fluid (44). Higher throughput 384-well MULTI-SPOT (and 1536-well MULTI-ARRAY) plates are also available, but only in lower-plex configurations.

2.3. Comparisons and Considerations of Multiplex Cytokine Assays

Overall, cytokine multiplex technologies hold several advantages over conventional ELISA, the most obvious and important being the ability to multiplex or run multiple parallel assays in single, small-volume samples. Simultaneous cytokine measurement is highly desirable in the context of network-based approaches to biomarker discovery, wherein major emphasis is placed not only on identifying candidate biomarkers, but understanding the interplay between the various cytokine family members (45). From a practical perspective, multiplexing becomes particularly advantageous when quantifying sample that is either precious or limited in volume. Indeed, compared to running multiple separate ELISAs, multiplex assays require far less sample, reagent (especially antibodies), and labor time (parallel assays that are highly amenable to automation); and therefore have the potential to dramatically reduce costs (7). Yet, any improvement in cost and time efficiencies ought certainly to be balanced against the generally higher capital equipment costs for high-density multiplexing systems.

Importantly, multiplex cytokine assays are able to maintain these advantages over traditional ELISA without sacrificing performance (sensitivity, specificity) or throughput (46), although several studies have raised questions about the reliability of these assays (see below) (47). Moreover, the linear dynamic range exhibited by multiplex assays is much wider than a typical sandwich ELISA (by ~2 orders of magnitude), enabling accurate cytokine quantification with minimal dilution. While dilution helps to reduce matrix effects in biological samples, it can also introduce substantial error and bias into cytokine/analyte measurement, especially when large dilution steps are required for samples that contain proteins across a wide dynamic range of concentrations (e.g., serum, plasma). Indeed, since dilution reduces the concentrations both of target cytokine/analyte and soluble cytokine receptors (as well as other circulating cytokine-binding proteins), the relative amount of receptor-bound vs. "free" cytokine available for detection can potentially be altered (7, 48).

While comparison studies with ELISA have generally established the validity of multiplex assays for cytokine quantitation in biological specimens (reliability concerns notwithstanding) (49–51), a number of recent studies reported significant differences in assay reproducibility and performance between the various multiplex platforms and even between commercial kits for the same system. For instance, Dabitao et al. (52) compared the performance of a 9-plex ECL-based MSD plate and a 6-plex Becton Dickinson CBA kit for measuring pro-inflammatory cytokines in the serum of HIV-infected patients and healthy controls. While the two systems displayed comparable sensitivities (based on standard curves), the MSD assay was superior in terms of accuracy (spike recovery of cytokine) and detection frequency of endogenous circulating cytokines. Earlier studies using serum or plasma of healthy donors likewise reported a significant performance advantage of MSD's ECL-based assays (number of species detected, dynamic range, lower, and upper limits of quantification) over bead-based systems (xMAP-based and FlowCytomix) and other planar arrays (FASTQuant) (53, 54). Despite significant variation in absolute cytokine values, similarities in the relative expression patterns of cytokines between the different multiplex systems were, however, generally noted in these studies (52, 54). Moreover, in a direct comparison of 10-plex kits (human cytokine) from MSD and Luminex (Invitrogen), Chowdhury et al. (54) showed that the Luminex system had better precision compared to the more sensitive MSD platform. Indeed, bead-based assays should theoretically have improved precision compared to planar arrays on account of the ~50–100 individual measurements made for each assay in the mutliplex (corresponding to the ~50–100 microspheres per bead population) (34). Yet, Hanley et al. (55) demonstrated that variation in microsphere diameter (arising from inadequate manufacturing quality control) is a likely significant source of stochastic variance (and hence, imprecision) in bead-based assays.

Similar to the findings reported by Dabitao et al. (52), a recent multi-site comparison study by Breen et al. (56) revealed marked performance differences between MSD and Luminex-based assays (different kits from three suppliers) in the measurement of cytokines in the serum of HIV-infected patients and healthy controls. The authors also reported finding significant inter-laboratory and inter-kit variation, the latter of which probably reflects the confounding influence of supplier differences in antibody pairs and potentially other reagents (42). Yet, as was noted in previous studies reporting discrepant cytokine values between same-platform kits (47, 57), analogous patterns of cytokine perturbation were obtained using the different xMAP panels (56).

Using LPS- and phytohemagglutinin-stimulated sodium heparin plasma of healthy volunteers and a custom-conjugated 15-plex Luminex assay, de Jager et al. (48) showed that ostensibly trivial processes such as sample handling (freeze-thawing) and storage (duration, temperature) could significantly influence the reliability and reproducibility of cytokine detection. While most cytokines remained stable at −80 °C for ~2 years, degradation of certain cytokines was apparent as early as 1 year after storage. Within 4 years of storage, 10 of the 15 cytokines had degraded at least 40% of baseline values, half of them by ~75% (48). Since Breen et al. (56) used archival clinical plasma samples that were collected as early as 2001 (10 years before the study's publication) and no later than 2006, significant degradation of cytokines during storage (and to differing degrees depending on when samples were collected) may have contributed to the noted substantial intra- and inter-assay variability. However, it should be mentioned that plasma and not serum was analyzed in the study by Breen et al. (56); an important point to consider given that detection of at least some cytokines can be influenced by the type of biological matrix analyzed (e.g., plasma vs. serum), particularly when multiplex tools are used (7, 58).

To summarize, most studies to date have reported good correlation among bead-based and planar cytokine arrays and between multiplex assays and traditional ELISA (comparable relative changes), thus recommending the continued and expanded use of multiplexing systems in high-throughput screening applications (e.g., early and differential disease detection). The choice between multiplex assays is not obvious, however, and will surely reflect the nature of the clinical or research application. Factors such as desired plex level, assay sensitivity, dynamic range, flexibility, and throughput; as well as the cost of both consumables and equipment will likely factor in any decision (42). For instance, while MSD's ECL-based systems were found to excel in key performance measures, xMAP technology-based systems offer a higher degree of multiplexing capacity. Yet, common to all multiplex immunoassay systems are technological and operational issues relating to assay interference (antibody cross-reactivity, nonspecific binding, compatibility of diluents and assay buffers, other matrix effects); quality control (algorithms, protocols); protein vs. nucleic acid analysis (protein denaturation, costly and time-consuming antibody development process); and data analysis and interpretation (complex bioinformatics and computational models). These and other challenges have been recently discussed in considerable detail elsewhere (7, 34, 45, 59).

3. Cytokine Multiplexing for Biomarker Analysis in PD

It has been exceedingly difficult to bridge the gap between basic experimental research and the generation of usable serological biomarkers of PD. This largely stems from the fact that neuropathological states are so highly complex and heterogeneous in terms of etiology and mechanisms at play. According to stringent inclusion criteria stipulated by the German Society of Experimental and Clinical Neurotherapeutics, biomarkers for measuring PD progression and treatment efficacy should, among other things: (1) reflect core mechanisms of neurodegeneration; (2) show good correlation with disease progression as measured by established clinical rating scales (e.g., UPDRS; Hoehn and Yahr scale); and (3) be validated in preclinical animals models and replicated by at least two independent studies (1). Unfortunately, these strict requirements have not yet been met by any proposed biomarkers for early PD or the evaluation of its treatment. However, the experimental literature in general has suggested a number of potential PD biomarker candidates, most notably α-synuclein and DJ-1, but these have still not been rigorously tested in the clinical arena or else have been met with conflicting or ambiguous/nonspecific results (60).

Clinical rating scales, especially in the hands of experienced and specialized practitioners, can be very useful tools for diagnosing and tracking the progression of CNS disease; however, the early stages of neurological illnesses such as PD and AD can be extremely difficult to detect and are often missed on clinical intake. Hence, finding reliable biomarkers that can be objectively used for early (differential) diagnosis, as well as assessing the course of primary disease and likelihood of the development of certain co-morbid symptom clusters would be invaluable (1). Specifically, detecting pre-symptomatic or prodromal stages of disease could provide sufficient time to implement emerging new neuroprotective treatments such as the neurotrophic factor inducer, Cogane (PYM50028), or the antioxidant agent, coenzyme Q10, both of which are currently in clinical trials for the treatment of early stage PD (although preliminary findings from the CoQ10 study are not promising). Indeed, the results of several preclinical studies using different toxin models of PD suggested that pharmacologic attenuation or prevention of DA neuron loss required the application of putative neuroprotective agents during a relatively narrow time window before or after lesion induction, and definitely prior to onset of motor symptoms (61, 62). However, other animal studies have pointed to the surprisingly robust neuroreparative and neurorestorative potential of some of these agents, even at times far removed from initial toxin insult (62, 63). Nonetheless, a majority of studies seem to agree that once neuroinflammatory and oxidative stress cascades (and other degenerative brain processes) reach a certain threshold momentum for neurodegeneration, further cell loss will in all likelihood prove to be extremely difficult to arrest or even slow down (let alone reverse). Thus, prophylactic neuroprotective drug treatment strategies might be most useful, but would obviously necessitate the development and implementation of highly effective early biomarkers of disease.

It should also be underscored that PD is a very heterogeneous illness and that certain sub-types or endophenotypes of the disease likely require specific tailored treatment regimens. Biomarker identification could conceivably provide a better means of stratifying such diverging categories of disease. Indeed, given the substantial co-morbidity evident in PD, biomarker profiles would go a long way in helping to establish a means of identifying which individuals are most likely to develop specific sub-categories of co-morbid symptoms, ranging from affective (depression, anxiety) and cognitive disturbances (executive function deficits, dementia) to potentially even sleep (insomnia, difficulty falling asleep) and autonomic problems (gastrointestinal, genitourinary, and sexual dysfunction). As cytokines are considered key players in the pathogenesis of both neurological and psychiatric diseases, they may be ideally positioned as candidate biomarkers of PD and its neuropsychiatric co-morbidities. It is our belief that multiplex array technology may be particularly well suited for assessing the potential of blood-borne cytokines to fulfill this role. The strength of this method lies in its ability to detect simultaneous levels of multiple cytokine species in small amounts of sample (presumably serum or plasma), which is imperative given that cytokine impact is dependent on the coordinated activity of the varied members of the cytokine families. Our notion of a cytokine/biomarker-based risk stratification schema for the co-morbid presentations of PD is presented in Fig. 3.

Using an ultrasensitive 8-plex ECL-based assay from MSD, Scully et al. (64) found that female patients with "pure" irritable Bowel syndrome (IBS), a non-life-threatening functional Bowel disorder characterized primarily by abdominal pain, bloating, and discomfort could be differentiated from IBS patients with extra-intestinal co-morbidities (fibromyalgia, premenstrual dysmorphic disorder, and chronic fatigue syndrome). Indeed, while IBS patients displayed increased overall concentrations of the pro-inflammatory cytokines, IL-6 and IL-8, relative to an age- and gender-matched control group, additional elevations of IL-1β and TNF-α further distinguished IBS patients with extra-intestinal co-morbid conditions. The multiplexed cytokine profiles were unable, however, to differentiate between various clusters of co-morbid symptoms (e.g., fibromyalgia vs. chronic fatigue syndrome). While IBS is clearly not a CNS disorder per se (nor is it per se a "disease") it does involve significant dysregulation of brain, gut, immune, and endocrine systems (65). Moreover, psychiatric co-morbidity has been estimated to approach 60% in IBS patients (66). This study

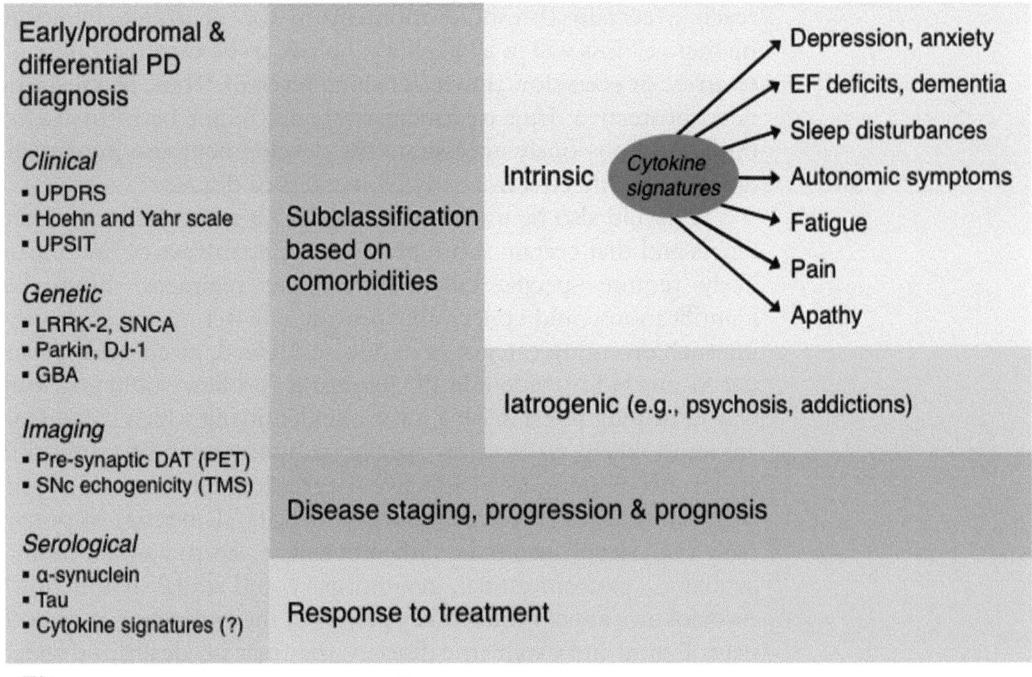

Fig. 3. Biomarker-based risk stratification schema for the co-morbid presentations of PD. *UPDRS* unified Parkinson's disease rating scale; *UPSIT* University of Pennsylvania smell identification test; *LRRK-2* leucine-rich repeat kinase 2; *SNCA* synuclein, alpha (non A4 component of amyloid precursor); *GBA* β-glucocerebrosidase; *DAT* dopamine transporter; *PET* positron emission tomography; *TMS* transcranial magnetic stimulation.

thus aptly demonstrates the potential of emerging multiplex technologies to identify disease-relevant cytokine signatures in blood and probably other bodily fluids, which can in turn be used to help refine co-morbidity-based risk stratification schema and expand our understanding of immunomechanisms subserving the development of co-morbid psychiatric illness.

4. Conclusion

PD is typically diagnosed at a late stage of disease progression, after ~70% loss of SNc dopaminergic neurons. Diagnosis at earlier, pre-symptomatic stages would permit development of preventative, as opposed to palliative therapies, with the potential of dramatically slowing or otherwise altering disease progression. Given the high rates of co-morbidity in PD and the detrimental effects these symptoms can have on quality of life and potentially even primary disease progression, identification, and treatment of PD patients at very early stages or increased risk of co-morbid illness is another worthwhile goal. It is our contention that using multiple serological biomarkers, allowing one to obtain a sort of "signature" or profile of biochemical mediators, would be a valuable addition to the clinical work-up and follow-up of PD. In fact, when multiple blood and/ or CSF markers are combined and analyzed together rather than independently, significant improvements in sensitivity and specificity can often be realized. Still greater improvements could conceivably be achieved by combining serological parameters with markers from other modalities (e.g., clinical, imaging, genetic) (67).

The search for blood cytokine signatures of specific diseases or subgroups of disease requires the development and implementation of highly sensitive and reliable screening tools capable of performing medium-to-high-density and high-throughput applications. It is in this capacity that we advocate the use of cytokine multiplex assays such as those discussed in this chapter. While recent advances in mass spectrometry-based quantitative proteomics (e.g., isobaric tags for relative and absolute quantitation, multiple reaction monitoring) figure to play an increasingly important role in (ultra-) high-density biomarker profiling, high-throughput affinity-based protein arrays should remain invaluable tools for biomarker analysis and validation, especially for diseases in which cytokines are hypothesized or known to be primary players in disease pathogenesis.

Acknowledgements

This work was supported by funds from the Canadian Institutes of Health Research (D.L. and S.H.) and Parkinson Society Canada (S.H.). S.H. is a Canada Research Chair in Neuroscience. Thanks to Neville Ko for creating the schematic in Fig. 2.

References

1. Gerlach M et al (2012) Biomarker candidates of neurodegeneration in Parkinson's disease for the evaluation of disease-modifying therapeutics. J Neural Transm 119(1):39–52. doi:10.1007/s00702-011-0682-x
2. Morgan JC, Mehta SH, Sethi KD (2010) Biomarkers in Parkinson's disease. Curr Neurol Neurosci Rep 10:423–430
3. Tolosa E, Wenning G, Poewe W (2006) The diagnosis of Parkinson's disease. Lancet Neurol 5:75–86
4. Schlossmacher MG, Mollenhauer B (2010) Biomarker research in Parkinson's disease: objective measures needed for patient stratification in future cause-directed trials. Biomark Med 4:647–650
5. Litteljohn D et al (2010) Inflammatory mechanisms of neurodegeneration in toxin-based models of Parkinson's disease. Parkinsons Dis 2011:713517. doi:10.4061/2011/713517
6. Anisman H, Merali Z, Hayley S (2008) Neurotransmitter, peptide and cytokine processes in relation to depressive disorder: comorbidity between depression and neurodegenerative disorders. Prog Neurobiol 85:1–74
7. Leng SX et al (2008) ELISA and multiplex technologies for cytokine measurement in inflammation and aging research. J Gerontol A Biol Sci Med Sci 63:879–884
8. Leentjens AF et al (2003) Higher incidence of depression preceding the onset of Parkinson's disease: a register study. Mov Disord 18: 414–418
9. Stefanova E et al (2006) Depression predicts the pattern of cognitive impairment in early Parkinson's disease. J Neurol Sci 248:131–137

10. McDonald WM, Richard IH, DeLong MR (2003) Prevalence, etiology, and treatment of depression in Parkinson's disease. Biol Psychiatry 54:363–375
11. Temel Y (2007) Inhibition of 5-HT neuron activity and induction of depressive-like behavior by high-frequency stimulation of the subthalamic nucleus. Proc Natl Acad Sci U S A 104:17087–17092
12. Frisina PG et al (2008) The effects of antidepressants in Parkinson's disease: a meta-analysis. Int J Neurosci 118:667–682
13. Berg D (2008) Biomarkers for the early detection of Parkinson's and Alzheimer's disease. Neurodegener Dis 5:133–136
14. Trew M, Suchowersky O (2005) Anxiety and Parkinson's disease. In: Pfeiffer RF, Ebadi M (eds) Parkinson's disease. CRC Press, Boca Raton, FL, pp 339–346
15. Nagatsu T, Sawada M (2005) Inflammatory process in Parkinson's disease: role for cytokines. Curr Pharm Des 11:999–1016
16. Mangano EN et al (2012) Interferon-gamma plays a role in paraquat-induced neurodegeneration involving oxidative and proinflammatory pathways. Neurobiol Aging 33(7):1411–1426. doi:10.1016/j.neurobiolaging.2011.02.016
17. Tansey MG et al (2008) Neuroinflammation in Parkinson's disease: is there sufficient evidence for mechanism-based interventional therapy? Front Biosci 13:709–717
18. Reale M et al (2009) Peripheral cytokines profile in Parkinson's disease. Brain Behav Immun 23:55–63
19. Chen H et al (2008) Peripheral inflammatory biomarkers and risk of Parkinson's disease. Am J Epidemiol 167:90–95
20. O'Brien SM et al (2007) Plasma cytokine profiles in depressed patients who fail to respond to selective serotonin reuptake inhibitor therapy. J Psychiatr Res 41:326–331
21. Domenici E et al (2010) Plasma protein biomarkers for depression and schizophrenia by multi analyte profiling of case-control collections. PLoS One 5(2):e9166. doi:10.1371/journal.pone.0009166
22. Alesci S et al (2005) Major depression is associated with significant diurnal elevations in plasma interleukin-6 levels, a shift of its circadian rhythm, and loss of physiological complexity in its secretion: clinical implications. J Clin Endocrinol Metab 90:2522–2530
23. Dhabhar FS et al (2009) Low serum IL-10 concentrations and loss of regulatory association between IL-6 and IL-10 in adults with major depression. J Psychiatr Res 43:962–969
24. Hannestad J, Dellagioia N, Bloch M (2011) The effect of antidepressant medication treatment on serum levels of inflammatory cytokines: a meta-analysis. Neuropsychopharmacology 36(12):2452–2459. doi:10.1038/npp. 2011.132
25. Diamond M, Kelly JP, Connor TJ (2006) Antidepressants suppress production of the Th1 cytokine interferon-gamma, independent of monoamine transporter blockade. Eur Neuropsychopharmacol 16:481–490
26. Raison CL et al (2005) Depression during pegylated interferon-alpha plus ribavirin therapy: prevalence and prediction. J Clin Psychiatry 66:41–48
27. Kaneko N et al (2006) Suppression of cell proliferation by interferon-alpha through interleukin-1 production in adult rat dentate gyrus. Neuropsychopharmacology 31:2619–2626
28. Ishikawa J, Ishikawa A, Nakamura S (2007) Interferon-alpha reduces the density of monoaminergic axons in the rat brain. Neuroreport 18:137–140
29. Anisman H et al (2007) Interferon-alpha effects are exaggerated when administered on a psychosocial stressor backdrop: cytokine, corticosterone and brain monoamine variations. J Neuroimmunol 186:45–53
30. Litteljohn D et al (2010) Interferon-gamma deficiency modifies the effects of a chronic stressor in mice: implications for psychological pathology. Brain Behav Immun 24:462–473
31. Ling MM, Ricks C, Lea P (2007) Multiplexing molecular diagnostics and immunoassays using emerging microarray technologies. Expert Rev Mol Diagn 7:87–98
32. Young HA (2009) Cytokine multiplex analysis. Methods Mol Biol 511:85–105
33. Shi M, Caudle WM, Zhang J (2009) Biomarker discovery in neurodegenerative diseases: a proteomic approach. Neurobiol Dis 35:157–164
34. Ellington AA et al (2010) Antibody-based protein multiplex platforms: technical and operational challenges. Clin Chem 56:186–193
35. Braeckmans K et al (2002) Encoding microcarriers: present and future technologies. Nat Rev Drug Discov 1:447–456
36. Mangano EN, Hayley S (2009) Inflammatory priming of the substantia nigra influences the impact of later paraquat exposure: neuroimmune sensitization of neurodegeneration. Neurobiol Aging 30:1361–1378
37. Gibb J et al (2011) Effects of stressors and immune activating agents on peripheral and central cytokines in mouse strains that differ in stressor responsivity. Brain Behav Immun 25:468–482

38. Luminex Corp (2010) Overcoming the cost and performance limitations of ELISA with xMAP technology. xMAP technology technical note [white paper]. http://www.luminexcorp.com/prod/groups/public/documents/lmnxcorp/308-xmap-vs.-elisa-white-paper.pdf
39. Sista RS et al (2008) Heterogeneous immunoassays using magnetic beads on a digital microfluidic platform. Lab Chip 8:2188–2196
40. Hartmann M et al (2009) Protein microarrays for diagnostic assays. Anal Bioanal Chem 393:1407–1416
41. Luminex Corp (2010) Equivalent analytical performance between the new MAGPIX system and the Luminex 100/200 system. xMAP technology technical note [white paper). http://www.luminexcorp.com/prod/groups/public/documents/lmnxcorp/314-magpix-vs-lx200-white-pape.pdf
42. Lash GE, Pinto LA (2010) Multiplex cytokine analysis technologies. Expert Rev Vaccines 9:1231–1237
43. Wu G (2010) Assay development: fundamentals and practices. Wiley, Hoboken, NJ, pp 43–53
44. Fichorova RN et al (2008) Biological and technical variables affecting immunoassay recovery of cytokines from human serum and simulated vaginal fluid: a multicenter study. Anal Chem 80:4741–4751
45. Vistnes M, Christensen G, Omland T (2010) Multiple cytokine biomarkers in heart failure. Expert Rev Mol Diagn 10:147–157
46. Dupont NC et al (2005) Validation and comparison of luminex multiplex cytokine analysis kits with ELISA: determinations of a panel of nine cytokines in clinical sample culture supernatants. J Reprod Immunol 66:175–191
47. Djoba Siawaya JF et al (2008) An evaluation of commercial fluorescent bead-based luminex cytokine assays. PLoS One 3(7):e2535. doi:10.1371/journal.pone.0002535
48. de Jager W et al (2009) Prerequisites for cytokine measurements in clinical trials with multiplex immunoassays. BMC Immunol 10:52. doi:10.1186/1471-2172-10-52
49. Elshal MF, McCoy JP (2006) Multiplex bead array assays: performance evaluation and comparison of sensitivity to ELISA. Methods 38:317–323
50. Dossus L et al (2009) Validity of multiplex-based assays for cytokine measurements in serum and plasma from "non-diseased" subjects: comparison with ELISA. J Immunol Methods 350:125–132
51. Codorean E et al (2010) Correlation of XMAP and ELISA cytokine profiles; development and validation for immunotoxicological studies in vitro. Roum Arch Microbiol Immunol 69:13–19
52. Dabitao D et al (2011) Multiplex measurement of proinflammatory cytokines in human serum: comparison of the Meso Scale Discovery electrochemiluminescence assay and the Cytometric Bead Array. J Immunol Methods 372(1–2):71–77. doi:10.1016/j.jim.2011.06.033
53. Fu Q, Zhu J, Van Eyk JE (2010) Comparison of multiplex immunoassay platforms. Clin Chem 56:314–318
54. Chowdhury F, Williams A, Johnson P (2009) Validation and comparison of two multiplex technologies, Luminex and Mesoscale Discovery, for human cytokine profiling. J Immunol Methods 340:55–64
55. Hanley BP, Xing L, Cheng RH (2007) Variance in multiplex suspension array assays: microsphere size variation impact. Theor Biol Med Model 4:31. doi:10.1186/1742-4682-4-31
56. Breen EC et al (2011) Multisite comparison of high-sensitivity multiplex cytokine assays. Clin Vaccine Immunol 18:1229–1242
57. Nechansky A et al (2008) Comparison of the calibration standards of three commercially available multiplex kits for human cytokine measurement to WHO standards reveals striking differences. Biomark Insights 3:227–235
58. Prabhakar U et al (2004) Validation and comparative analysis of a multiplexed assay for the simultaneous quantitative measurement of Th1/Th2 cytokines in human serum and human peripheral blood mononuclear cell culture supernatants. J Immunol Methods 291:27–38
59. Master SR, Bierl C, Kricka LJ (2006) Diagnostic challenges for multiplexed protein microarrays. Drug Discov Today 11:1007–1011
60. Mollenhauer B et al (2011) α-Synuclein and tau concentrations in cerebrospinal fluid of patients presenting with parkinsonism: a cohort study. Lancet Neurol 10:230–240
61. Peterson AL, Nutt JG (2008) Treatment of Parkinson's disease with trophic factors. Neurotherapeutics 5:270–280
62. Yasuda T, Mochizuki H (2010) Use of growth factors for the treatment of Parkinson's disease. Expert Rev Neurother 10:915–924
63. Visanji NP et al (2008) PYM50028, a novel, orally active, nonpeptide neurotrophic factor inducer, prevents and reverses neuronal damage induced by MPP+ in mesencephalic neurons and by MPTP in a mouse model of Parkinson's disease. FASEB J 22:2488–2497
64. Scully P et al (2010) Plasma cytokine profiles in females with irritable Bowel syndrome and

extra-intestinal co-morbidity. Am J Gastroenterol 105:2235–2243
65. Ohman L, Simrén M (2010) Pathogenesis of IBS: role of inflammation, immunity and neuroimmune interactions. Nat Rev Gastroenterol Hepatol 7:163–173
66. Folks DG (2004) The interface of psychiatry and irritable Bowel syndrome. Curr Psychiatry Rep 6:210–215
67. Eller M, Williams DR (2009) Biological fluid biomarkers in neurodegenerative parkinsonism. Nat Rev Neurol 5:561–570

Chapter 8

Exploring the Diagnostic Potential of Immune Biomarker Coexpression in Gulf War Illness

Gordon Broderick, Mary Ann Fletcher, Michael Gallagher, Zachary Barnes, Suzanne D. Vernon, and Nancy G. Klimas

Abstract

Complex disorders like Gulf War Illness (GWI) often defy diagnosis on the basis of a single biomarker and may only be distinguishable by considering the coexpression of multiple markers measured in response to a challenge. We demonstrate the practical application of such an approach using an example where blood was collected from 26 GWI, 13 healthy control subjects, and 9 unhealthy controls with Chronic Fatigue at three points during a graded exercise challenge. A 3-way multivariate projection model based on 12 markers of endocrine and immune function was constructed using a training set of $n = 10$ GWI and $n = 11$ healthy controls. These groups were separated almost completely on the basis of two coexpression patterns. In a separate test set these same features allowed for discrimination of new GWI subjects ($n = 16$) from unhealthy ($n = 9$) and healthy control subjects with a sensitivity of 70% and a specificity of 90%.

Key words: Cytokine profile, Coexpression patterns, Exercise response, Gulf War Illness, Regression model, Diagnostic classification, Partial least squares, Batch partial least squares

1. Introduction

Gulf War Illness (GWI) is a complex multisymptom illness of unknown etiology associated with deployment to the Persian Gulf between 1990 and 1991. Symptom presentation shows a strong overlap with the case definition for Chronic Fatigue Syndrome (CFS) with 4.9% of the 693,826 Gulf War troops deployed satisfying the latter (1). Our work and the work of others strongly suggest that the pathogenesis of GWI and CFS includes both a neuroendocrine (2–5) and an immunologic component (6–11). Earlier work in this area has lead to debates over the pro-inflammatory (12, 13) or anti-inflammatory (14, 15) nature of these disorders and more recent results suggest that they may not fit easily into either of these conventional descriptive categories.

Qing Yan (ed.), *Psychoneuroimmunology: Methods and Protocols*, Methods in Molecular Biology, vol. 934,
DOI 10.1007/978-1-62703-071-7_8, © Springer Science+Business Media, LLC 2012

Common to the majority of existing studies is a focus on the difference in expression of individual cytokines, hormones, and neurotransmitters. Even though the nervous, endocrine, and immune systems are highly integrated their biomarkers continue to be analyzed individually leaving patterns of coordinated response largely unexplored. In addition, investigations have focused on immune status in patients at rest and have not sought to actively probe the immune response. Used recently to investigate CFS (16), exercise can be used to elicit a coordinated "fight or flight" response in the nervous, endocrine and immune systems. We chose a similar standardized exercise challenge to amplify immune and neuroendocrine response in GWI patients (9–11, see Notes 1–3). In an initial analysis of the data we found that the patterns of association linking immune and endocrine biomarkers differed very significantly in GWI patients. Under effort a characteristic remodeling of the association network occurred around nodes for CD19+ B cell abundance, IL-5 and IL-6 responsiveness in culture as well as soluble CD26 (11). Further analysis indicated that initial IL-1a concentration and CD2+/CD26+ cell abundance strongly influenced the course of this remodeling.

Though key in gaining new insight into the basic disease mechanisms of GWI, this type of analysis requires at least 15–30 samples to support the mathematical assembly of association networks in each illness group. Therefore with current technology such an approach is impractical for use as a clinical assay for the diagnosis of individual patients. Even though the association patterns linking immune biomarkers differ from one illness group to the next, we ask the inverse question in this work in order to reduce the sample burden. Namely, is there a subset of associations shared somewhat consistently by all subjects that might be preserved to a different extent in GWI, vs. CFS and healthy controls? This question requires much less data to answer making this yardstick a more plausible tool to deploy in clinic. Constructing a multivariate statistical model to capture patterns of change shared by various cytokines, cortisol and neuropeptide Y (NPY) across the entire time course we show that such patterns can indeed serve in distinguishing GWI subjects from controls. More importantly, we formally test the predictive performance of this approach using a separate validation set where we show that cytokine patterns identified in the training set also distinguish new GWI subjects from patients with CFS, an illness with significant overlap in clinical presentation.

2. Materials

The use of multivariate statistical models in defining molecular phenotypes for complex illness is the principal focus of this chapter. The foundation for conducting such an analysis is a dataset consisting of a large number of candidate biomarkers. In general these biomarkers are substantially cross-correlated or partially redundant. They will have been measured in samples collected from an appropriately recruited cohort of subjects (Subheading 2.1) assigned to clinically relevant diagnostic groups using standard assessment tools (Subheading 2.2). Typically samples of blood, saliva, or other fluids will have been collected and analyzed using industry standard assays (Subheading 2.3).

2.1. A Standardized Case Definition and Psychometric Tools

In this example, subject inclusion criteria was derived from Fukuda et al. (17), and consisted in identifying veterans deployed to the theater of operations between August 8, 1990 and July 31, 1991, with one or more symptoms present after 6 months from at least two of the following: fatigue; mood and cognitive complaints; and musculoskeletal complaints (joint pain, stiffness or muscle pain). The suitability of the Fukuda definition for identifying GWI patients is supported by the work of Collins et al. (18).

In support of the case definition psychometric questionnaires used to assess illness severity included the Multidimensional Fatigue Inventory (MFI) (19), a 20-item self-report instrument designed to measure fatigue, and the Medical Outcomes Study 36-item short-form survey (SF-36) (20) assessing health-related quality of life. Typically all subjects also receive a physical examination and provided a medical history including the GWI symptom checklist as per the case definition.

2.2. Instruments for Assessment of Exercise Response

Considering the response to a physiological challenge can enhance the expression of candidate biomarkers. In this case a Graded eXercise Test (GXT) was administered using a Vmax Spectra 29c Cardiopulmonary Exercise Testing Instrument, Sensor-Medics Ergoline 800 fully automated cycle ergometer, and SensorMedics Marquette MAX 1 Sress ECG (SensorMedics Corp., Yorba Linda, CA).

2.3. Standard Assays for Measuring Immune Markers in Blood

The data used here to illustrate the identification of biomarkers coexpression patterns is based on measurements of immune cell signaling. Peripheral blood mononuclear cells (PBMCs) were recovered from heparinized samples of whole blood and cultured for 48 h with phytohemaglutinin at 37 °C, 5% CO_2. Following incubation, culture supernatants were collected and frozen at −70 °C until analyzed for concentrations of IL-1α, IL-5, IL-6, IL-10, TNFα, and IFNγ. Levels of IL-6, IL-10, and TNFα were also determined in plasma samples that were separated with 2 h, stored at −70 °C and not thawed prior to analysis. In all cases measurement was performed using commercial ELISA kits (Immunotech, Miami, FL), quality-controlled using National Institute for Biological Standards and Control/World Health Organization cytokine reference standards. Plasma sCD26 was also measured by ELISA (Bender Med Systems, Burlingame, CA) and NPY was measured using a RIA from Alpco Diagnostics (Salem, NH). Salivary cortisol was determined by immunoassay using the Salimetrics high sensitivity kit (State College, PA). This measure has been shown to correlate well with cortisol in blood during exercise (21).

2.4. Computational Tools

2.4.1. Standard Hypothesis Tests

Differences in the expression of individual markers were assessed using the nonparametric Wilcoxon rank sum test and the significance of first-order trends was based on the Friedman test for repeated measures. A parametric two-way ANOVA was also used to test for the significance of group and time effects as well as the time-group interaction effect. Statistical significance was set at $p<0.05$. All hypothesis testing was performed using the MatLab Statistics Toolbox (MathWorks, Natick, MA).

2.4.2. Multivariate Regression Analysis

In this example we used a projection to latent structures technique (22, 23), also called partial least squares (PLS), to identify patterns of cytokine coexpression that could classify GWI subjects. This method enables the construction of A composite features each consisting of different weighted sums of the original variables. Like the basic model for principal component analysis (PCA) these A features are computed for the input space X (Eq. 1) described by k markers measured in n subjects. However in PLS composite features are also computed simultaneously for an output space Y (Eq. 2) described by m response markers measured in the same n subjects. These composite features are defined by the loading parameters P and C (Eqs. 1 and 2) that describe the contribution of each variable to each feature. These loading parameters are then adjusted iteratively by exchanging information between the new feature spaces T and U with residual error H using the inner relation in Eq. 3. This is done to maximize correspondence of the input features with the features summarizing the responses. The objective is to identify a set of features that best capture the variability in the input marker space X by controlling for residual error E while also maximizing their relevance to the response variables Y by minimizing residual error F. The NIPALS algorithm (nonlinear iterative partial least squares) (24) was used to solve for the optimal set of parameter values in Eqs. 1, 2, and 3 presented here in standard matrix form i.e., subscript being row dimension, superscript being column dimension. Importantly these features are computed with the constraint that they be mutually orthogonal or statistically uncorrelated. This basic property supports the estimation of unbiased parameter estimates with minimal error and the decomposition of output variability into fractions directly assignable to each model component.

$$ {}_n[X]^k = {}_n[T]^A {}_A[P']^k + {}_n[E]^k \quad (1) $$

$$_n[Y]^m =_n [U]^A{}_A[C']^m +_n [F]^m \tag{2}$$

$$_n[U]^A =_n [T]^A +_n [H]^A \tag{3}$$

Here the objective of the analysis is to assign a subject to either the GWI or the healthy control group on the basis of their profile in 12 markers of neuroendocrine and immune function. This requires a variant of PLS called PLS discriminant analysis (PLS-DA) (25) where a dummy outcome variable Y is created that describes membership to diagnostic class. In this case two such binary variables were created assigning membership y_{ik} of each subject i to the control group $k=1$ and the GWI group $k=2$ respectively with $y_{ik} \in [0,1]$. Each feature $a \leq A$ is expressed as a linear combination of the original cytokine, hormone and neurotransmitter concentrations x_k each weighted by a loading coefficient p_{ka}.

Uncertainty in the estimation of the feature weights expressed in terms of their standard error was computed using leave-one-out cross validation (26, 27) where the model is repeatedly estimated with each subject omitted in turn. These multiple cross-validation models provide populations of parameter estimates from which significance may be estimated. For example the significance of the difference between a feature score for two individual subjects was based on the dispersion of score values obtained during cross-validation for each subject.

All multivariate methods such as PCA, PLS, and partial least squares discriminant analysis (PLS-DA) calculations were conducted with the SimcaP software (Umetrics, Kinnelon, NJ).

2.4.3. Statistical Tools for Assessing the Diagnostic Performance

Classification performance statistics and receiver operating characteristic (ROC) curves were calculated using functions found in the SPSS Statistics software package (IBM, Armonk, NY) and the MatLab Statistics Toolbox software (MathWorks, Natick, MA).

3. Methods

The analysis that is the focus of this chapter is best described by working through the following example involving the recruitment and assessment of a suitable subject group (Subheading 3.1), the measurement of a relevant physiological response (Subheading 3.2), the collection and analysis of biological samples (Subheading 3.3), and finally the identification and assessment of diagnostic markers (Subheading 3.4, also see Notes 4–6).

Application of the above-mentioned tools, protocols, and assays resulted in the creation of a dataset consisting of 58 human subjects distributed across 3 diagnostic groups and both genders. In the data subset of interest each subject was described by 12 markers of neuroendocrine and immune function assessed in blood collected at three points in time during a standard exercise challenge.

3.1. Recruitment of a Study Cohort

In this example, a first subset of 10 GWI and 11 control subjects described previously (9) were recruited from the Miami Veterans Administration Medical Center and studied. Subjects were male and ranged in age between 30 and 55. Subjects were in good health prior to 1990, and had no current exclusionary diagnoses that could reasonably explain the symptoms and their severity. Subjects taking medications that may impact immune function were excluded (e.g., steroids, immunosuppressive agents). Control subjects consisted of Gulf War era sedentary veterans and were matched to GWI subjects by age, gender, body mass index (BMI) and ethnicity. Controls were also selected and matched to patients on the basis of their general fitness level, estimated a priori from their history of activity and confirmed during exercise challenge. Consistent with these criteria and specific to this analysis a second group was subsequently recruited consisting of an additional 16 male and 10 female GWI subjects as well as 9 male CFS subjects and 2 new male control subjects. This new group of subjects was used as a separate validation set in this example.

3.2. Applying Standard Exercise Challenge

The McArdle protocol (28) for graded exercise was used to elicit an immune-endocrine response. Subjects pedal at an initial output of 60 W for 2 min, followed by an increase of 30 W every 2 min until the subject reaches: (1) a plateau in maximal oxygen consumption (VO2); (2) a respiratory exchange ratio above 1.15; or (3) the subject stops the test.

3.3. Sample Collection and Analysis

Prior to the exercise challenge a first blood draw was conducted after subjects sat quietly for 30 min. Second and third blood draws were conducted upon reaching peak effort (VO2 max) and at 4-h post exercise, respectively. At each blood draw, five 8-mL tubes of blood were collected in CPT vacutainers (B-D-Biosciences, San Jose, CA). Importantly, diurnal variations in this and other indicators were controlled by conducting assessments at the same time of day for all subjects. Blood samples were processed and markers recorded as described in Subheading 2.3.

3.4. Numerical Analysis

3.4.1. Assessing Changes in the Expression of Individual Biomarkers

1. Calculate the change in median expression of each cytokine occurring between the GWI and the healthy control subjects and test for significance. A standard Mann–Whitney nonparametric test can be used for this purpose and applied at each time point separately.

   Although results presented in Table 1 suggest a general over-expression of cytokines in the GWI group only a subset of these achieved statistical significance. In particular we observed

Table 1
Changes in the expression of signaling molecules in GWI

Signal molecule	GWI(t0) -Ctrl(t0)	GWI(t1) -Ctrl(t1)	GWI(t2) -Ctrl(t2)
Saliva			
Cortisol	0.13 (0.15)	-0.04 (0.49)	0.07 (0.06)
PHA-stimulated Blood Culture			
IL-1α	-3.40 (0.66)	9.00 (0.95)	3.00 (0.68)
IL-5	81.00 (0.00)	30.00 (0.00)	41.50 (0.00)
IL-6	-111.00 (0.38)	1185.50 (0.10)	2398.50 (0.19)
IL-10	-19.00 (0.96)	-177.50 (0.42)	269.50 (1.00)
TNFα	206.50 (0.05)	53.00 (0.68)	167.50 (0.10)
INFγ	100.00 (0.07)	170.70 (0.02)	158.20 (0.02)
Plasma			
IL-6	10.75 (0.01)	11.85 (0.03)	9.50 (0.02)
IL-10	-1.80 (0.27)	-3.10 (0.50)	-1.65 (0.43)
TNFα	2.00 (0.49)	-1.30 (0.95)	1.75 (0.21)
sCD26	-85.50 (0.11)	-12.00 (0.81)	14.50 (0.86)
NPY	-5.03 (0.65)	3.95 (0.55)	11.69 (0.97)
Composite Features			
Level 1 Feature 1	0.39 (0.01)	0.62 (0.01)	0.46 (0.00)
Level 1 Feature 2	-0.01 (0.81)	0.06 (0.86)	-0.31 (0.38)

Difference in median expression values (significance p-value, Mann–Whitney) between GWI and healthy controls (Ctrl) prior to exercise ($t0$), at peak effort ($t1$) and 4-h post-exercise ($t2$). PHA-stimulated ex vivo culture cytokines are reported as pg/10^5 lymphocyte cells. All signals measured in plasma are expressed in pg/mL. Salivary cortisol is reported in μg/dL

significantly higher response to PHA stimulation in GWI subjects for IL-5 at all 3 sample times ($p \leq 0.001$) and in IFNγ with challenge ($p = 0.02$, 0.02). Marginally higher TNF-α responsiveness was also observed ($p = 0.05$) in PHA-stimulated culture but only at rest ($t0$). This was accompanied by significantly higher concentrations of IL-6 in plasma ($p \leq 0.03$) both prior to and throughout the challenge. Interestingly, no significant differences were observed in salivary cortisol, NPY, and in ex vivo-stimulated culture for IL-1, IL-6, and sCD26. The same applies to IL-10 measured both in culture and in plasma.

2. Evaluate significance of trends in the expression of each marker across time. The nonparametric Friedman test for repeated measures and the standard 2-way ANOVA were used for this purpose.

In this example the majority of significant trends were found in the response of healthy control subjects. A systematic progression across time was found for IL-1α ($p = 0.01$) and IL-5 ($p = 0.05$) in

PHA-stimulated culture for healthy controls as well as in the expression of IL-10 in culture ($p=0.04$) and in plasma ($p=0.05$). Similar exercise-induced changes in NPY ($p \leq 0.001$) were also observed. In comparison GWI subjects as a group displayed a lower responsiveness to exercise. Only IL-5 concentrations in PHA-stimulated culture showed any significant trend ($p=0.03$) in GWI and produced a significant group × time interaction effect based on a parametric two-way ANOVA. Though trends in both salivary cortisol ($p=0.06$ controls; 0.15 GWI) and TNF-α ($p=0.10$ controls; 0.08 GWI) failed significance under the Friedman test, results from the two-way ANOVA showed a significant interaction of diagnostic group with time for these markers ($p=0.04$, 0.01).

3.4.2. Isolating Patterns of Biomarker Coexpression

The nervous, immune, and endocrine systems are generally recognized as being highly integrated regulatory networks. As a result, even though there were relatively few differences in the absolute expression of individual markers, there may still be coregulatory imbalances. Because the basic PLS algorithm described in Subheading 2.4.2 can be applied to all data points independently of sample time the dynamics of the immune response are not captured. To address this we applied a two-step analysis commonly referred to as 3-way PLS or batch-PLS (29, 30). This model is described in Fig. 1.

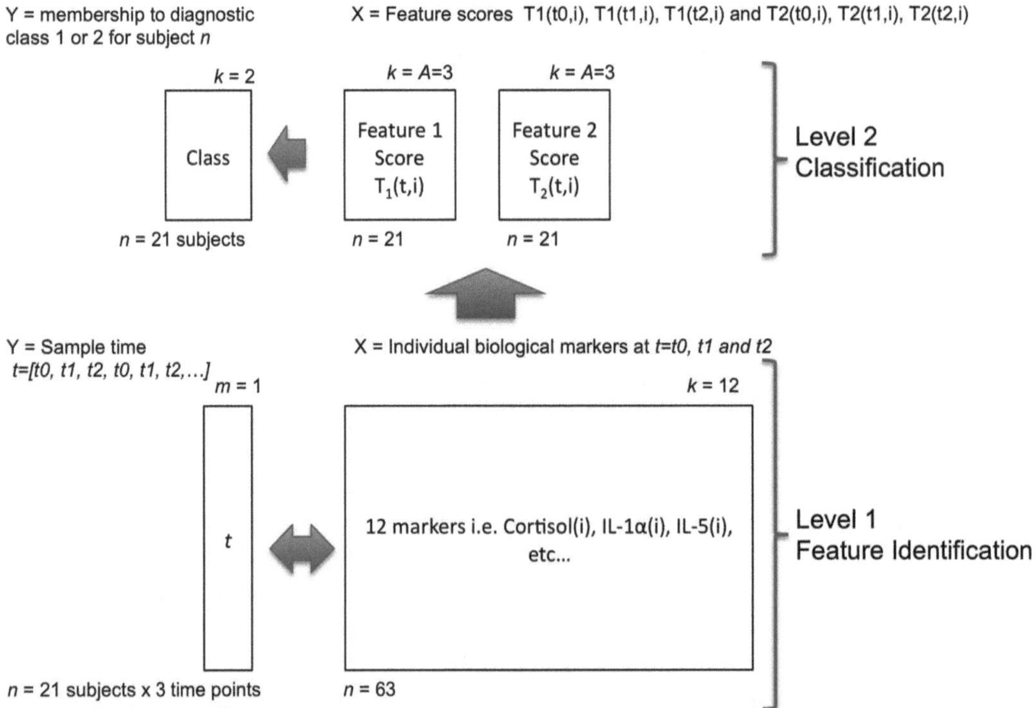

Fig. 1. PLS-DA classification model structure. Diagram of the input and output relationships defined at each level of the PLS model for classification of subjects to the GWI or healthy control class.

1. First PLS was applied to all measurements across all individual markers using sample time t as a response Y in level 1 of the model (steps 1 and 2). This was done to enforce the sequence of values when identifying the features that best described the patterns of coexpression linking the 12 markers (X in level 1). In a preprocessing step all regressor variables in the X block were log transformed. Each log-transformed variable was then scaled by dividing with the corresponding standard deviation computed about zero instead of the mean. The response variable Y describing the progression of each batch or exercise challenge was not transformed nor was it centered. To capture the unequal spacing in time of the three observations made during each trial we used an approximate time vector of $[t0, t1, t2] = [0, 30, 270]$ in minutes. In addition, the training set used here contains roughly 8% missing array elements. Missing data was handled implicitly by the NIPALS algorithm using an extension to the original computation proposed by Christoffersson (31) that consists essentially in iteratively substituting missing values with their model predictions. This approximate method performs well with up to 10–20% missing data and has been implemented in the Simca software package mainly because of its rapid and robust convergence properties. A comparison with alternate approaches more suitable for higher fractions of missing data may be found in Grung and Manne (32).

   In the current example each sample is described by 12 biomarkers, 6 of which were measured in culture, 5 in plasma and one in saliva. This level 1 analysis produced a base model supported by 2 significant features that captured approximately 89% of the total variability ($R_x^2 = 0.89$) in the data (Table 2).

Table 2
PLS model fit and structure

Model	Component a	R^2_X	R^2_X(cum)	Eigenvalues	R^2_Y	R^2_Y(cum)	Q^2	Q^2(cum)
Level 1 Model								
Observations (N)=69	1	0.83	0.83	9.91	0.40	0.40	0.40	0.40
K=12 Biomarkers vs Time	2	0.07	0.89	0.81	0.06	0.46	0.04	0.42
Level 2 Model								
Observations (N)=21	1	0.53	0.53	3.19	0.38	0.38	0.33	0.33
2 Level-1 features at 3 times (K=6)	2	0.32	0.85	1.93	0.09	0.46	0.04	0.36

R^2_x and R^2_y are Pearson correlation coefficients or total sum of squared regression (SSR) captured by the partial least squares (PLS) model for the regressor X (molecular signals) and predicted variable Y (diagnostic class) spaces respectively. The value $Q^2 = 1\text{-PRESS/SST}$ expresses overall model performance in terms of reduction in the predicted residual sum of squared errors (PRESS) in leave-one-out cross validation

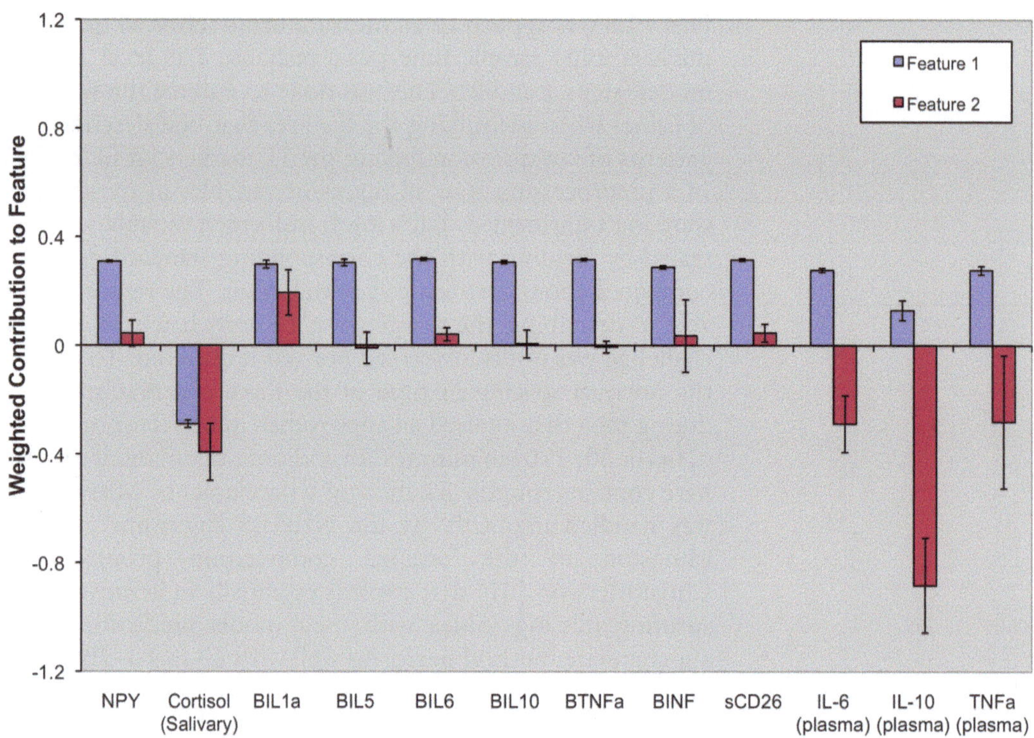

Fig. 2. Structure of composite features. The relative contribution p_{ka} of each biomarker k to each of the two level-1 model features ($a = 1, 2$) that optimally separate the subjects into their respective diagnostic groups. The first feature captures a broad-spectrum disturbance across all biomarkers. The second feature captures a pattern of co-expression whereby increases in IL-1a are offset by a corresponding increase in cortisol, IL-6, and IL-10. *Whiskers* represent the standard error in estimation for each weight p_{ka}. All level-1 feature 1 weights are significant at $p \leq 0.001$. Only the feature 2 weights for cortisol ($p \leq 0.001$), IL-1a ($p = 0.024$), IL-6 ($p = 0.008$) and IL-10 ($p \leq 0.001$) were significant at $p < 0.05$.

The contribution of each biomarker to these features is shown in Fig. 2. Accounting for 82% of the variability, the first feature described a broad-spectrum response to exercise. Expression of NPY and cytokines measured in plasma as well as in ex vivo culture all correlated positively with one another and negatively with salivary cortisol. Accounting for 7% of the overall variability, a second pattern was defined by the coexpression of salivary cortisol, IL-6, and IL-10 in plasma and an opposite IL-1α response in culture.

2. Features identified in step 1 are then used to define a new input array for level 2 of the analysis. At level 2 the input variables to the classification model were the scores $T_a(t,i)$ in each feature a evaluated for each subject i at each time point t in step 1 of the analysis namely $T_1(t0,i)$, $T_1(t1,i)$, $T_1(t2,i)$, $T_2(t0,i)$, $T_2(t1,i)$, $T_2(t2,i)$. These feature scores were not transformed and were scaled to unit variance before estimation of the level-2 model. PLS-DA was then applied (see Subheading 2.4.2) to manage the temporal relationships linking feature scores at each sample

point in this new level-2 feature space. Because PLS-DA carries information about the diagnostic classes, the time course features extracted in level 2 are those that provide optimal discrimination of GWI patients from the control subjects.

This second step produces a set of level-2 features each consisting of weighted sums in $T_1(t0,i)$, $T_1(t1,i)$, $T_1(t2,i)$, $T_2(t0,i)$, $T_2(t1,i)$, $T_2(t2,i)$. In this way the full time course in each coexpression pattern (T_1 and T_2) identified in level 1 is captured for each subject. Moreover by weighting individual elements of the time course it is possible to emphasize or diminish the contribution of a level-1 score at specific phases of the challenge. Scores produced at level 2 of the analysis now summarize for each subject the complete progression across all time points for all 12 markers. The position of a subject's profile in this new level-2 feature space is then used by the PLS-DA model to predict a degree of membership to the GWI illness class.

In this example two level-2 features were identified, each summarizing almost exclusively the corresponding time course from the first level of the model. The progression in time of all 12 markers for each subject may now be expressed in terms of only two level-2 scores (Fig. 3). Together they summarized roughly 85% of the variation across time of both level-1 features (Table 2). They also captured close to half of the total variability in diagnostic class membership ($R_y^2 = 0.46$) even though a relatively narrow assessment of immune function was used. Leave-one-out cross-validation indicated that this model was also reasonably robust in predicting diagnostic class for data excluded from model fitting ($Q^2 = 0.36$). Close to 40% of variability in class membership was accounted for by broad-spectrum changes across time (feature 1). Another 9% was captured by the progression in feature 2. Interestingly this sequential set of scores contributed positively to the classification model's performance ($Q^2 = 0.04$) even though no statistically significant separation of individual median values was found for feature 2. This underscores the fact that feature 2 as computed in the PLS regression model adds important detail to feature 1 and should be used in conjunction with the latter.

3. Using model cross validation as an estimate of variability in individual time course profiles we can now compare one subject to another on the basis of changes in level-1 patterns across time.

To illustrate this we compared the progression of level-1 feature scores in a case-matched (age, BMI and % of predicted maximum VO2) pair of GWI patients and healthy controls: CS201 and PC 105 (Fig. 4a, b). While these subjects separate on the basis of feature 1 alone, controlling for other sources of variability by comparing a matched pair now reveals significant differences in feature

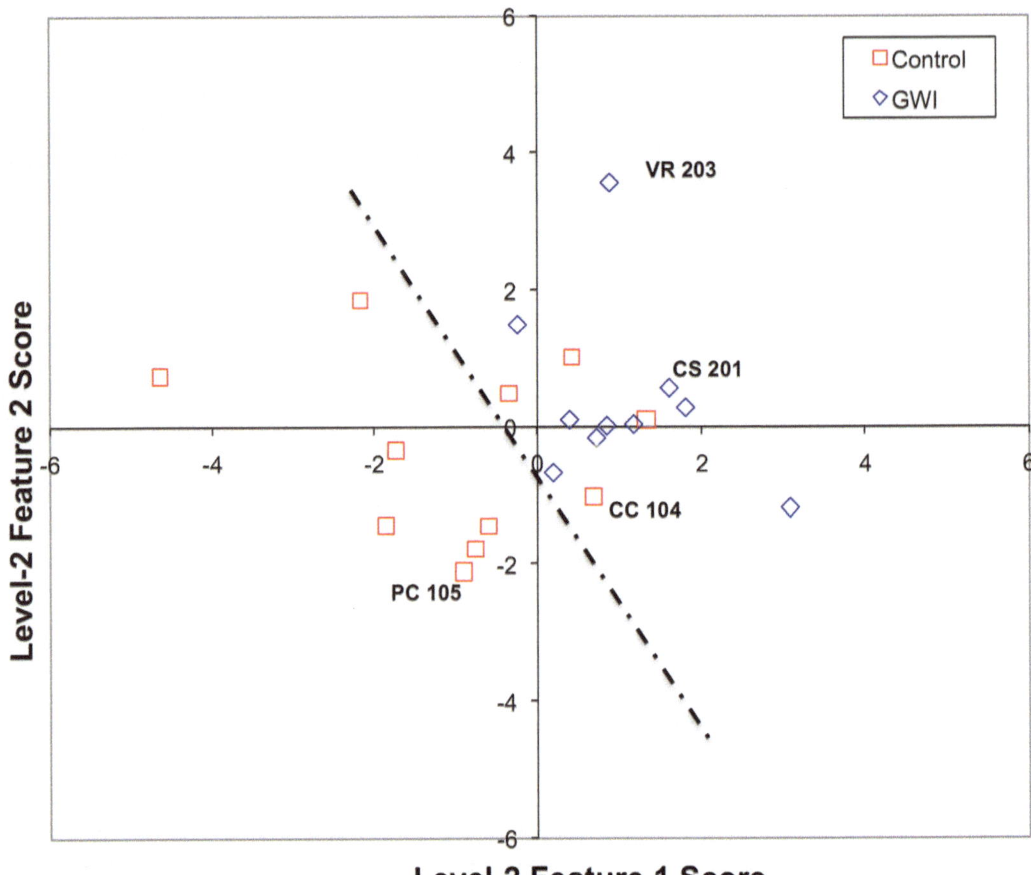

Fig. 3. Separation of subjects in feature space. Distribution of GWI and control subjects in a feature space defined by the co-expression of 12 biomarkers of neuroendocrine-immune status. Each axis is defined by a specific linear combination of biomarkers and the evolution in these patterns over the course of a graded exercise challenge. Each point captures the entire time course recorded for that subject. In this feature space 4 of 11 control subjects appear to group with the 10 GWI subjects.

2 especially at peak effort ($t1$) ($p = 0.05$). Examination of the level-2 classification model revealed that the contribution of feature 2 scores at time $t1$ were weighted an order of magnitude higher (0.180 $t1$) than those at time $t0$ and $t2$ (0.016 $t0$, 0.017 $t2$). In fact only at $t1$ were feature 2 scores weighted similarly to those for feature 1 (0.278 $t0$, 0.227 $t1$, 0.299 $t2$).

The important detail added by feature 2 can also be visualized further by comparing two individuals who share very similar feature 1 scores: GWI subject VR 203 and control subject CC 104. Though these individuals share a very similar broad-spectrum baseline immune activation (feature 1), they differ dramatically in their expression of feature 2 scores across time (Fig. 4c, d). Both these examples and the structure of the classification model suggest that differences in feature 2 score, in particular at peak effort, may be of

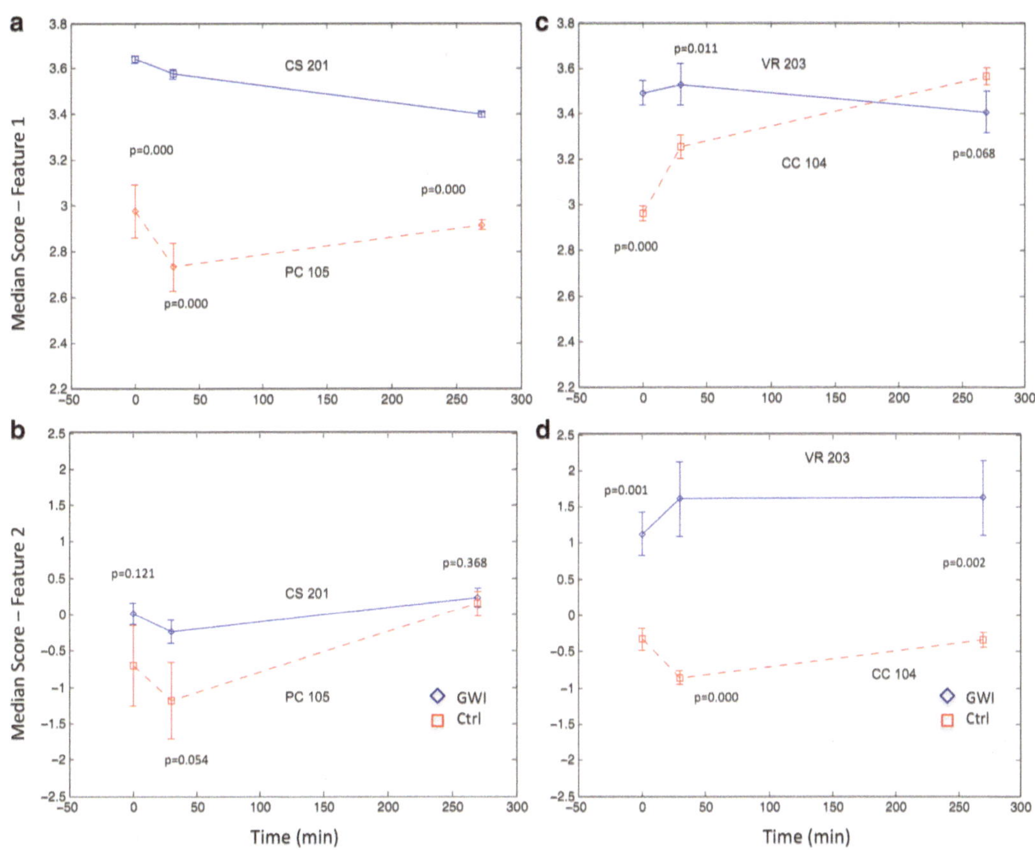

Fig. 4. Evolution of feature scores in time for matched pairs. Median expression of level-1 feature 1 (**a**) and feature 2 (**b**) prior to exercise (*t0*), at peak effort (*t1*) and 4-h post-exercise (*t2*) are shown in (**a**, **b**) for GWI subject CS 201 (*blue diamonds*) and case matched control subject PC 105 (*red squares*). (**c**, **d**) Shows data for GWI subject VR 203 (*blue diamonds*) and control subject CC 104 (*red squares*). Error bars display the median absolute deviation from median as computed from repeated cross-validation for these observations. In (**a**, **b**) time and illness effects can be seen in both level-1 feature 1 and feature 2. Significant deviations at peak effort in feature 2 illustrate why this time point is highly weighted in the level-2 model. In (**c**, **d**) we observe significant time effects in level-1 feature 1 and while illness results in a persistent offset in the expression of feature 2.

specific diagnostic value and that this contribution may be obscured by high within group dispersion. Interestingly feature 2 scores summarized at level 2 of the model correlated significantly with differences in physical fatigue ($p<0.01$) and to a lesser extent general fatigue ($p=0.06$) among GWI subjects but not in control subjects ($p=0.38$, 0.11 respectively). No significant correlation with either physical or general fatigue was found in GWI for feature 1 ($p=0.27$, 0.85). In contrast while these were borderline significant in healthy controls ($p=0.05$, 0.05). This would suggest that feature 2 might serve as an indicator of relative illness severity in GWI.

3.4.3. Exercise Response as a Basis for Classification

To assess classifier performance the continuous scale for class membership can be transformed to a discrete class assignment by

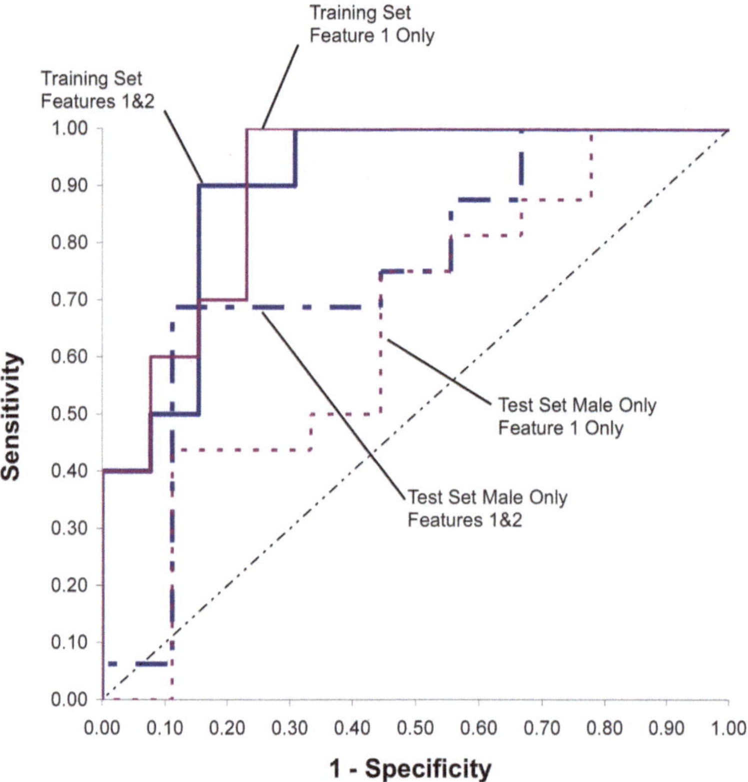

Fig. 5. Linear classifier performance. Receiver-operator characteristic (ROC) curves for a linear discriminant model constructed from cytokine, NPY and cortisol co-expression in 10 GWI and 11 male control subjects. Sensitivity and specificity of classification obtained at various membership threshold values is presented for the original training set as well as for a validation test set consisting of 9 male CFS patients as well as 16 new GWI and 2 new male control cases.

applying a membership threshold. Detection sensitivity and assignment specificity values can then be computed using these binary assignments. This is repeated over a range of threshold values to produce a receiver-operator characteristic (ROC) curve (33).

1. In this example separate receiver-operator characteristic (ROC) curves were computed for classification using the broad-spectrum disturbance alone (feature 1) as well as classification including the inflammatory imbalance pattern (feature 2) (Fig. 5, Table 3). Both classifiers performed similarly on the training set of 10 male GWI and 11 male healthy control subjects each producing an area under the curve (AUC) significantly better than random assignment ($p=0.001$ Table 3). Nonetheless, at 85% specificity the use of both features delivers a sensitivity of 90% rather than 70% possible with one feature alone.
2. Performance differences became very noticeable when these models were applied to a test set. Our first validation set

Table 3
Receiver-operator characteristics (ROC) for PLS-DA classifiers

Model	Data set	Positive:Negative	Area under curve	Std. Error(a)	Asymptotic Sig.(b)	Asymptotic 95% Conf. Int. Upper Bound	Lower Bound
Feature 1 Only	Training set	10 : 11 ctrl	0.900	0.064	*0.001*	0.774	1.026
Feature 1 and 2	Training set	10 : 11 ctrl	0.900	0.065	*0.001*	0.772	1.028
Feature 1 Only	Test set (male only)	16 : 9 CFS, 2 ctrl	0.646	0.122	0.234	0.407	0.885
Feature 1 and 2	Test set (male only)	16 : 9 CFS, 2 ctrl	0.750	0.110	*0.042*	0.534	0.966
Feature 1 Only	Test set (male and female)	26 (incl. 10 female): 9 CFS, 2 ctrl	0.615	0.117	0.308	0.387	0.844
Feature 1 and 2	Test set (male and female)	26 (incl. 10 female): 9 CFS, 2 ctrl	0.679	0.113	0.113	0.458	0.901

Detailed statistics for receiver-operator curves (ROC) describing the sensitivity as a function of 1-specificity obtained in classification models based on partial least squares discriminant analysis (PLS-DA). These include the area under the curve (AUC) with the associated standard error of estimation, the corresponding significance p-value as well as the upper and lower confidence limits at the 0.05 significance level. Statistics are reported for classification in the training set, a male only test set and a mixed gender seta. Under the nonparametric assumption

[a] Under the nonparametric assumption

[b] Null hypothesis: true area = 0.5

consisted of 16 new male GWI subjects, 9 male CFS controls, and 2 new male healthy controls. The corresponding ROC curves for the 1- and 2-feature classifiers are shown in Fig. 5. When tested on these new male subjects, classification using only the first feature does not differ significantly from a random assignment ($p = 0.23$ AUC). Inclusion of the second feature delivered a significant increase in AUC ($p = 0.04$ Table 3) with 90% specificity available at 70% sensitivity. Recall that the training set contained only male GWI and control subjects. To test the impact of gender we constructed a second validation set by adding ten female GWI cases to the first set. Classification performance decreased drastically. Neither model performed better than random assignment although two features were still preferable ($p = 0.11$) to one ($p = 0.31$) (Table 3).

3. We intentionally included CFS subjects in the validation set as a disease control group since CFS is clinically similar to GWI. Using the ROC analysis performed on the training set we

choose a predicted membership threshold of 0.35 above which we assigned a given case to the GWI group. This corresponded in the training set to a sensitivity of 100% and a specificity of 70% or the correct assignment of 7 of 11 healthy controls and all 10 GWI subjects. Among the GWI test cases, we found correct assignment of 11 out of 16 male cases but only 3 of 10 female cases. With regard to the CFS control subjects, only two of nine subjects were classified as GWI with the other seven classified correctly as non-GWI. Recall that no CFS controls were used to train this classifier. Therefore these patterns of immune marker coexpression appear reasonably specific to GWI in male patients even when presented with clinically similar CFS subjects.

4. Notes

1. In recent work (11) we demonstrated that while the expression of individual immune and endocrine markers provides some diagnostic information in the study of GWI, the patterns through which these markers coordinate their expression offer significant new insight into this illness. Indeed while relatively few individual markers changed significantly in expression, the coexpression network linking these markers underwent widespread changes in organization and structure in GWI.
2. While structural changes in the patterns of biomarker coexpression offer a highly discriminatory fingerprint the sample burden required for identifying these changes in individual patients is substantial and an alternative method must be considered if molecular phenotyping is to be deployed clinically. Here we have attempted to identify a subset of immune marker associations that are preserved across all subjects but might be expressed to a different extent and perhaps in a different direction in GWI patients. We have also focused on linear interactions to make the problem even more tractable.
3. The analysis presented here identified two such shared patterns linking 12 immune mediators measured in blood and saliva. The majority of GWI subjects separated from healthy controls on the basis of a common trend whereby a higher than expected expression of most immune markers coincided with a lower than expected concentration of salivary cortisol (feature 1). As reported previously (11) this broad-spectrum response included the joint over-expression of individual inflammatory markers, Th1 and Th2 cytokines namely IL-6 in plasma as well as IL-5, TNF-α, and INF-γ in PHA-stimulated culture. Recent evidence suggests that sensitization with a

foreign antigen mimicking self can induce a similar mixed Th2/Th1 cytokine profile (34). Human proteins with structural similarity to exogenous allergens can cross-react with allergen-specific IgE antibodies, inducing sustained inflammation and lymphocyte proliferation (35–38). Among these Hom s 2 (37) and Hom s 4 (36) are known to induce IgE reactivity as well as a strong IFN-γ response.

4. While an offset in baseline immune status (feature 1) was sufficient to identify most GWI subjects, a subset of these could not be distinguished on this basis alone. This subset supported the identification of a second coexpression pattern (feature 2). This pattern suggests that GWI subjects might differ from controls in their acute-phase regulation of cortisol, IL-6, IL-10, and possibly TNFα. This was accompanied by an altered lymphocyte IL-1α responsiveness to PHA stimulation, a cytokine associated with "sickness behavior" (39). Because of the high degree of heterogeneity in this preliminary cohort, differences in this second coexpression pattern achieved significance only in case-matched GWI and control subjects. This was especially true at peak effort where the contribution of feature 2 was significantly weighted.

5. Though subtle, small changes in feature 2 were nonetheless instrumental in maintaining high specificity and sensitivity in the classification of new test subjects with GWI as well as subjects suffering from CFS (90% specificity and 70% sensitivity). Interestingly this signature involves important myokines, metabolically active cytokines, such as IL-6 and TNF-α with key roles in energy metabolism. IL-6 has been called a true "exercise factor" as levels of this cytokine increase exponentially up to 100-fold during exercise (40). This is generally followed by a compensatory expression of the anti-inflammatory cytokine IL-10 and cortisol. The release of cortisol is also mediated in part by IL-6 via feedback to the HPA axis (41). Independent of this, IL-6 is known to activate one of the principal regulators of cellular energy status: the AMP-activated protein kinase (AMPK) pathway. IL-6 has also been recently reported to have an insulin-sensitizing effect (42–44). Conversely increases in TNFα promote insulin resistance (45) and expression of this cytokine is inhibited by IL-6 (46). Availability of metabolic energy stores therefore relies at least in part on a balance of these hormones and cytokines.

   In this respect it was interesting to note that subjects with CFS, another fatiguing illness, did not manifest this pattern of cytokine coexpression to the same extent as GWI subjects. Indeed only 2 of the 9 CFS controls were assigned to the GWI group by the classification model. Consequently even though metabolic repercussions may be similar, the basic mechanisms driving neuroendocrine-immune dysfunction might be quite different in GWI and these illnesses may constitute very distinct regulatory regimes (47).

6. Though our results appear to extrapolate well to new subjects in a separate validation cohort the overall number of subjects examined remains relatively small. Therefore we suggest this analysis be considered preliminary even though the group size is consistent with that used recently in related studies (4, 5). In addition the panel of cytokines used was relatively narrow and by no means constituted a complete survey of the immune response. In recognition of this a simple linear classification model was chosen as a more conservative approach to guard against over-fitting the data.

Acknowledgements

This work was supported by grants from the NIAAA: R21AA016635 (PI MA Fletcher); NIAID: R01AI065723 (PI MA Fletcher); CFIDS Assoc. of America (2): (PI N Klimas, PI G Broderick); NIAID: UO1 AI459940 (PI N Klimas); NIAMSD R01 AR057853-01A1 (PI N Klimas); VA merit awards (PI N Klimas); Dynamic Modeling in GWI,CFS/ME; GW080152 (PI N Klimas), and the University of Alberta (PI G Broderick).

References

1. Kang HK, Natelson BH, Mahan CM et al (2003) Post-traumatic stress disorder and chronic fatigue syndrome-like illness among Gulf War veterans: a population-based survey of 30,000 veterans. Am J Epidemiol 157: 141–148
2. Unwin C, Blatchley N, Coker W et al (1999) Health of UK servicemen who served in Persian Gulf War. Lancet 353:169–178
3. Crofford LJ, Young EA, Engleberg NC et al (2004) Basal circadian and pulsatile ACTH and cortisol secretion in patients with fibromyalgia and/or chronic fatigue syndrome. Brain Behav Immun 18:314–325
4. Golier JA, Schmeidler J, Legge J et al (2006) Enhanced cortisol suppression to dexamethasone associated with Gulf War deployment. Psychoneuroendocrinology 31(10): 1181–1189
5. Golier JA, Schmeidler J, Legge J et al (2007) Twenty-four hour plasma cortisol and adrenocorticotropic hormone in Gulf War veterans: relationships to posttraumatic stress disorder and health symptoms. Biol Psychiatry 62(10): 1175–1178
6. Maher K, Klimas NG, Fletcher MA (2003) Immunology. In: Jason LA, Fennell PA, Taylor RR (eds) Handbook of chronic fatigue syndrome. Wiley, Hoboken, pp 124–151
7. Vojdani A, Thrasher JD (2004) Cellular and humoral immune abnormalities in Gulf War veterans. Environ Health Perspect 112(8): 840–846
8. Siegel SD, Antoni MH, Fletcher MA et al (2006) Impaired natural immunity, cognitive dysfunction, and physical symptoms in patients with chronic fatigue syndrome: preliminary evidence for a subgroup? J Psychosom Res 60(6):559–566
9. Whistler T, Fletcher MA, Lonergan W et al (2009) Impaired immune function in Gulf War illness. BMC Med Genomics 2:12
10. Broderick G, Fuite J, Kreitz A et al (2010) A formal analysis of cytokine networks in chronic fatigue syndrome. Brain Behav Immun 24(7): 1209–1217

11. Broderick G, Kreitz A, Fuite J et al (2011) A pilot study of immune network remodeling under challenge in Gulf War illness. Brain Behav Immun 25(2):302–313
12. Moss RB, Mercandetti A, Vojdani A (1999) TNF-alpha and chronic fatigue syndrome. J Clin Immunol 19(5):314–316
13. Gaab J, Rohleder N, Heitz V et al (2005) Stress-induced changes in LPS-induced proinflammatory cytokine production in chronic fatigue syndrome. Psychoneuroendocrinology 30:188–198
14. Skowera A, Cleare A, Blair D et al (2004) High levels of type 2 cytokine-producing cells in chronic fatigue syndrome. Clin Exp Immunol 135(2):294–302
15. ter Wolbeek M, van Doornen LJ, Kavelaars A et al (2007) Longitudinal analysis of pro- and anti-inflammatory cytokine production in severely fatigued adolescents. Brain Behav Immun 21(8):1063–1074
16. Light AR, White AT, Hughen RW et al (2009) Moderate exercise increases expression for sensory, adrenergic, and immune genes in chronic fatigue syndrome patients but not in normal subjects. J Pain 10(10):1099–1112
17. Fukuda K, Nisenbaum R, Stewart G et al (1998) Chronic multisymptom illness affecting air force veterans of the Gulf War. JAMA 280:981–988
18. Collins JF, Donta ST, Engel CC et al (2002) The antibiotic treatment trial of Gulf War Veterans' Illnesses: issues, design, screening, and baseline characteristics. Control Clin Trials 23(3):333–353
19. Smets EM, Garssen B, Bonke B et al (1995) The multidimensional fatigue inventory (MFI) psychometric qualities of an instrument to assess fatigue. J Psychosom Res 39(3):315–325
20. Ware JE Jr, Sherbourne CD (1992) The MOS 36-item short-form health survey (SF-36). I. Conceptual framework and item selection. Med Care 30(6):473–483
21. Cadore E, Lhullier F, Brentano M et al (2008) Correlations between serum and salivary hormonal concentrations in response to resistance exercise. J Sports Sci 26(10):1067–1072
22. Wold S, Trygg J, Berglund A et al (2001) Some recent developments in PLS modeling. Chemom Intell Lab Syst 58:131–149
23. Eriksson L, Antti H, Gottfries J et al (2004) Using chemometrics for navigating in the large data sets of genomics, proteomics, and metabonomics (gpm). Anal Bioanal Chem 380(3):419–429
24. Wold S, Esbensen K, Geladi P (1987) Principal component analysis. Chemom Intell Lab Syst 2:37–52
25. Barker M, Rayens W (2003) Partial least squares for discrimination. J Chemom 17(3):166–173
26. Efron B, Gong G (1983) A leisurely look at the bootstrap, the jackknife, and cross-validation. Am Stat 37:36–48
27. Krzanowski WJ (1987) Cross-validation in principal component analysis. Biometrics 43: 575–584
28. McArdle WD, Katch FI, Katch VL (2007) Exercise physiology: energy, nutrition, and human performance. Lippincott Williams & Wilkins, London, p 954
29. Wold S, Kettaneh N, Friden H et al (1998) Modelling and diagnostics of batch processes and analogous kinetic experiments. Chemom Intell Lab Syst 44:331–340
30. Antti H, Bollard ME, Ebbels T et al (2002) Batch statistical processing of H-1 NMR-derived urinary spectral data. J Chemom 16: 461–468
31. Christoffersson A (1970) The one component model with incomplete data. Ph.D. thesis, Uppsala University
32. Grung B, Manne R (1998) Missing values in principal component analysis. Chemom Intell Lab Syst 42:125–139
33. Greiner M, Pfeiffer D, Smith RD (2000) Principles and practical application of the receiver-operating characteristic analysis for diagnostic tests. Prev Vet Med 45(1–2):23–41
34. Bünder R, Mittermann I, Herz U et al (2004) Induction of autoallergy with an environmental allergen mimicking a self protein in a murine model of experimental allergic asthma. J Allergy Clin Immunol 114(2):422–428
35. Fedorov AA, Ball T, Mahoney NM et al (1997) The molecular basis for allergen cross-reactivity: crystal structure and IgE-epitope mapping of birch pollen profilin. Structure 5(1):33–45
36. Aichberger KJ, Mittermann I, Reininger R et al (2005) Hom s 4, an IgE-reactive autoantigen belonging to a new subfamily of calcium-binding proteins, can induce Th cell type 1-mediated autoreactivity. J Immunol 175(2): 1286–1294
37. Mittermann I, Reininger R, Zimmermann M et al (2008) The IgE-reactive autoantigen Hom s 2 induces damage of respiratory epithelial cells and keratinocytes via induction of IFN-gamma. J Invest Dermatol 128(6): 1451–1459
38. Valenta R, Mittermann I, Werfel T et al (2009) Linking allergy to autoimmune disease. Trends Immunol 30(3):109–116
39. Dantzer R, O'Connor JC, Freund GG et al (2008) From inflammation to sickness and depression: when the immune system subjugates

the brain. Nat Rev Neurosci 9(1):46–56. Review

40. Pedersen BK, Akerström TC, Nielsen AR et al (2007) Role of myokines in exercise and metabolism. J Appl Physiol 103(3):1093–1098. Review
41. Steensberg A, Fischer CP, Keller C et al (2003) IL-6 enhances plasma IL-1ra, IL-10, and cortisol in humans. Am J Physiol Endocrinol Metab 285(2):E433–E437
42. Carey AL, Steinberg GR, Macaulay SL et al (2006) Interleukin-6 increases insulin-stimulated glucose disposal in humans and glucose uptake and fatty acid oxidation in vitro via AMP-activated protein kinase. Diabetes 55(10):2688–2697
43. Choy EH, Isenberg DA, Garrood T et al (2002) Therapeutic benefit of blocking interleukin-6 activity with an anti-interleukin-6 receptor monoclonal antibody in rheumatoid arthritis: a randomized, double-blind, placebo-controlled, dose-escalation trial. Arthritis Rheum 46(12):3143–3150
44. Wallenius V, Wallenius K, Ahrén B et al (2002) Interleukin-6-deficient mice develop mature-onset obesity. Nat Med 8(1):75–79
45. Plomgaard P, Bouzakri K, Krogh-Madsen R et al (2005) Tumor necrosis factor-alpha induces skeletal muscle insulin resistance in healthy human subjects via inhibition of Akt substrate 160 phosphorylation. Diabetes 54(10):2939–2945
46. Starkie R, Ostrowski SR, Jauffred S et al (2003) Exercise and IL-6 infusion inhibit endotoxin-induced TNF-alpha production in humans. FASEB J 17(8):884–886
47. Ben-Zvi A, Vernon SD, Broderick G (2009) Model-based therapeutic correction of hypothalamic-pituitary-adrenal axis dysfunction. PLoS Comput Biol 5(1):e1000273

Chapter 9

Neuroimmune Mechanisms of Depression in Heart Failure

Jessica A. Jiménez and Paul J. Mills

Abstract

Heart failure (HF) is a major and costly public health concern, and its prognosis is grim—with high hospitalization and mortality rates. It is well documented that HF patients experience disproportionately high rates of depression and that depressed HF patients have worse clinical outcomes than their non-depressed counterparts. The purpose of this chapter is to introduce the reader to the study of depression in HF, and how psychoneuroimmunologic principals have been applied to further elucidate the mechanisms (i.e., neurohormonal and cytokine activation) linking these co-morbid disorders.

Key words: Heart failure, Depression, Inflammation, Renin-angiotensin-aldosterone system, Sympathetic nervous system

1. Introduction

Heart failure (HF) is a major public health concern, especially in societies where a sizable proportion of the population is over 65 years of age. HF is often the last stage of cardiovascular disease, and its prognosis is grim—with high hospitalization and mortality rates. Interestingly, heart disease, including HF, is often accompanied by a psychological symptom complex, including low mood, hostility, anger, and poor quality of life (1).

In recent years, the study of depression in HF has garnered scientific interest due to its high prevalence in HF patients and its strong tendency to worsen medical prognosis (1–4). Although the etiology of depression in HF remains unclear, the disorders appear to share a similar pathogenesis, involving disturbance of the balance between sympathetic and parasympathetic tone, and increased inflammation, as evidenced by elevated circulating levels of proinflammatory cytokines (2). Considering that depression has also been associated with incident HF (5, 6), most scholars favor

Qing Yan (ed.), *Psychoneuroimmunology: Methods and Protocols*, Methods in Molecular Biology, vol. 934,
DOI 10.1007/978-1-62703-071-7_9, © Springer Science+Business Media, LLC 2012

a bidirectional pathophysiology, in which depression may precede or follow the development of HF.

The purpose of this chapter is to introduce the reader to the study of depression in HF, and how psychoneuroimmunologic principals have been applied to further elucidate the mechanisms linking these co-morbid disorders. We begin the chapter with a brief discussion of the epidemiology and pathophysiology of HF, then of the characteristics and consequences of depression in HF, and conclude with discussion and presentation of relevant psychoneuroimmunological findings concerning the shared pathophysiology of depression and HF.

2. Heart Failure

2.1. Epidemiology of Heart Failure

In the United States, the prevalence of HF is 2.42%, with higher rates found in older, male adults (7, 8). Despite significant advances in treatment, the prognosis for patients remains grim: 20–30% of HF patients die within a year of diagnosis, and 45–60% die within 5 years (9). Among older adults, HF is the most common condition for hospitalization (10), with 990,000 hospitalizations per year in the US (8) at an approximate cost of $39.2 billion (11).

2.2. Definition and Classification of Heart Failure

The American College of Cardiology (ACC) and American Heart Association (AHA) define HF as a complex clinical syndrome that can result from any structural or functional cardiac disorder that impairs the ability of the ventricles to fill with or eject blood (12). The upper chambers of the heart are composed of the right and left atria, and the lower chambers include the right and left ventricles. The ventricles are muscular chambers that contract to pump blood (*systole*). After systole, the ventricle muscles normally relax during *diastole*, allowing blood from the atria to fill the ventricles. The heart's ability to pump can be compromised via two mechanisms: (1) reduction in the volume of oxygenated blood ejected from the left ventricle (LV) as a result of diminished myocardial contractility; and (2) inadequate venous return to heart, resulting from impaired ventricle filling and relaxation.

Although HF varies in its etiologies and clinical features, it can be broadly classified into two categories: HF with systolic dysfunction (also known as "HF with reduced ejection fraction" (HFrEF)), characterized by a reduced left ventricle ejection fraction (LVEF), which is a measure of the percentage of blood that is ejected from the heart into the aorta with each systole; HF with preserved ejection fraction (HFpEF) is a complex disorder, where LVEF is normal or mildly abnormal. Other LV abnormalities include abnormal relaxation and filling, concentric remodeling, hypertrophy, increased

Table 1
Functional classifications and disease progression stages of heart failure

	Definition	Examples
New York Heart Association functional (NYHA) classes		
NYHA class I	No limitation of physical activity	Ordinary physical activity does not cause undue fatigue, palpitation, or dyspnea (shortness of breath)
NYHA class II	Slight limitation of physical activity	Comfortable at rest, but ordinary physical activity results in fatigue, palpitation, or dyspnea
NYHA class III	Marked limitation of physical activity	Comfortable at rest, but less than ordinary activity causes fatigue, palpitation, or dyspnea
NYHA class IV	Unable to carry out any physical activity without discomfort	Symptoms of cardiac insufficiency at rest. If any physical activity is undertaken, discomfort is increased
American College of Cardiology/American Heart Association Stages of Heart Failure		
Stage A	High risk for developing HF, but without structural heart disease or symptoms of HF	Hypertension, diabetes mellitus, CAD, family history of cardiomyopathy
Stage B	Structural heart disease, but asymptomatic	Previous myocardial infarction, left ventricular dysfunction, valvular heart disease
Stage C	Structural heart disease with previous or current symptoms, but managed with medical treatment	Structural heart disease, dyspnea and fatigue, impaired exercise tolerance
Stage D	Marked symptoms at rest despite maximal medical therapy	Advanced disease requiring hospital-based support, a heart transplant or palliative care

extracellular matrix, abnormal relaxation and filling, decreased diastolic distensibility, and abnormal calcium handling.

There are two primary scales that are used to classify HF. The New York Heart Association (NYHA) functional scale, which is based on symptoms, classifies HF in categories from I to IV (Table 1).

The other scale is the American College of Cardiology/American Heart Association (ACC/AHA) scale, a newer classification that stages patients as either A, B, C, or D (Table 1) (12). The ACC/AHA staging system classifies HF as a progressive disease, and once a particular stage is reached there is no opportunity to transition to a lower stage (e.g., a stage C HF patient cannot return to stage B). This system is often complemented by the NYHA functional classification system. In contrast, ACC/AHA Stage C patients can shift between Functional Classes I–IV at any given time. Movement up and down NYHA classes is common, depending on the clinical status of the patient during the time of assessment.

3. Pathophysiology of Heart Failure

HF is characterized by activation of the renin-angiotensin-aldosterone system (RAAS) and the sympathetic nervous system (SNS), as well as inflammatory pathways. Regardless of its etiology and classification, HF begins with injury to the myocardium (e.g., myocardial infarction), which reduces cardiac output. In response, the body engages in a series compensatory mechanisms, including: (1) maintaining perfusion pressure by increasing the circulation of blood volume; (2) activating immune and inflammatory pathways; and (3) restructuring cardiac muscle cells and reshaping the ventricle chamber. This systematic response involves complex interactions between the RAAS and SNS, which are collectively referred to as neurohormonal responses.

Neurohormonal activation and cytokine activation are designed for acute responses to injury, but prolonged activation of these compensatory mechanisms eventually leads to further declines in cardiac functioning. Currently, the most successful pharmacological therapies for HF block aspects of the body's compensatory responses to myocardial injury (12); thus, there is increasing scientific interest in understanding neurohormonal and cytokine activation in the context of HF.

3.1. Renin-Angiotensin-Aldosterone System

The RAAS system maintains renal blood flow after the myocardium has sustained injury via its effects on remodeling the vasculature and increasing plasma volume. Decreased renal perfusion pressure results in secretion of renin by juxtaglometer cells lining the afferent renal arterioles. Specifically, renin cleaves angiotensinogen to form decapeptide angiotensin-I. The angiotensin converting enzyme (ACE) cleaves two C terminal amino acids to form angiotensin-II, the primary effector of the system. Receptors for angiotensin-II are divided into subtypes, AT-1 and AT2. AT-1 is the predominate subtype in the vascular endothelium and a primary target for pharmacologic blockade. Binding of angiotensin-II to AT-1 receptors results in increases in the release of intracellular calcium from the sacroplasma reticulum via activation of protein kinase C. The binding of angiotensin-II in the vasculature results in an increase in systematic vasculature resistance and restoration of blood pressure.

Prolonged compensatory actions of the RAAS in HF bring adverse consequences, however, including increased vascular resistance. Increases in resistance create undue myocardial burden and decreased cardiac output, resulting in left ventricular hypertrophy. Angiotensin-II initiates apoptosis and interstitial fibrosis, which contribute to the remodeling of the extracellular matrix in the myocardium (e.g., myocyte hypertrophy). The effects of angiotensin-II on the myocardium and peripheral vasculature results in decreased cardiac output and renal perfusion. Angiotensin-II is also involved in the increase of plasma volume by initiating production of minerocorticoid aldosterone by the adrenal cortex. Aldosterone acts on the distal tubules of the renal nephron and activates a sodium-potassium exchange, which results in the retention of sodium and water. The increased plasma volume exacerbates fluid overload and peripheral edema. Chronic excess of aldosterone leads to increased fibrosis in the atria, ventricles, kidneys, and perivasculature.

3.2. Sympathetic Nervous System

Vascular baroreceptors respond to declines in cardiac output and stroke volume by increasing sympathetic nerve activity and consequent release of the catecholamine norepinephrine. Sympathetic activation improves cardiac output by increasing heart rate, myocardial contractility and stroke volume. Sympathetic activation also increases systematic resistance and blood pressure in the peripheral vasculature, and via catecholamines, increases renin release and angiotenin-II production, further increasing vascular resistance and afterload.

The direct effects of sympathetic activation on the myocardium itself is primarily mediated via two classes of β-adrenergic receptors, namely the β-1 and β-2 receptors. In a normal heart, β-1s comprise approximately 80% of the total β-adrenergic receptor pool (13); however, chronic sympathetic activation significantly downregulates β-1 receptors leaving a greater proportional presence of β-2 receptors of approximately 40% (13). While β-2 receptors are less downregulated, they are susceptible to inactivation from repetitive agonist stimulation, becoming less responsive to adrenergic agonists. Although the release of norepinephrine acutely increases myocardial contractility, chronic stimulation in HF worsens cardiac function (direct cytotoxic effects), resulting in progressive dysfunction of the LV, worsening pulmonary edema and potentially death. Higher levels of circulating norepinphrine have been associated with poorer survival, and greater functional decline in HF.

3.3. Systemic Inflammation

The "cytokine hypothesis" proposes that HF progression is an inflammatory process and that elevated levels of proinflammatory cytokines worsen LV dysfunction. There is a significant body of evidence to suggest that elevated levels of cytokines are associated with cardiac decline in HF. Particularly, the inflammatory cytokines tumor necrosis factor-alpha (TNF-α) and Interluekin-6 (IL-6) are among the most widely studied cytokines in HF.

TNF-α is a polypeptide that activates endothelial cells, recruits inflammatory cells, and enhances the production of other proinflammatory cytokines. TNF-α is secreted from immune cells during the early stages of HF; however, in the final stages, the cardiac myocytes secrete TNF-α in high quantities. TNF-α appears to be particularly important in the transition from compensated to acute decompensated HF; the latter being a state of exacerbated HF requiring hospitalization. TNF-α has been extensively studied in animal models, and overexpression of TNF-α by the cardiac myocytes leads to inflammatory myocarditis and subsequent mycocyte hypertyophy, LV dilatation, and progressive LV dysfunction. For example, exogenous administration of TNF-α at concentrations comparable to those observed in HF, produces significant declines in myocardial contractility, worsening LV dysfunction and increasing pulmonary endema.

IL-6 is also elevated in HF, particularly in the end-stages of the disease. Although IL-6 was initially thought to have only proinflammatory effects like those of TNF-α, research in murine models suggests that IL-6 also plays an immune modulatory role in response to secretion of TNF-α. IL-6 has direct effects on the myocardium, including decreasing contractility, activating matrix metalloproteinases, and contributing to LV remodeling. Like TNF-α, IL-6 is secreted from the myocardial cells during the end-stages of HF, but not during mild or moderate stages of the disease.

4. Depression in Heart Failure

4.1. Epidemiology of Depression in Heart Failure Patients

Depression in HF has been extensively studied because of its high prevalence in HF patients and its tendency to worsen medical prognosis (1–4). HF patients experience disproportionately high rates of depression compared to the general population, with a point prevalence of 21.5% (14) compared to 6.6% in the general population (15). Single depressive symptoms, however, can be detected in 24–85% of HF patients (2). Depression has also been associated with incident HF. In a community sample of 2,501 patients (mean follow-up 14 years), Williams and colleagues found that depression was an independent predictor of developing HF in women (HR = 1.96, 95% CI = 1.11, 3.46, $p = 0.02$), but not in men (5). In a study of 4,538 older adult patients enrolled in the Systolic Hypertension in the Elderly Program (SHEP), depressed patients were 2.82 times (95% CI = 1.71, 4.67; $p < 0.001$) more likely to develop HF over a 4.5-year-follow-up period (6). The association between depression and HF did not significantly vary by sex. Although not all studies have found gender effects, Williams et al.'s findings follow trends seen in depressed, non-HF populations: the National Comorbidity Survey, for example, reported a 1.7 greater odds of women developing depression at some point in their lifetime compared to men (15).

4.2. Patient Characteristics and Depression

The prevalence of depression in HF appears to significantly differ by health status, demographics, and social factors. In their meta-analysis of depression in HF, Rutledge et al. found that 11–25% of outpatients and 35–70% of inpatients were depressed (14). Rutledge and colleagues also found that depressive symptomatology increased with severity of HF diagnosis, ranging from 11% of patients with NYHA functional class I to 42% of NYHA class IV patients (14). Several studies have found higher depression in younger, as well as female HF patients (16). Social factors may contribute to incident depression in HF. In a study of 245 HF patients without depression at baseline, living alone, alcohol abuse, perception of medical care as being a substantial economic burden, and poor health status were independent predictors of developing depressive symptoms (17). The effects appear to be multiplicative in nature: 15.5% of patients developed depression when only one of the factors were present, 36.2% developed depression when two factors were present, and 69.2% developed depression when three or more were present.

4.3. Clinical Outcomes in Heart Failure Patients with Depression

Of great clinical significance, studies find that depression has adverse effects on the course and prognosis of HF. Increased psychological surveillance of HF patients over the past 15 years has highlighted the pivotal role of depression in HF (18). Sherwood et al. (19) reported that depressive symptomatology was associated with a 1.56 (95% CI; 1.07, 2.29; $p<0.001$) increased risk of death or hospitalization during a median 3-year follow-up period. In a sample of 374 patients hospitalized for HF, Jiang et al. (20) found that HF patients with major depression had 2.23 greater odds (95%CI 0.04, 4.77; $p=0.04$) of mortality and 3.07 (95%CI 1.41, 6.66; $p=0.005$) greater odds of readmission at 1 year compared to HF patients with no depression. In a sample of 1,006 hospitalized HF patients, Jiang et al. (21) found that patients whose Beck Depression Inventory (BDI) scores were 5–9, 10–18, and ≥19 were 21%, 53%, and 83%, respectively, more likely to die than patients whose BDI score was ≤5 ($p<0.001$). Vaccarino et al. (22) also found that there was a graded associated between the number of depressive symptoms and increased risk of death or decline of daily living at 6 months. In this prospective study of 391 patients with decompensated HF on admission to the hospital, patients with ≥11 depressive symptoms, compared with those with <6 depressive symptoms, had an 82% higher risk of either functional decline or death. In a study of longitudinal outcomes (mean follow-up 39 months) in HF patients with comordid atrial fibrillation, Frasure-Smith et al. (23) found that elevated depressive symptoms significantly predicted cardiovascular mortality (HR: 1.57; 95% CI 1.20, 2.07; $p<0.001$). The authors also commented that the increased risk of death was similar to risks associated with not taking standard medications to manage HF, such as anticoagulants and aldosterone antagonists. Worsening depressive symptomatology over time is also associated with increased risk of adverse outcomes. A study of 147 HF outpatients found that a 1-point change in BDI scores was associated 1.07 increased risk of death or cardiovascular hospitalization (95% CI 1.02, 1.12, $p=0.007$) (24). The results from these studies indicate that depression is an independent predictor of worse clinical outcomes in HF patients (18).

4.4. Quality of Life in Heart Failure Patients with Depression

In addition to its cardiotoxic effects, depressed HF patients suffer reduced physical functioning and worse quality of life. Depressed patients report poorer quality of life and greater functional impairment than non-depressed patients, even when compared with patients of a higher (i.e., worse) NYHA functional class, which may suggest that patient perceptions of physical functioning, rather than the clinical status itself, predicts quality of life outcomes (25, 26). In a small study ($n=58$) of associations between disease severity, functional status, depression, and daily quality of life, greater depression severity was positively associated with worse self-reported physical and emotional quality of life in HF patients. A recent study by Hallas et al. (27) conducted in 146 HF patients found that patients with more negative beliefs about the consequences of HF, and less perceived control were more anxious and depressed compared to patients with more positive beliefs. Greater depression ratings also predicted poorer quality of life. Patients with more negative beliefs also had more maladaptive behaviors and less coping resources, which may also have downstream affects on quality of life. In a study of 155 HF patients, Gottlieb et al. (16) found that depressed patients scored significantly worse than non-depressed patients on all components of the quality of life questionnaires. In a more recent study, Gottlieb et al. (28) demonstrated that depression is minimally related to objective assessments of HF severity, such as peak O_2 consumption, B-type natriuretic peptide levels or ejection fraction. However, depression significantly affects subjective measurements of HF severity, such as NYHA classification or 6-min walk test (8). Undoubtedly, depression negatively affects quality of life, but there is building evidence to also suggest that depression alters patient perceptions of physical functioning and disease severity, which may result in poorer ratings on subjective measures.

5. Psychoneuro-immunology: Understanding Pathophysiological Links Between Heart Failure and Depression

Given the adverse effects of depression on cardiac prognosis, understanding the biological pathways that link HF and depression may provide routes for pharmacological and behavioral interventions. The comorbid nature of HF and depression suggests that they share a similar pathophysiology: inflammation.

After more than a decade of research on this topic, although the mechanistic relationships between depression and inflammation are not fully understood, much progress has been made. Depressed patients without HF have significantly higher levels of IL-1β, IL-6, TNF-α, and Interferon-gamma (IFN-γ) (29). Potential sources of inflammatory activation in HF include SNS activation and hyperactivity of the hypothalamic-pituitary-adrenal axis (30, 31).

5.1. Lessons Learned on Inflammatory and Other Immune Responses in Depression in HF

One of the main lines of investigation in our laboratory has been the application of the cytokine model and other theoretical models of broader immune activation in the context of depression in HF. We have conducted several studies that lend support to the theory that systematic inflammation, as well as broader dysregulation of immune system, may underlie the relationship between depressive symptoms and progression of HF. Our approach to the study of these topics has been the use of both cross-sectional and prospective studies. For the former, we have assessed a broad range of inflammatory and cell adhesion biomarkers in patients with established HF and with a range of depressive symptomatology. For the latter, we are studying with ACC/AHA Stage B patients, individuals who are at risk for developing symptomatic HF but who at present are not symptomatic. In these individuals, we are again assessing a broad range of inflammatory and cell adhesion biomarkers, as well as depression, but repeatedly over the course of several years. The intention is to temporally model inflammation as it relates to the onset and offset of depression and to the onset and progression from non-symptomatic to symptomatic HF. Here we present some of our cross-sectional findings.

5.2. Assessing Depressive Symptoms

In our studies we have primarily measured depression via the Beck Depression Inventory (version–IA; BDI-IA), which a 21-item self-administered assessment of extent to which patients experience depressive symptoms (32). Scores of 0–9 indicate minimal or no depression, 10–18 indicate mild–moderate depression, 19–29 moderate–severe depression, and 30–63 severe depression. The reliability of this measure in our samples has been $\alpha > 0.90$. Since there has been some evidence to suggest cognitive/affective and somatic aspects of depression differentially relate to clinical course in HF (33), we are also examining these BDI sub-scales of depression in our studies: (1) the cognitive/affective subscale assesses symptoms such as sadness and dissatisfaction (13 items, score range 0–39); and (2) the somatic subscale assesses features such as changes in appetite and feelings of fatigue (7 items, score range 0–21).

5.3. Assessing Cyokines and Cellular Adhesion Molecules

Circulating TNF-α, IL-6, and IL-1β levels are determined in plasma by commercial ELISA. For IL-6, the intraassay CV (%) is 2.2, the inter-assay CV (%) is 3.9, and the assay sensitivity <0.71 pg/mL; for TNF-α, the intraassay CV (%) is 8.0, the inter-assay CV

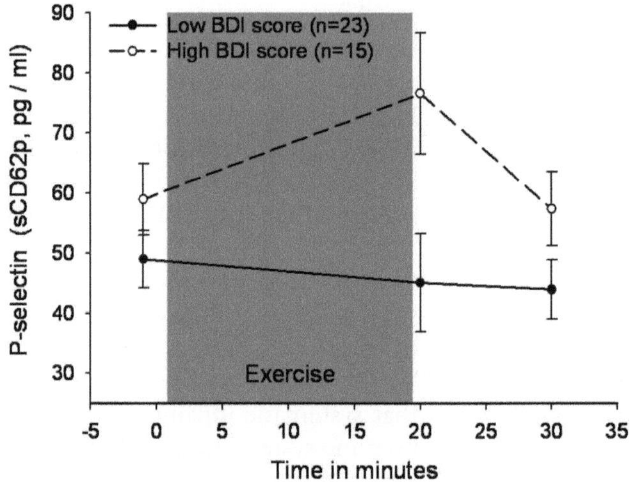

Fig. 1. Changes in sP-selectin in response to acute exercise in HF patients with high (>10, $n=15$) and low (≤10, $n=23$) BDI scores.

(%) is 16.3, and the assay sensitivity <0.18 pg/mL; for IL-1β, the intraassay CV (%) is 6.8, the inter-assay CV (%) is 8.3, and the assay sensitivity <0.1 pg/mL.

Circulating C-reactive protein (CRP) levels are determined in plasma using the High Sensitive CRP Reagent Set (DiaSorin; Stillwater, MN) using the Roche Cobas Mira Plus analyzer (Roche, Palo Alto, CA). Intra- and inter-assay coefficients of variation are <5%. Precision and sensitivity performance values are excellent: intra-assay CV (%) <1.0, inter-assay CV (%) = 1.6, sensitivity <0.05 mg/L.

Soluble intercellular adhesion molecule-1 (sICAM-1, sCD54) and sP-selectin (sCD62P) are determined by commercial ELISA. The precision and sensitivity performance values are as follows: sICAM-1 (intra-assay CV (%) = 4.6, inter-assay CV (%) = 6.6, sensitivity <0.35 ng/mL); sCD62P (intra-assay CV (%) = 5.1, inter-assay CV (%) = 8.8, sensitivity <0.5 ng/mL).

Proinflammatory cytokines, such as TNF, IL-6, and CRP, have been associated with cardiac dysfunction in both human and animal models. However, in 2009 Wirtz et al. (34) in our group provided the first study investigating whether depressive symptoms were associated with exercise-induced increases in circulating levels of adhesion molecules expressed on endothelial cells (sP-selectin and soluble sICAM-1), leukocytes (sICAM-1), and platelets (sP-selectin). Using data from 39 middle-aged male HF patients and 19 male control subjects, the authors found that higher depression symptomatology moderated greater increases in sP-selectin levels in response to an acute exercise challenge over time in HF patients as compared with control subjects ($F=3.25$, $p=0.05$). Post hoc testing revealed that in HF patients, higher depression scores (BDI) were significantly associated with greater increases in sP-selectin levels over time in response to the exercise (Fig. 1).

Also, in HF patients, higher BDI scores were associated with higher sP-selectin levels at pre-exercise and post-exercise time points (main effect of BDI: $F=4.86$, $p=0.035$). These effects were not found for the control subjects. These findings suggest that levels of sP-selectin are higher before and after exercise and have greater increases in response to exercise in male HF patients with increasing depressive symptom severity. These findings could have implications for acute coronary syndromes associated with exercise and thereby may impact mortality.

While it is widely acknowledge that indictors of inflammation are cross-sectionally associated with both depression and HF severity, our laboratory was among the first to explore whether different types of inflammatory markers prospectively predict depressive symptom in HF patients. Wirtz et al. (35) assessed the relationship of proinflammatory cytokines and cellular adhesion molecules on depressive symptoms at 12 months following initial study of 30 HF patients. The authors found that sICAM-1—but not IL-6 or CRP—was associated with depression scores 12 months later ($r=0.38$, $p=0.045$). Hierarchical linear regression models revealed that sICAM-1 significantly predicted depression scores at the 12-month follow-up, with sICAM-1 independently explaining between 7% ($\beta=0.26$, $p=0.040$) and 10% ($\beta=0.35$, $p=0.045$) of the total variance in depression scores. These findings suggest that the adhesion molecule sICAM-1 is an independent, prospective predictor of depressive symptoms in HF. The prospective nature of these findings support the suggested role for inflammation in increasing the severity of future depressive symptomatology.

5.4. Assessing Chemotaxis and Cellular Immunity

Until recently, immune cell migration, particularly chemotaxis, has been largely ignored in respect to depression symptoms and HF. Chemokines are essential for providing signaling to leukocytes for extravasation from the blood and directing locomotion (36, 37). When overexpressed, recruitment and migration factors are injurious to the cardiovascular system (38) and can generate angiogenesis and fibrous tissue deposition, which can lead to myocardial dysfunction in HF (39, 40). Particularly, studying acute physiologic responses to controlled challenges serve as a window into the complex physiologic processes involved in cardiac diseases (41).

One of the members of our group therefore developed an in vitro chemotaxis assay to assess functional capacity of peripheral blood mononuclear cells (PBMCs). PBMCs are separated from whole blood using Ficoll-Hypaque, washed, and then re-suspended in RPMI 1,640 with 20 mmol/L HEPES (serum-free media). In a modified Boyden chamber, the patient's PBMCs are then incubated with either the bacterial peptide f-met leu phe (fMLP), the physiologic chemokine stromal cell derived factor-1 (SDF-1), or the adrenergic agonist isoproterenol, or chemotaxis buffer. Chemotaxis responsiveness of PBMCs to the bacterial peptide fMLP is commonly used to measure nonspecific natural immune activity. The chemokine SDF-1 binds to its specific receptor CXCR4, and subsequently stimulates lymphocyte adhesion and transendothelial migration, playing a role in adaptive cellular immunity. Levels of SDF-1 and CXCR4 are elevated in patients with HF and have been found to attenuate cardiac myocyte contractility (27). PBMCs are incubated with these agents for 2 h at 37 °C, then the top of the membrane is then gently rinsed with phosphate-buffered saline and the non-migrated cells are removed. The membrane is then removed from the plate and briefly submerged in phosphate-buffered saline. Once dry, the membrane is read by a fluorescence plate reader (CytoFluor) at an excitation of 485 nm and emission of 530 nm.

Redwine et al. (42) studied the relationship between depressive symptoms and PBMC chemotaxis both at rest and in response to a moderate acute exercise challenge in 65 middle-aged HF patients and 45 non-HF control subjects. Chemotaxis of PBMCs was examined in vitro to either fMLP or SDF-1 immediately before and after the exercise. The author found that HF patients had reduced chemotaxis to SDF-1 compared with non-CHF subjects ($p<05$). The authors also found that higher BDI scores were significantly associated with reduced baseline chemotaxis to SDF-1 in both CHF and non-CHF subjects ($p=0.025$). In contrast, higher BDI scores were associated with increased chemotaxis to fMLP and SDF-1 in response to exercise in the HF patients ($p=0.027$; Fig. 2).

The authors also found that cognitive depressive symptoms, but not somatic depressive symptoms were inversely associated with baseline chemotaxis to fMLP and SDF-1 in HF and controls. When stratified by HF diagnosis, these associations persisted when controlling for covariates. However, neither cognitive nor somatic symptoms were associated with changes in chemotaxis from pre-to-post exercise task.

The results from the study suggested a shift in immune cell mobility in HF patients with greater depressive symptom severity, with reduced chemotaxis to a physiologically specific chemokine at rest but increased chemotaxis to both nonspecific and specific chemical attractants in response to physical activity. Findings could have implications for cardiac repair and remodeling in HF patients and therefore disease progression.

A second chemotaxis study conducted by Redwine et al. (43) investigated if depressive symptoms were related to alterations in the sensitivity of PBMCs to the β-adrenergic agonist isoproterenol in patients at rest and after acute exercise in 77 patients with HF and 44 controls. As mentioned previously, sympathetically modulated immune dysregulation is a part of the pathophysiology of HF; however, this process may be exacerbated in the presence of depression. The study results indicated that depressive symptom severity ($p=0.001$) and higher resting levels of plasma norepinephrine

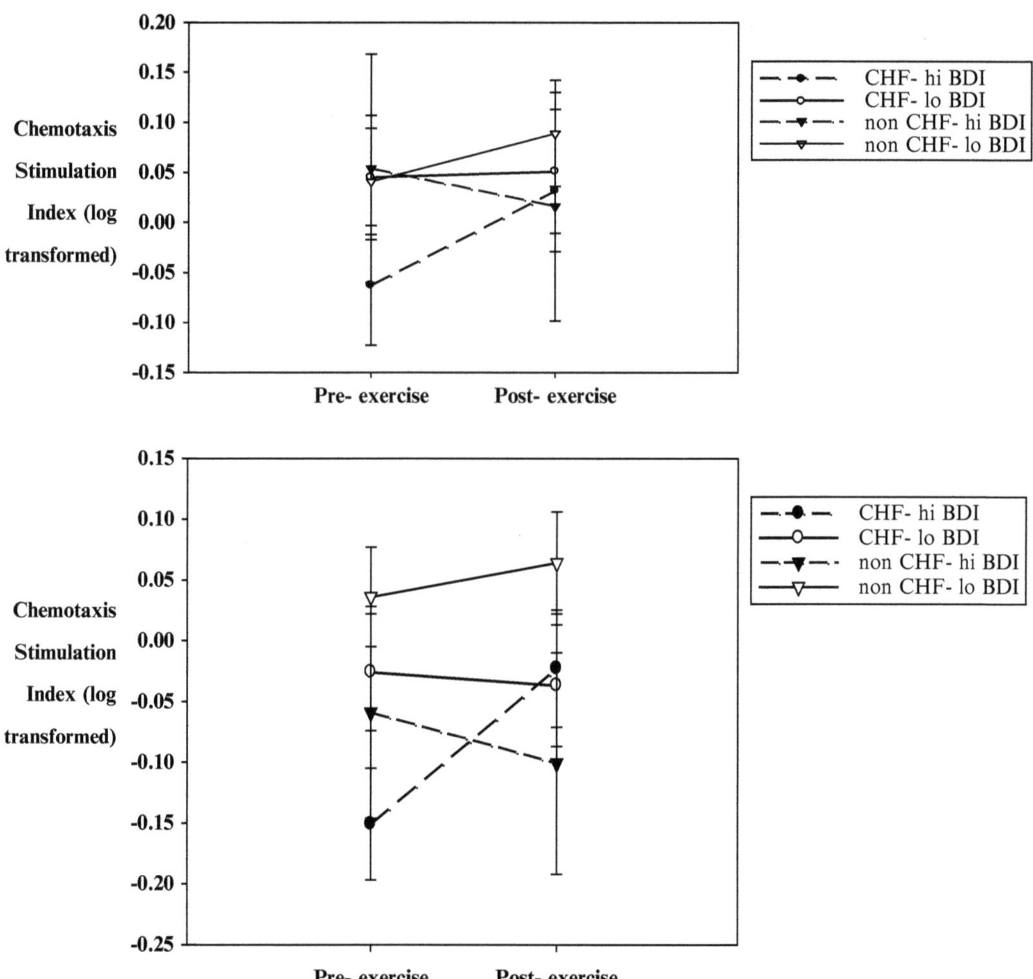

Fig. 2. Changes in a logarithmic transformed stimulation index (SI) of chemotaxis to fMLP (*top panel*) and the chemokine SDF-1 (*bottom panel*) in HF patients and non-HF controls with high (hi) and low (lo) Beck Depression Inventory (BDI) scores in response to exercise. Data are expressed as means ± SEM.

($p = 0.003$) were associated with greater chemotaxis after exercise in patients with HF (Fig. 3).

The authors concluded that patients with HF with higher depressive symptoms and plasma norepinephrine exhibit increased circulating immune cell chemotaxis to isoproterenol, suggesting greater adrenergic sensitivity. Increased immune cell migration in patients with HF who have elevated depressive symptoms could be associated with cardiac remodeling and HF disease progression.

5.5. Assessing Th1/Th2 Ratios

Although, as we have discussed, inflammatory cytokines have been implicated as a possible mediator of psychological symptoms of depression and HF, it has been unclear if systematic inflammation represents a broader dysregulation of the immune system.

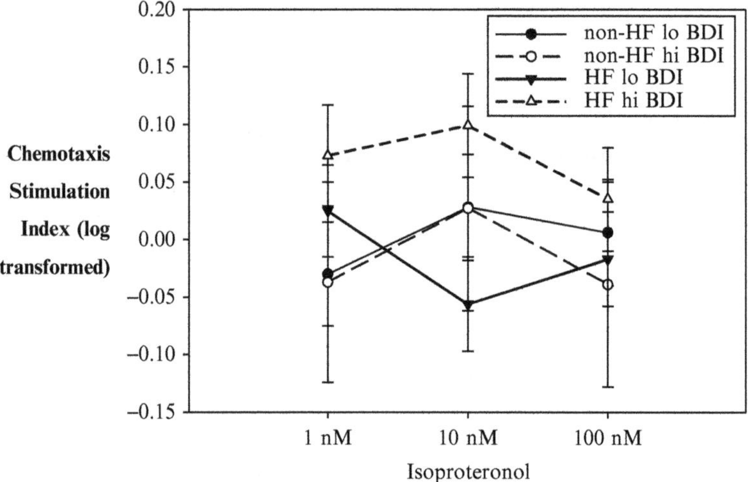

Fig. 3. Change scores (pre- minus post-exercise) and chemotaxis to three concentrations of isoproteronol (1 nM, 10 nM, and 100 nM/L) in HF patients and non-HF controls. High (hi) vs. low (lo) depression are determined by scores ≥10 and <10 on the BDI. Data expressed as means ± SEM.

Particularly, cellular immunity is important for protection against infection. Th1 cells promote cellular immunity by rapidly producing a range of cytokines such as IFN-γ that activate other Th1 cells to fight infectious agents. Th1 cells also exert a negative regulatory role on Th2 cells that produce cytokines such as IL-4 and IL-10. Th2 cytokines, on the other hand, attenuate immune defenses if they are locally over-expressed, by decreasing activities of major effectors such as Th1 cells (44, 45). A Th2 shift may have a profound effect on the susceptibility of the organism to infection (46), increase inflammation, and lead to dilated cardiomyopathy and HF (47). Maintaining Th1/Th2 homeostasis is important for preserving health. Thus, examining Th1/Th2 ratios can provide information on the balance of cellular immune activation vs. negative regulation of cellular immunity.

Redwine et al. (48) examined the relationship of depressive symptoms with cellular immune activity measured by the Th1/Th2 ratio and cardiac rehospitalization and/or death in 18 HF patients (mean age = 62, NYHA classes II–IV). The authors found that higher baseline depression scores were associated with a prospective increase in incidence of cardiac-related hospitalizations and/or death ($p = 0.037$). Lesser IFN-γ/IL-10 expressing CD4+ T cell ratios were related to higher depressive symptom scores at baseline ($p = 0.005$, Fig. 4) and a prospective increased incidence of cardiac-related hospitalization or death over a 2-year period ($p = 0.05$). The results suggest that a shift in the Th1/Th2 ratio may play a role in the association between depressive symptoms

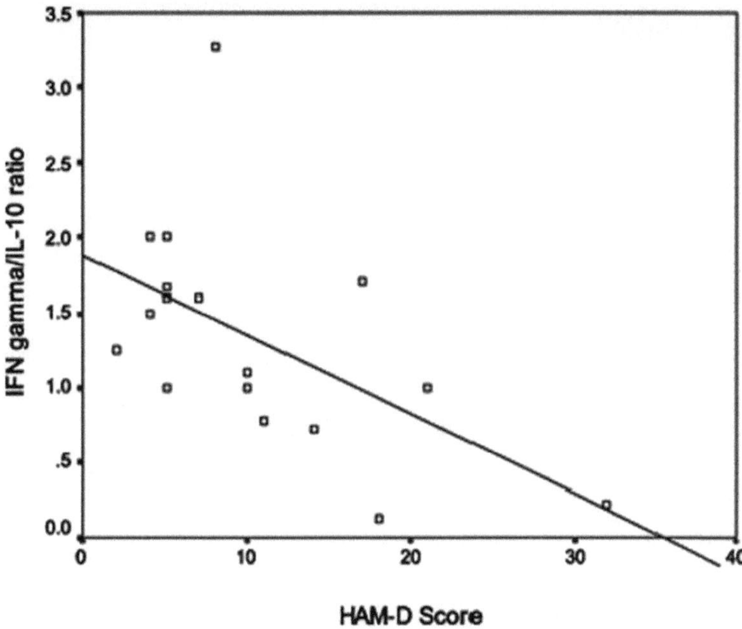

Fig. 4. Relationship between IFN-γ/IL-10 ratios and Hamilton depression scores in HF patients.

and morbidity and mortality in HF patients, suggesting broader immune dysregulation.

5.6. Other Pathways and Explanations

The cytokine and immune dsyregulation models are only two potential explanations for the link between HF and depression. The most widely discussed behavioral pathway is medication adherence (34). Cardiac patients, including those with HF, who have co-morbid depression have three times higher risk of cardiac medication non-adherence compared to non-depressed patients (35). The management of HF relies on a complex regimen of medications and self-care practices, and patients who do not adhere may suffer worse cardiac prognosis (34).

Another potential explanation for the link between depression and HF may be inherent due to the diagnosis of depression, and measure of its severity. The diagnostic criteria for major depressive disorder as well as screening for depressive symptoms, includes both cognitive and somatic symptoms. Thus, depressive symptomatology, such as fatigue, loss of energy, problems concentrating, weight loss or gain, and sleep disturbance, may be the result of underlying cardiac dysfunction (3). More recent studies have recognized this overlap, and now it is favored to report somatic and cognitive symptomatology separately as we have done in our studies.

6. Conclusions

HF is a major and costly public health concern, and its prognosis is grim—with high hospitalization and mortality rates. It is well documented that HF patients experience disproportionately high rates of depression and that depressed HF patients have worse clinical outcomes than their non-depressed counterparts. Thus, understanding mechanisms that link HF and depression has become a major area of scientific interest. A psychoneuroimmunological approach to examining these relationships is proving fruitful and merits increasing attention. The work conducted thus far in our laboratory group, as well as other groups, suggests that HF and depression may be linked by increased neuroimmune activation.

References

1. Kent LK, Shapiro PA (2009) Depression and related psychological factors in heart disease. Harv Rev Psychiatry 17:377–388
2. Norra C, Skobel EC, Arndt M et al (2008) High impact of depression in heart failure: early diagnosis and treatment options. Int J Cardiol 125:220–231
3. Watson K, Summer KM (2009) Depression in patients with heart failure: clinical implications and management. Pharmacotherapy 29: 49–63
4. Shapiro P (2009) Treatment of depression in patients with congestive heart failure. Heart Fail Rev 14:7–12
5. Williams SA, Kasl SV, Heiat A et al (2002) Depression and risk of heart failure among the elderly: a prospective community-based study. Psychosom Med 64:6–12
6. Abramson J, Berger A, Krumholz HM et al (2001) Depression and risk of heart failure among older persons with isolated systolic hypertension. Arch Intern Med 161:1725–1730
7. Bui AL, Horwich TB, Fonarow GC (2010) Epidemiology and risk profile of heart failure. Nat Rev Cardiol 8:30–41
8. Roger VL, Go AS, Lloyd-Jones DM et al (2010) Heart disease and stroke statistics—2011 update: a report from the American Heart Association. Circulation 123:18–209
9. Levy D, Kenchaiah S, Larson MG et al (2002) Long-term trends in the incidence of and survival with heart failure. N Engl J Med 347:1397–1402
10. DeFrances CJ et al (2008) 2006 National hospital discharge survey. Natl Health Stat Report 5:1–20
11. Lloyd-Jones D, Adams RJ, Brown TM et al (2010) Heart disease and stroke statistics—2010 update: a report from the American Heart Association. Circulation 121:e46–e215
12. Hunt SA, Abraham WT, Chin MH et al (2009) 2009 Focused update incorporated into the ACC/AHA 2005 guidelines for the diagnosis and management of heart failure in adults: a report of the American College of Cardiology Foundation/American Heart Association Task Force on Practice Guidelines Developed in Collaboration with the International Society for Heart and Lung Transplantation. J Am Coll Cardiol 53:e1–e90
13. Bristow MR (2000) ß-adrenergic receptor blockade in chronic heart failure. Circulation 101:558–569
14. Rutledge T, Reis VA, Linke SE et al (2006) Depression in heart failure: a meta-analytic review of prevalence, intervention effects, and associations with clinical outcomes. J Am Coll Cardiol 48:1527–1537
15. Kessler RC, Berglund P, Demler O et al (2003) The epidemiology of major depressive disorder: results from the National Comorbidity Survey Replication (NCS-R). JAMA 289:3095–3105
16. Gottlieb SS, Khatta M, Friedmann E et al (2004) The influence of age, gender, and race on the prevalence of depression in heart failure patients. J Am Coll Cardiol 43:1542–1549
17. Havranek EP, Spertus JA, Masoudi FA et al (2004) Predictors of the onset of depressive symptoms in patients with heart failure. J Am Coll Cardiol 44:2333–2338
18. Tousoulis D, Antonopoulos AS, Antoniades C et al (2010) Role of depression in heart

failure—choosing the right antidepressive treatment. Int J Cardiol 140:12–18

19. Sherwood A, Blumenthal JA, Trivedi R et al (2007) Relationship of depression to death or hospitalization in patients with heart failure. Arch Intern Med 167:367–373
20. Jiang W, Alexander J, Christopher E et al (2001) Relationship of depression to increased risk of mortality and rehospitalization in patients with congestive heart failure. Arch Intern Med 161:1849–1856
21. Jiang W, Kuchibhatla M, Clary GL et al (2007) Relationship between depressive symptoms and long-term mortality in patients with heart failure. Am Heart J 154:102–108
22. Vaccarino V, Kasl SV, Abramson J et al (2001) Depressive symptoms and risk of functional decline and death in patients with heart failure. J Am Coll Cardiol 38:199–205
23. Frasure-Smith N, Lesperance F, Habra M et al (2009) Elevated depression symptoms predict long-term cardiovascular mortality in patients with atrial fibrillation and heart failure. Circulation 120:134–140
24. Sherwood A, Blumenthal JA, Hinderliter AL et al (2011) Worsening depressive symptoms are associated with adverse clinical outcomes in patients with heart failure. J Am Coll Cardiol 57:418–423
25. Sullivan M, Levy WC, Russo JE et al (2004) Depression and health status in patients with advanced heart failure: a prospective study in tertiary care. J Card Fail 10:390–396
26. Jiang W, Kuchibhatla M, Cuffe MS et al (2004) Prognostic value of anxiety and depression in patients with chronic heart failure. Circulation 110:3452–3456
27. Hallas CN, Wray J, Andreou P et al (2011) Depression and perceptions about heart failure predict quality of life in patients with advanced heart failure. Heart Lung 40:111–121
28. Gottlieb SS, Kop WJ, Ellis SJ et al (2009) Relation of depression to severity of illness in heart failure (from Heart Failure and a Controlled Trial Investigating Outcomes of Exercise Training (HF-ACTION)). J Am Coll Cardiol 103:1285–1289
29. Maes M (2001) Psychological stress and the inflammatory response system. Clin Sci 101: 193–194
30. Penninx BW, Kritchevsky SB, Yaffe K et al (2003) Inflammatory markers and depressed mood in older persons: results from the health, aging and body composition study. Biol Psychiatry 54:566–572
31. Bremmer MA, Beekman AT, Deeg DJ et al (2008) Inflammatory markers in late-life depression: results from a population-based study. J Affect Disord 106:249–255
32. Beck A, Steer RA (1987) Manual for the revised Beck Depression Inventory. Psychological Corportation, San Antonio
33. Linke SE, Rutledge T, Johnson BD et al (2009) Depressive symptom dimensions and cardiovascular prognosis among women with suspected myocardial ischemia: a report from the National Heart, Lung, and Blood Institute-Sponsored Women's Ischemia Syndrome Evaluation. Arch Gen Psychiatry 66:499–507
34. Wirtz PH, Hong S, Redwine LS et al (2009) Depressive symptoms are associated with soluble P-selectin reactivity to acute exercise in heart failure. Biol Psychiatry 65:801–807
35. Wirtz PH, Redwine LS, Mills PJ (2010) Response regarding inflammation as a predictor of depression in heart failure. Brain Behav Immun 24:174–175
36. Szabo MC, Butcher EC, McIntyre BW et al (1997) RANTES stimulation of T lymphocyte adhesion and activation: role for LFA-1 and ICAM-3. Eur J Immunol 27:1061–1068
37. Chen J, Fujimoto C, Vistica BP et al (2006) Active participation of antigen-nonspecific lymphoid cells in immune-mediated inflammation. J Immunol 177:3362–3368
38. Adamopoulos S, Parissis J, Kroupis C et al (2001) Physical training reduces peripheral markers of inflammation in patients with chronic heart failure. Eur Heart J 22:791–797
39. Pyo RT, Sui J, Dhume A et al (2006) CXCR4 modulates contractility in adult cardiac myocytes. J Mol Cell Cardiol 41:834–844
40. Frangogiannis NG, Dewald O, Xia Y et al (2007) Critical role of monocyte chemoattractant protein-1/CC chemokine ligand 2 in the pathogenesis of ischemic cardiomyopathy. Circulation 115:584–592
41. Linden W, Gerin W, Davidson K (2003) Cardiovascular reactivity: status quo and a research agenda for the new millennium. Psychosom Med 65:5–8
42. Redwine LS, Wirtz PH, Hong S et al (2009) Potential shift from adaptive immune activity to nonspecific inflammatory activation associated with higher depression symptoms in chronic heart failure patients. J Card Fail 15:607–615
43. Redwine LS, Wirtz PH, Hong S et al (2010) Depression as a potential modulator of beta-adrenergic-associated leukocyte mobilization in heart failure patients. J Am Coll Cardiol 56: 1720–1727
44. Bot A, Smith KA, von Herrath M (2004) Molecular and cellular control of T1/T2 immunity at the interface between antimicrobial

defense and immune pathology. DNA Cell Biol 23:341–350

45. Elenkov IJ (2004) Glucocorticoids and the Th1/Th2 balance. Ann N Y Acad Sci 1024:138–146
46. Fairweather D, Frisancho-Kiss S, Yusung SA et al (2004) Interferon-γ protects against chronic viral myocarditis by reducing mast cell degranulation, fibrosis, and the profibrotic cytokines transforming growth factor-β1, Interleukin-1β, and Interleukin-4 in the Heart. Am J Pathol 165:1883–1894
47. Afanasyeva M, Georgakopoulos D, Belardi DF et al (2005) Impaired up-regulation of CD25 on CD4+ T cells in IFN-γ knockout mice is associated with progression of myocarditis to heart failure. Proc Natl Acad Sci USA 102:180–185
48. Redwine LS, Mills PJ, Hong S et al (2007) Cardiac-related hospitalization and/or death associated with immune dysregulation and symptoms of depression in heart failure patients. Psychosom Med 69:23–29

Chapter 10

A Reinterpretation of the Pathogenesis and Cure of Cancer According to the Psychoneuroimmunological Discoveries

Paolo Lissoni

Abstract

The recent discoveries in the oncological researches have demonstrated that the prognosis of the neoplastic diseases depends on not only the biological characteristics of tumors, including oncogene expression and growth factor receptor activity, but also on the immune status of cancer patients. This is because the well-documented importance of the anticancer immunity in the initiation of the tumor that is mainly modulated by lymphocytes. In addition, the knowledge on the interactions between the immune and neuroendocrine systems has demonstrated that the immune responses are physiologically under a psychoneuroendocrine control. In particular, it has been confirmed that the activation of the brain opioid tone may suppress the generation of an effective anticancer immunity, whereas it is stimulated by other neuroendocrine structure, namely the pineal gland, through the release of at least two indole hormones with anticancer activity, melatonin and 5-methoxytryptamine, exerting both antiproliferative and immunostimulatory effects. By investigating the immune and neuroendocrine functions in cancer patients, it has been observed that cancer progression is associated with a progressive decline in the pineal function, which would constitute the main cancer-related endocrine deficiency, and the occurrence of the irreversible immune alterations. The most prognostically important factors would consist of a diminished endogenous production of anticancer cytokines, such as IL-2 and IL-12, as well as an abnormally enhanced secretion of cytokines provided by suppressive effect on the anticancer immunity, namely IL-14, TGF-beta, and IL-6. The psychoneuroimmunotherapeutic approach in the treatment of cancer would simply consist of the corrections of the various endocrine and immune cancer-related alterations in an attempt to re-establish the neuroimmune condition of the health status.

Key words: Neuroimmunomodulation, Psychoneuroimmunology, Psychoncology

1. Introduction

The recent advances in the discoveries of the chemical bases mediating the influence of the psychospiritual status on the immune system, the so-called Psychoneuroendocrinoimmunology (PNEI), allowed the possibility to reinvestigate the pathogenesis of the

Qing Yan (ed.), *Psychoneuroimmunology: Methods and Protocols*, Methods in Molecular Biology, vol. 934, DOI 10.1007/978-1-62703-071-7_10, human neoplasms as a systemic disease, characterized by a progressive alteration of the physiological psychoneuroimmune interactions responsible for the modulation of the immune responses, including the anticancer immunity (1–3). Then, in contrast to the strategies commonly followed in the treatment of cancer that aim at the destruction of cancer cells independently of the immune status of cancer patients, the proposal of PNEI in the treatment of human neoplasms is consisting of the correction of the major immune and neuroendocrine alterations occurring during the clinical course of the neoplastic disease, in an attempt to restore the neuroimmune status of health. Therefore, the PNEI strategy in the treatment of cancer is simply consisting of an exogenous substitutive administration of those natural anticancer hormones, such as the pineal indole hormones (4), neuroactive substances, and antitumor cytokines, namely IL-2 and IL-12 (5, 6), whose endogenous production is abnormally and progressively reduced in the neoplastic disease, in association with strategies capable to counteract the enhanced production of hormones and cytokines provided by an immunosuppressive activity.

2. The Physiology of the Anticancer Immunity

Obviously, a correct elaboration of psychoneuroimmune strategies to cure cancer by restoring the natural immune resistance against tumor growth requires well-defined knowledge of the physiological mechanisms involved in the anticancer immunity, as well as an adequate analysis of the immune status of the single cancer patient before the proposal of an immunotherapeutic strategy. At present, it is known that the human anticancer immunity is substantially an IL-2-dependent phenomenon (7) and that lymphocytes are the main immune cells responsible for tumor cell destruction through a cytotoxic mechanism (8).

IL-2 is the main growth factor for T lymphocytes, which is able to transform NK cells into lymphokine-activated killer cells (LAK) that are capable of destroying fresh human cancer cells independently of their antigenicity, whereas in basal conditions NK cells are only able to destroy laboratory artificial cancer cell lines (5). On the other hand, T cytotoxic lymphocytes ($CD8^+$ cells) mediate an antigen-dependent anticancer cytotoxicity after their activation by IL-12 released from the dendritic cells (6), which play also a fundamental role in the anticancer immunity by presenting tumor antigens in association with class I and class II histocompatibility antigens, with a following activation of T cytotoxic lymphocytes ($CD8^+$ cells) and T helper ($CD4^+$ cells) lymphocytes, respectively (9, 10).

In any case, despite the great complexity of the mechanisms involved in generating an effective antitumor immune reaction, the anticancer immunity is synthetically founded on the three main subtypes of $CD4^+$ lymphocytes, which include the $CD4^+CD25^-$ (5), the $CD4^+CD25^+$ (11), and the $CD4^+CD17^+$ T cells (12). The $CD4^+CD25^-$ cells are defined as T helper (TH) lymphocytes, with two further cell subtypes, the TH1 and TH2 cells on the basis of their cytokine production, IL-2 or IL-4, IL-5, IL-10, and IL-13, respectively. The TH1 cells are the main producer of IL-2. The $CD4^+CD25^+$ T cells are the so-called T regulatory lymphocytes (T reg) (11), which play an immunosuppressive activity by inhibiting the production of the two main anticancer cytokines in humans, IL-2 and IL-12, through either a direct cell contact, or a secretion of suppressive cytokines, namely TGF-beta (13) and IL-10 (14). Finally, the $CD17^+$ cells, which are simply defined as $CD17^+$ cells, would play a stimulatory effect on the anticancer immunity by counteracting the generation of T reg lymphocytes. Other immunosuppressive cytokines are consisting of IL-6, namely produced by macrophages and responsible for the induction of the inflammatory response (15), and IL-1, TNF-alpha, IL-8, and IL-13. An antitumor immunostimulatory effect is also at least in part exerted by IL-15 and IL-18, with activities respectively similar to those of IL-2 and IL-12, as well as by IL-17, which suppresses T reg generation, and IL-23, which stimulates $CD17^+$ cell differentiation (12). IL-2 has also appeared to stimulate T reg cells (16), but it is not correct to reduce the role of IL-2 to the simple action of T reg cell growth factor, since IL-2-induced stimulation of T reg cells has been proven to be evident only in the patients who did not respond to IL-2 cancer immunotherapy (17).

It is known that host–tumor interaction mainly depends on three biological events, consisting of the efficacy of the anticancer immunity, the angiogenesis of tumor mass, and oncogene expression by cancer cells. In any case, from a physiopathological point of view, it would not be correct to separate these events, since an effective anticancer immune reaction has appeared to be also able to control the genetic characteristics of cancer cells and the angiogenic processes (18), as well as on the other hand angiogenic factors, such as VEGF, that have been proven to be also capable of inducing an immunosuppressive status by inhibiting the maturation of dendritic cells and their IL-12 production (19).

2.1. The Theoretical Bases of PNEI and the Psychoneuroendocrinoimmune System

PNEI is the most recent medical science that studies the neuroendocrinoimmune biochemistry, which mediates the emotions and the states of consciousness and their influence on the status of health through a regulation of the immune responses (1–3). The discoveries of PNEI would have not only a medical and scientific significance, but also a philosophic relevance, since they offer an answer to the problem of the relationship between biological body and spirit, as considered as the self-consciousness, by proposing a reciprocal influence of the neuroimmunobiochemistry on the status of consciousness and of the psychospiritual status on the neuroimmune interactions.

According to the recent advances in the areas of the neurosciences and PNEI itself, it is possible to identify in the complex brain neuronal interactions a pyramidal functional structure, consisting of three fundamental levels of neuron relationships, represented by the neurotransmission, the neuromodulation, and the psychoneuromodulation, which are the expression of three different grades of brain neuronal integration.

The neurotransmission is characterized by the existence of five main neurotransmitters, represented by noradrenalin, serotonin, dopamine, acetylcholine, and histamine. Acetylcholine is responsible for the maintenance of the status of awake, the memory processes, and the ethical behavior. Noradrenalin is involved in activating the mechanisms of stress and anxiety. Serotonin plays a major role in the control of mood. Dopamine is responsible for the perception of pleasure and for the expansion of consciousness and the extrasensorial sensitivity, including the hallucinatory experience. Finally, histamine exerts an inhibitory action on food intake and a stimulatory activity on the awake status. The neuromodulation is founded on the existence of two fundamental neuronal regulatory systems, consisting of gabaergic-type A and glutamate neurons, provided by an inhibitory and an excitatory action on the neuronal functions, respectively. The excessive glutamate-induced neuronal excitation may allow a neuron death due to the activation of the apoptotic mechanisms.

Finally, the third superior integrative system, which realizes the psychoneuromodulation, is constituted by three fundamental brain functional units, consisting of opioid system, cannabinergic system, and nitric oxide (NO) system. The opioid system has three main types of opioid receptors, -mu, -delta, and -kappa receptor, with beta-endorphin, met-enkephalin, and dinorphin as endogenous agonists, and it is involved in mediating the unconscious life, including stress, depression, and anxiety conditions (20). On the other hand, the cannabinergic system, which produces two main cannabinoid agonists, *N*-arachidonylethanol-amide (anandamide) and 2-arachidonylglycerol (2-AG), is responsible for the perception of pleasure and the expansion of consciousness (21). Finally, the NO system is mainly involved in regulating the interactions between opioid and cannabinergic systems, which are linked to the two fundamental psychic principles proposed by Freud (22), Eros and Thanatos, which are the expression of the spiritual consciousness, love and sexual pleasure and of the unconscious life and self-destruction, respectively.

2.2. The Psychoneuroendocrine Regulation of the Anticancer Immunity

The PNEI results have demonstrated that the psychoneuroendocrine functions related to the perception of sexual pleasure and spiritual life play a direct anticancer activity due to either antiproliferative action exerted by both pineal indoles and cannabinoid agents, or stimulation of the antitumor immunity (4, 21).

Finally, by considering the relation between the two major brain systems of the psychoneuromodulation and the endocrine glands, the opioid system is more linked to the pituitary gland, as demonstrated by its activation in stress conditions (20), whereas the cannabinergic system, which is functionally linked to the pineal (22), is activated in conditions of pleasure and spiritual perception (21). The two most investigated pineal indole hormones, melatonin (MLT) and 5-methoxytryptamine (5-MTT), have appeared to exert an anticancer antiproliferative activity (4, 23). MLT and 5-MTT are mainly secreted during the night and during the day, respectively, with a following well-defined light/dark circadian rhythm in their secretion.

In vivo, the immune responses, including the anticancer immunity, depend not only on immune factors, but also on their psychoneuroendocrine modulation, because the existence of a physiological brain central regulation of the immune system (1–3), which represents the biochemical basis of psychological and spiritual influences on the immune reactivity. The opioid system has been proven to inhibit the anticancer immune response (20), whereas the cannabinoid-pineal functional unit plays a stimulatory role on the antitumor immunity (4, 21), mainly due to a direct stimulatory action of MLT itself on IL-2 production from TH1 lymphocytes by acting on specific cell surface MLT receptors, as well as on IL-12 secretion from dendritic cells. In contrast, the activation of the opioid system allows an inhibition of the secretion of both IL-2 and IL-12 (20), and this finding could explain the stimulatory influence of stress, depression, and pain on tumor onset and development.

2.3. The Psychoneuroimmune Pathogenesis of Cancer as a Systemic Disease

The application of PNEI knowledge to the interpretation of cancer pathogenesis has allowed us to identify those immune and neuroendocrine alterations, which may explain the failure of cancer patients to destroy their tumor. These cancer-related immunoendocrine alterations are not a simple epiphenomenon, but on the contrary they represent the cause responsible at least in part for cancer progression related to the immunosuppressive status of patients. Then, cancer-related immunosuppression would mainly depend on an altered psychoneuroendocrine regulation of the immune system, rather than to be the expression of a primary damage of immune cells themselves (1–3).

Unfortunately, the common oncologic management of cancer patients does not include the evaluation of their immune and neuroendocrine status within the clinical investigations carried out before proposing a therapy of cancer.

It is a common opinion that cancer patients do not immunologically react against their tumors, but on the contrary the recent advances in the knowledge of the anticancer immunity have demonstrated that cancer patients have an immune reaction in the presence of tumor, which, however, is consisting of the induction of an immunosuppressive status rather than an effective anticancer immune response, and this finding would be the consequence of the great variety of immune and neuroendocrine alterations, which characterize the progression of the neoplastic disease (24–27).

Cancer-related immune dysfunctions may be classified into two essential types, consisting of alterations of cytokine blood concentrations and anomalies in immune cell and lymphocyte subsets, which may be summarized, as follows:

1. Cytokine alterations: the main disorders in cytokine blood concentrations, provided by a potential negative prognostic significance, are consisting of:
   - Low levels of IL-2.
   - Low levels of IL-12 in the very disseminated disease.
   - High levels of TGF-beta and IL-10.
   - High levels of inflammatory cytokines, including IL-6, IL-1, and TNF-alpha.
2. Immune cell alterations:
   - Low number of $CD4^+$ T helper cells.
   - Low number of dendritic cells.
   - Increased number of T reg cells.
   - Possible low number of $CD17^+$ cells.

As far as cancer-related endocrine and psychoneuroendocrine alterations are concerned, the progressive decline in the nocturnal production of the pineal hormone MLT would represent the most common cancer-related endocrine deficiency, which could at least in part explain cancer progression because of its anticancer activity. Another frequent endocrine alteration occurring in the advanced neoplastic disease is represented by the evidence of hypercortisolemia and of a lack of the physiological cortisol circadian rhythm, which has been proven to negatively influence the prognosis of several tumor histotypes, including lung and breast carcinomas (28).

As far as the status of the psychoneuromodulation in cancer patients is concerned, the neoplastic disease is generally characterized by an enhanced brain opioid tone associated with a diminished brain cannabinergic tone, which would be responsible for the progressive decline in the capacity of feeling pleasure, the so-called anaedonia, with the progression of cancer.

Obviously, cancer-related immune and neuroendocrine alterations are linked in a reciprocal way. Then, cancer-related hypercortisolemia could be due to the enhanced production of IL-6, which is able to directly stimulate cortisol secretion from the adrenal gland, and on the other hand, the progressive decline in IL-2 production could depend at least in part on the concomitant progressive decline in the pineal function, namely in MLT secretion.

The systemic nature of the neoplastic disease is confirmed by the evidence of a profound damage involving the psychoneuroendocrinoimmune system in patients with advanced neoplastic disease, as documented by the great variety of alterations of the immune, endocrine, and neuroendocrine functions and their relationships, which may occur during the clinical course of the neoplastic disease (24–27).

3. The Neuroimmunotherapy of Cancer

The neuroimmunotherapy (NIT) of cancer constitutes a new potential approach in the biological treatments of cancer, whose aim is the correction of cancer-related immune and neuroendocrine alterations, in an attempt to restore the immunoendocrine status of health. In fact, because of the physiological existence of a neuroendocrine regulation of the immune responses, a manipulation of the immune system would have to be constantly associated with a concomitant modulatory action of the neuroendocrine system. In more detail, the PNEI approach in cancer therapy is consisting of three major objectives:

1. The substitute therapy of cancer-related endocrine deficiency of the pineal gland through the administration of pharmacological doses of MLT during the night and of 5-MTT during the day, at least 20 mg/day for MLT and 5 mg/day for 5-MTT.
2. The correction of the main immune alterations by the exogenous injection of the two main anticancer cytokines in humans, IL-2 and IL-12, by using low-dose IL-2 ranging from 1.5 to 3 million IU/day through a subcutaneous injection, because of its less toxicity with respect to the intravenous route of administration, for 5 days/week for 4 consecutive weeks or by an alternating schedule consisting of 2 weeks of therapy followed by 2-week rest period for at least 3 months (29–31).
3. The inhibition of cancer-related inflammatory response, because of its negative influence on the anticancer immunity.

The application of NIT in the treatment of human neoplasms has to be constantly preceded by an adequate analysis of the immune and endocrine status of cancer patients, in an attempt to put into evidence their main anomalies and to know what has to be corrected by the various therapeutic strategies.

The history of the clinical cancer therapies according to a PNEI approach may be chronologically synthetized, as follows:

1. Neuroimmune therapy with MLT alone as a palliative treatment in metastatic cancer patients, for whom no other standard effective therapy was available: it is extremely rare to observe objective tumor regressions with MLT alone, which, however, may occur in a percentage generally less than 3 % and with a percentage of 1-year survival of 30 % in untreatable cancer patients with life expectancy less than 1 year, with promising results particularly in non-small cell lung cancer, pancreatic cancer, and melanoma (32). In addition, MLT has been proven to be effective in the palliative therapy of the neoplastic cachexia, asthenia, and thrombocytopenia, because of its thrombopoietic properties.
2. NIT with MLT plus subcutaneous low-dose IL-2 in untreatable metastatic solid tumor patients with life expectancy less than 1 year: this schedule is justified by the fact that MLT has appeared to enhance the efficacy of IL-2 in most solid tumor histotypes, namely in non-small cell lung cancer, hepatocarcinoma, melanoma, gastric cancer, and pancreatic cancer. This biological regimen has been shown to induce objective tumor regressions in a percent of about 20 % and with a percent of survival at 1- and at 3-years of about 50 % and 9 %, respectively (30).
3. Chemoneuroendocrine therapy with the conventional chemotherapies plus pharmacological doses of MLT in cancer patients with poor clinical status: the association with MLT may reduce the toxicity of chemotherapy, by resulting as effective in the prevention of cardiotoxicity, neurotoxicity, and thrombocytopenia, whereas no efficacy was seen in the prevention of anemia, neutropoenia, vomiting, and alopecia (32). Moreover, MLT has also appeared to enhance the efficacy of chemotherapy itself, and this evidence is not surprising, since it has been demonstrated that the anti-oxidant agents, as well as MLT itself, may enhance the cytotoxic potency of the chemotherapeutic drugs (33).
4. NIT with MLT, subcutaneous low-dose IL-2 and the long-acting mu-opioid receptor antagonist naltrexone (NTX) (34): another neuromodulatory strategy could be represented by a block of cancer-related enhanced brain opioid tone, because of its immunosuppressive effect. The results, however, are very preliminary, and in particular it has to be established the optimal schedule of NTX administration, in terms of either dosage and/or times of administration.
5. NIT with subcutaneous low-dose IL-2 plus MLT and plus subcutaneous low-dose IL-12 injected before the onset of IL-2

administration to stimulate the TH1 cell differentiation: the association between IL-2 and IL-12 has been proven to induce the maximal lymphocytosis described up to now in the literature (35). Since the efficacy of immunotherapy depends on the increase in lymphocyte number, the association between IL-2 and IL-12 could constitute the best future immunotherapeutic combination in the treatment of advanced human neoplasms.

4. Conclusions

According to the recent oncological discoveries, it is physiopathologically incorrect to separate the investigation of the genetic and growth factor receptor expression by cancer cells from the analysis of the endocrine and immune status of cancer patients. This statement I justified by the fact that the immune system may not only inhibit cancer cells but also control their characteristics, as well as the angiogenic processes, and the biological degree of malignancy. Therefore, the grade of malignancy of cancer cells would simply represent a consequence of a cancer-related immunosuppressive status. So, the correction of all the great number of alterations in the endogenous production of cytokines occurring during the clinical history of the neoplastic disease represent a fundamental aim in cancer therapy. Unfortunately, the development of anticancer therapeutic strategies with monoclonal antibodies has diminished the interest for cancer immunotherapy with cytokines.
Then, the most effective cancer immunotherapeutic schedule described in the literature up to now still remains that with IL-2 plus IL-12, already proposed more than 10 years ago. A further improvement could be achieved by activating IL-17 in an attempt to counteract T- regulatory lymphocytes to have the anticancer immunity.

References

1. Rubinow DR (1990) Brain, behaviour and immunity: an interactive system. J Natl Cancer Inst Monogr 10:79–82
2. Jankovic BD (1994) Neuroimmunomodulation. From phenomenology to molecular evidence. Ann N Y Acad Sci 741:3–38
3. Lissoni P, Cangemi P, Pirato D et al (2001) A review on cancer-psychospiritual status interactions. Neuroendocrinol Lett 22: 175–180
4. Maestroni JGM (1993) The immunoneuroendocrine role of melatonin. J Pineal Res 14:1–10
5. Grimm EA, Mazumder A, Zhang HZ, Rosenberg SA (1982) Lymphokine-activated killer cell phenomenon. J Exp Med 155:1823–1841
6. Banks R, Patel PM, Selby PJ (1995) Interleukin-12: a new clinical player in cytokine therapy. Br J Cancer 71:655–659
7. Chouaib S, Fradelizi D (1982) The mechanism of inhibition of human IL-2 production. J Immunol 129:2463–2467
8. Atzpodien J, Kirchner H (1990) Cancer, cytokines and cytotoxic cells. Klin Wochenschr 68:1–11

9. Rosenberg SA (1992) The immunotherapy and gene therapy of cancer. J Clin Oncol 10:180–199
10. Woijtowicz-Praga S (1997) Reversal of tumor-induced immunosuppression: a new approach to cancer therapy. J Immunother 20:165–177
11. Zou W (2006) Regulatory T cells, tumour immunity and immunotherapy. Nat Rev Immunol 6:295–307
12. Battelli E, Oukka M, Kuchroo VK (2007) TH-17 cells in the circle of immunity and autoimmunity. Nat Immunol 8:345–350
13. Kasid A, Bell GI, Director EP (1988) Effects of transforming growth factor-beta on human lymphokine-activated killer cell precursors: autocrine inhibition of cellular proliferation and differentiation to immune killer cells. J Immunol 141:690–695
14. Moore KW, O'Garra A, de Waal-Malefyt R et al (1993) Interleukin-10. Annu Rev Immunol 11:165–172
15. Kishimoto T (1989) The biology of interleukin-6. Blood 74:1–10
16. Kunutso KL, Disis ML, Salazar LG (2007) CD4 regulatory T cells in human cancer pathogenesis. Cancer Immunol Immunother 556:2471–2485
17. Cesana GC, De Raffaele G, Cohen S et al (2006) Characterization of CD4+CD25+ regulatory T cells in patients treated with high-dose interleukin-2 for metastatic melanoma or renal cell carcinoma. J Clin Oncol 24: 1169–1177
18. Foon KA (1989) Biological response modifiers: the new immunotherapy. Cancer Res 49:1621–1627
19. Gabrilovich SI, Chen HL, Girgis KR et al (1996) Production of vascular endothelial growth factor by human tumor inhibits the functional maturation of dendritic cells. Nat Med 2:1096–1103
20. Plotnikoff NP, Miller GC (1983) Enkephalins as immunomodulators. Int J Immunopharmacol 5:437–442
21. Grotenhermen F (2004) Pharmacology of cannabinoids. Neuroendocrinol Lett 25:14–22
22. Regelson W, Pierpaoli W (1987) Melatonin: a rediscovered antitumor hormone? Cancer Invest 5:379–385
23. Sze SF, Ng TB, Liu WK (1993) Antiproliferative effect of pineal indoles on cultured tumor cell lines. J Pineal Res 14:27–33
24. Riesco A (1970) Five-year cancer cure: relation to total amount of peripheral lymphocytes and neutrophils. Cancer 25:135–140
25. Broder S, Muul L, Waidmann TA (1978) Suppressor cells in neoplastic disease. J Natl Cancer Inst 61:5–11
26. Sacerdote P, Panerai A (1999) Role of opioids in the modulation of TH1/TH2 responses. Neuroimmunomodulation 6:422–423
27. Schwartz RH (2005) Natural regulatory T cells and self-tolerance. Nat Immunol 6:326–330
28. Mormont MC, Levi F (1997) Circadian system alterations during cancer processes: a review. Int J Cancer 70:241–247
29. Wittington R, Fauldsm D (1993) Interleukin-2. Drugs 46:4466–4483
30. Lissoni P, Brivio F, Fumagalli L et al (2008) Neuroimmunomodulation in medical Oncology: application of psychoneuroimmunology with subcutaneous low- dose IL-2 and the pineal hormone melatonin in patients with untreatable metastatic solid tumors. Anticancer Res 28:1377–1382
31. Recchia F, Saggio G, Nuzzo A et al (2006) Multicentric phase 2 study of interleukin-2 and 13-cis retinoic acid as maintenance therapy in advanced non-small cell lung cancer. J Immunother 29:87–94
32. Lissoni P (2000) Is there a role for melatonin in supportive care? Support Care Cancer 10: 110–116
33. Conti A, Maestroni GJM (1995) The clinical neuroimmunotherapeutic role of melatonin in Oncology. J Pineal Res 19:103–110
34. Lissoni P, Malugani F, Bordin V et al (2002) A new neuroimmunotherapeutic strategy of subcutaneous low-dose interleukin-2 plus the long-acting opioid antagonist naltrexone in metastatic cancer patients progressing on interleukin-2 alone. Neuro Endocrinol Lett 23:255–258
35. Lissoni P, Pittalis S, Rovelli F et al (1995) Interleukin-2, melatonin and interleukin-12 as a possible neuroimmune combination in the biotherapy of cancer. J Biol Regul Homeost Agents 9:63–66

Chapter 11

Aging Microglia: Relevance to Cognition and Neural Plasticity

Rachel A. Kohman

Abstract

Over the years it has become evident that the immune system can affect the function of the central nervous system (CNS), including altering cognitive processes. The impact of immune activation on the CNS is particularly important for aged individuals, as the brain's resident immune cells, microglia, acquire a pro-inflammatory profile. The low-grade chronic neuroinflammation that develops with normal aging likely contributes to the susceptibility to cognitive deficits and a host of age-related pathologies. Understanding why microglia show increased inflammatory activity (i.e., neuroinflammation) and identifying effective treatments to reduce microglia activation is expected to have beneficial effects on cognitive performance and measures of neural plasticity. However, microglia also promote regeneration after injury. Therefore, effective treatments must dampen inflammatory activity while preserving microglia's neuroprotective function. Discovering factors that induce neuroinflammation and investigating potential preventative therapies is expected to uncover the ways of maintaining normal microglia activity in the aged brain.

Key words: Aged, Neuroinflammation, Learning, Memory, Neurogenesis, Long-term potentiation, Exercise, Nutrition, Microglia, Cytokine

1. Introduction

Increased emphasis is being placed on the immune system's ability to impact health and functioning of the brain. While transient immune activation is generally beneficial, chronic and/or heightened immune activity can disrupt cognitive processes and even be neurotoxic (1). The impact of immune activation on the central nervous system (CNS) is particularly important for aged individuals, as normal aging is associated with development of low-grade chronic inflammation in the CNS. A key player in the development of the age-related increase in neuroinflammation is microglial cells, the brain's resident macrophages. Microglia acquire a pro-inflammatory profile during the aging process and mount a heightened inflammatory response to

Qing Yan (ed.), *Psychoneuroimmunology: Methods and Protocols*, Methods in Molecular Biology, vol. 934,
DOI 10.1007/978-1-62703-071-7_11, © Springer Science+Business Media, LLC 2012

immune activation. These changes in microglia activity are proposed to contribute to age-related cognitive decline, the incidence of neurodegenerative diseases, as well as exaggerate the behavioral and cognitive deficits following infection. As the number of individuals surviving into old age continues to increase, the need to identify the mediating factors of the age-related changes in immune activity and potential treatments to slow or prevent its onset is crucial for ensuring healthy aging and reducing health care costs.

The present chapter reviews age-related changes in microglia activity with an emphasis on the neural alterations and functional consequences of increased microglia activity associated with aging, as these changes have been suggested to contribute to age-related cognitive decline, frailty, disease progression, and alterations in mood. Additionally, we discuss how changes in immune activity in the brain may exacerbate the behavioral and cognitive effects of immune activation. Lastly, we explore the utility of non-drug based therapies (i.e., aerobic exercise and diet) to attenuate chronic neuroinflammation. The potential benefits of developing efficacious treatments for reducing neuroinflammation are vast. In the context of aging, anti-inflammatory treatments are expected to improve an individual's quality of life by improving general health, reducing the incidence of cognitive deficits, and decreasing the risk of neurodegeneration.

2. Microglia Phenotypes and Functional Roles

Microglial cells are the primary mediators of the innate immune response within the brain. They are estimated to make up approximately 10% of the total glial cell population in the mouse brain (2). Though microglia are distributed throughout the brain, certain regions such the hippocampal formation, striatum, and olfactory telencephalon have the highest densities in adulthood (3, 4). For example, in the mouse brain cortical areas showed densities around 9–13% while the dentate gyrus showed more than 15% of the total area was occupied by microglia (2). Whether the differences in microglia distribution are related to cell function is unknown, but may suggest that brain regions with higher densities may be more vulnerable to inflammatory events.

In a normal (i.e., uninjured) adult brain, microglial cells remain in a "resting" state. Resting microglia display a ramified morphology, consisting of many fine processes and a small cell body (5). In contrast to the name, resting microglia are not inactive, but rather the cellular processes are constantly surveying the surrounding extracellular space for any indication of infection or injury (6). Though we are far from understanding the complete role of microglial cells in the healthy brain, extensive research has focused on microglia that have undergone "activation." Microglia are a plastic group of cells that rapidly respond to changes in the environment by undergoing morphological changes and the release of cytoactive agents (5). For the sake of brevity, we will discuss activated microglia in two categories: classical activation and alternative activation. Classically activated cells express a proinflammatory phenotype whereas alternatively active cells participate in regenerative processes. Microglia activation should be conceived of as a range of activation rather than a simple on/off process, as cells may display some but not all characteristics associated with the classic or alternative phenotype. Under some condition cells may be able to express features of both phenotypes (7). How readily microglia can switch phenotypes has not been fully determined.

Classically activated microglia mediate the inflammatory response in the brain. In response to an injury or infection microglia acquire a reactive inflammatory phenotype, proliferate, and release inflammatory molecules. One of the initial features of the microglia inflammatory response is increased proliferation to ensure sufficient numbers of microglia to combat the threat. Additionally, microglia undergo morphological changes, as the processes are reacted and thicken and the cells become amoeboid-like in appearance (8, 9). Substantial changes in the expression of membrane-bound proteins accompany this transformation, as microglia upregulate expression of the major histocompatibility complex (MHC) molecules I and MHC II. Many of the activation-associated molecules are expressed at low levels in the resting state but are upregulated following activation such as MHC II, ionized calcium binding adaptor (Iba1), cluster of differentiation 86 (CD86), CD11b, CD68, and CD45 (4). As a means of coordinating the immune response, microglia secrete a host of signaling molecules including the proinflammatory cytokines interleukin-1β (IL-1β), IL-6, tumor necrosis factor-α (TNF-α) as well as chemokines, reactive oxygen species, nitric oxide, and prostaglandins (4, 10). Once the threat has been eliminated, microglia return to the resting surveillance state and reduce in numbers via programmed cell death (11, 12). While the inflammatory response mounted by microglia has the potential to be neurotoxic, particularly if prolonged, transient activation of microglia is generally beneficial and helps restore brain homeostasis by eliminating threats that could damage the brain.

In the alternatively activated form, microglia participate in wound healing, regenerative processes and can actively suppress inflammatory processes (13). Often the expression of the alternative phenotype is a compensatory response that follows the initial inflammatory response following injury as an attempt to restore homeostatic balance and facilitate repair (5, 13). The anti-inflammatory cytokines interleukin-4 (IL-4) and interleukin-13 (IL-13) are primary stimuli for inducing the alternative phenotype (7, 13–15).

Much of what we know about the alternative phenotype is based on work with macrophage cells, microglia's peripherally located relatives, and many of the identifying markers/antigens of alternative activation are common to both macrophages and microglia. For instance, increased expression of arginase 1 (AG1), mannose receptor (MRC1), peroxisome proliferation activation receptor gamma (PPAR-γ), Ym1 (Chitinase 3-like 3), and found in inflammatory zone 1 (FIZZ1) are markers of alternative activation (7, 13, 14, 16–18). Further, alternative activation is associated with increased expression of the anti-inflammatory cytokines interleukin-10 (IL-10), transforming growth factor-β (TGF-β), and growth factors such as insulin-like growth factor (IGF), nerve growth factor (NGF), and brain-derived neural growth factor (BDNF) (13, 17, 19, 20). The collective release of these factors fosters repair and reconstructive processes through regulating activity of the immune system, metabolic processes, and stimulating growth.

Recent work using animal disease models indicates alternatively activated microglia are important for limiting neurodegeneration (7, 21). For example, in a mouse model of multiple sclerosis (MS) deficiencies in IL-4 levels, the stimulus for alternative activation lead to faster onset of symptoms, increased numbers of infiltrating lymphocytes and classically activated microglia (7). Additionally, alternatively activated microglia may be protective in models of Alzheimer's disease (13, 21, 22). For example, Jimenez et al. (22) reported that alternatively activated microglia congregate around β-amyloid (Aβ) plaques in a transgenic mouse model of Alzheimer's disease and concluded that these cells may aid in removing Aβ plaques. Reducing the Aβ load may help limit inflammation and cell death, as Aβ can induce an inflammatory response from microglia (4). Given the protective role alternatively activated microglia play, identifying ways of enhancing the expression of the alternative microglia phenotype may be beneficial for slowing the progression of multiple sclerosis and potentially other diseases.

3. Age-Associated Changes in Microglia Phenotype

A large body of research has established that microglia from healthy aged animals express features associated with the classic inflammatory phenotype (10, 23–26). For instance, aged animals in the absence of any obvious neural pathology show increased expression of MHC II molecules; this increase has been observed in rodents, monkeys, and humans (24, 26–29). Though increases in MHC II molecules can occur in alternatively activated microglia, the additional evidence of increased basal expression of the proinflammatory cytokines IL-1β, IL-6, and TNF-α confirms that aging enhances the inflammatory phenotype (23, 24, 26, 30–32). Additionally, microglia from aged animals show increased expression of ED1 macrophage antigen, CD4, and leukocyte common antigen (26, 33, 34). It is important to note that the magnitude of microglia activation in aged animals is lower than microglia activation induced by an immune challenge. However, the chronic nature of the age-related activation likely contributes to the deleterious effects.

As noted, one feature of microglia activation is an increase in cell proliferation. While the data are limited, there is evidence that aging increases microglia proliferation. For example, Rozovsky et al. (35) found that cultured microglial cells isolated from the cerebral cortex of aged rats show increased proliferation relative to young rats. Similarly in the retina, microglia proliferation was increased in 10-month-old mice compared to 4-month-old mice (36). In a model of peripheral nerve injury, aged rats showed a similar increase in microglia proliferation during the first 3 days following injury relative to young rats. However, on the fourth day postinjury young rats showed a reduction in microglia proliferation, whereas aged rats showed higher rates of proliferation, indicating that aged animals take longer to terminate the proliferation response once initiated (37). In agreement, work from our laboratory found increased microglia proliferation in the dentate gyrus of aged mice compared to adult mice (38). Whether this age-related increase in microglia proliferation results in an increase in the total number of microglia in the brain or particular regions is a matter of debate. One study reported that stereological analysis revealed no age-related differences in the number of microglia in the hippocampus of C57BL/6J male mice, as less than a 10% increase was found in the aged compared to young mice (39). However, a separate study conducted by the same group of researchers found approximately a 20% increase in the number of new microglia in the dentate gyrus and CA1 region of the hippocampus in female C57BL/6JNNIA mice (40). These data indicate that sex differences exist, but whether strain differences also exist has not been investigated. Further work is needed to clarify whether the total number of microglia increases in the aged brain. Alternatively, age-related increases in proliferation may be accompanied by increased microglial cell death; indicating that the turn-over of microglia may increase in the aged while the total number would remain relatively similar to younger subjects. Regardless, the age-associated increase in microglia proliferation provides additional evidence that microglia undergo a host of changes in response to aging.

Lastly, aging is reported to induce morphological changes in microglia. For example, microglia in aged animals show increased volume of their cytoplasm as well as an increase in the density of lectin staining (37). Research has demonstrated that microglia take on the characteristics of activated microglia, namely, shorter processes and increased cytoplasm (37, 41). Microglia from aged animals also show increased number of vacuoles and inclusion bodies in the processes containing partially degraded material, indicating that microglia may be engaged in phagocytosis (41–43). It is important to note that morphological features alone is neither necessary nor sufficient to reveal activation status, as microglia can release cytoactive agents in the absence of morphological changes (44) though the observation in conjunction with other measures of activation is convincing evidence that aging primes microglia toward the classically activated phenotype.

3.1. Age-Related Changes in Microglia Regulation

Currently, the stimulus or events responsible for initiating microglia priming during aging is unknown. One possibility is that the lifelong removal of cellular debris is the underlying cause of microglia priming, as microglia may be activated by factors released by dying cells in the brain (10). Alternatively, irregular protein assembly can initiate microglia activation, a common feature of many neurodegenerative diseases (45). Microglia may be subject to senescence like majority of cells in the body. Streit (46) has proposed the microglia dysfunction hypothesis that suggests that one impact of aging is an increase in microglia dystrophy, as microglia show an increase in abnormal morphology such as twisted processes and cytoplasmic irregularities. These abnormal microglia have been observed in the brain of non-demented aged individuals, but the numbers of dystrophic microglia increase substantially when ongoing neurodegeneration is taking place (46). The age-related sensitization may result from one or a combination of these events that increase the release of inflammatory molecules or impair the ability of microglia, possibly via microglial cell death, to effectively defend the CNS. Ultimately creating an environment characterized by inflammation.

The age-related increase in microglia activity may also relate to deficiencies in regulatory mechanisms that normally inhibit microglia. Given the potential damaging effects of inflammation within the brain, regulatory mechanisms exist to maintain microglia in the "resting" state and inhibit activation. For instance neurons and astrocytes release substances that actively inhibit microglia activation. The best characterized example is CD200, a member of the immunoglobulin superfamily of membrane glycoproteins, which is considered a neuroimmune regulatory molecule. CD200 is released by neurons as well as astrocytes and subsequently binds to it cognate receptor CD200R that is expressed by microglia (47). Neurons are able to help maintain microglia in their quiescent or resting state through activation of the CD200R (47, 48). Mice deficient for CD200 show increased microglia division, as measured by co-labeling with the cellular proliferation marker Ki67 (49). Additionally, microglia from these CD200 deficient mice display characteristics associated with classic activation (48), indicating that CD200 is an important molecule in controlling microglia activation. Aged mice show reduced expression of CD200 (24), indicating that neurons have less regulatory control over microglia activation.

In addition to CD200, other neuroimmune regulators show reduced expression with aging. For instance, the chemokine CX3CL1 (also known as fractalkine and neurotactin) is present at reduced levels in aged mice compared to adult mice (50). Similar to CD200, fractalkine is released by neurons and its receptor is expressed on microglia (51). Fractalkine represents another system through which neurons can regulate immune activity within the brain. However, the effectiveness of this pathway seems to decline with age as aged animals show reduced expression of fractalkine within the brain that correlates with increased microglia activation (50, 52, 53). Administering fractalkine to aged mice has been shown to reduce microglia activation, indicating that the reduction in fractalkine levels is a key component of the age-induced changes in microglia. Further, blocking the activity of fractalkine by administering a fractalkine receptor antibody increases expression of MCH II and IL-1β in adult animals, confirming that reducing fractalkine activity increases microglia activation. Additional work has shown that in response to an immune challenge aged mice produce reduced amounts of fractalkine compared to adult mice (50). Immune activation reduces expression of the fractalkine receptor on microglia, but in aged mice there is a prolonged decrease in receptor expression (50). The prolonged decrease in the fractalkine receptor coupled with the reduced levels of the fractalkine ligand creates a weak regulatory mechanism, leaving microglia to continue to express an inflammatory phenotype. Knockout mice that lack the receptor for fractalkine show exaggerated cell death following administration of the neurotoxin, MPTP (1-methyl-4-pheny;-1,2,3,6-tetra-hydropyridine) as well as an enhanced neuroinflammatory response from microglia. These findings potentially indicate that the heightened neuroinflammatory response from microglia contributed to the increase in cell death. Taken together, evidence indicates that the aging brain loses strength in controlling microglia activation, leaving microglia primed toward the inflammatory phenotype that in response to an immune insult results in an exaggerated response.

Microglia show an age-related decrease in sensitivity to substances that regulate microglia activity. For instance, Rozovsky et al. (35) reported that, in culture, microglia from aged rats showed decreased responsiveness to the anti-inflammatory cytokine TGF-β that normally inhibits microglia activation and proliferation. Aged animals have increased basal expression of TGF-β, which may be an attempt to overcome resistance or functional deficiencies in receptor signaling (23). Further, aged mice show reduced hippocampal expression of the anti-inflammatory cytokine IL-4 and increased expression of interferon-γ (IFN-γ) that acts to activate microglia and induce proliferation (54, 55). The imbalance in pro- and anti-inflammatory cytokines that develops with age likely contributes to the deregulated activity of microglia leading to over activation of these cells in the aged brain. Decreases in the inhibitory control from neurons and changes in sensitivity to regulatory factors likely culminate to impair the ability of microglia to maintain normal homeostasis in the aged brain, creating cells that have defaulted or have been induced to express an inflammatory phenotype. We know that neuroinflammation has the potential to profoundly impact normal brain function. Identifying the agent(s) that initiate the age-associated microglia priming and discovering ways to strengthen the compromised regulatory mechanisms will represent a large step forward in the field and will aid in identifying targets for novel pharmaceutical treatments.

4. Behavioral and Cognitive Deficits Following Immune Activation

The communication between the brain and the peripheral immune system allows the body to orchestrate a physiological and behavioral response that facilitates recovery from infection. The behavioral alterations are collectively termed sickness behaviors and include development of a fever and reductions in locomotor activity, social interactions, sexual behavior, and food intake (56–59). The expression of sickness behavior is an adaptive response that reflects a shift in an animal's motivation that aids in recovery from illness, as reducing activity levels help conserve energy.

In addition to inducing sickness behavior, activation of the immune system impairs learning and memory processes (60–64). A host of work has demonstrated that administration of the bacterial endotoxin lipopolysaccharide (LPS) or administration of a live bacterium (e.g., *E. coli*) in adults disrupts acquisition and/or consolidation of new information. Reichenberg et al. (65) report that administration of LPS to human participants disrupts memory, as participants treated with LPS showed an impaired ability to learn a 15 item list of words, remember information from a story, and recall features of the figure compared to control participants. A more recent study reported that administration of LPS has no effect on human memory performance (66). However, this study administered half of the dose of LPS used in the Reichenberg study, indicating that the effects may be dose dependent.

Studies conducted with non-human animals reveal that tasks that engage the hippocampus are particularly sensitive to disruption following an immune challenge. Two commonly used behavioral tasks are auditory and context fear conditioning and the Morris water maze. In the fear conditioning paradigm, a novel context or a tone is paired with a mildly aversive footshock. Animals that have learned the task will display a fear response (i.e., freezing) when presented with the tone or placed back into the shock-paired context. The hippocampus is involved in learning the association between the context and footshock, but plays no role in learning the tone-shock association. Pugh et al. (63) report that LPS administration selectively impaired memory consolidation in a contextual fear conditioning task, but had no effect on auditory fear conditioning an effect later replicated by Thomson et al. (64). Additionally, several reports observed deficits in spatial learning in the water maze following immune activation (62, 67, 68). The water maze is a hippocampus-dependent task, in which animals must learn to locate a submerged platform by using spatial cues located around the testing room. Collectively the data suggest that immune activation disrupts performance on tasks that engage the hippocampus.

Caution must be taken when interpreting the cognitive effects of immune activation, as the accompanying sickness behaviors may influence performance in behavior tests independent of cognitive ability. Though researchers must be mindful many papers have convincingly demonstrated that cognitive deficits cannot be completely explained by sickness behavior. For instance, in adult animals sickness behavior persists for approximately 24 h after LPS administration whereas cognitive deficits are observed well beyond this time frame (60). Additionally, LPS administration was shown to disrupt acquisition of an autoshaping task, in which rats learned to press a lever for food. However, if the rats were allowed to acquire the task prior to LPS administration LPS has no effects on performance, indicating that sickness behavior cannot fully explain the performance decrements (69).

The cognitive deficits associated with immune activation have been attributed to increased levels of proinflammatory cytokines, particularly IL-1β, within the brain that are primarily released by microglia (70, 71). Inhibiting cytokine activity in the brain of adult animals has been found to block some of the cognitive deficits that result from an immune stimulus (63, 72). Additionally, similar deficits are observed following direct administration of cytokines (70). Interestingly, basal levels of cytokines are required for normal cognitive function, as inhibiting basal IL-1β levels disrupt memory formation (71, 73). These data indicate that there is an optimal range of cytokine levels in the brain and if the levels drop below or exceed the normal levels cognitive performance may be at risk.

4.1. Aging Exaggerates the Behavioral and Cognitive Response to Immune Activation

One consequence of the age-related priming of microglial cells is alterations in the response to infection. As noted, activation of microglia and the behavioral changes induced by the cytokines they release are generally beneficial and facilitate recovery. However, if the microglia response becomes abnormal (inhibited or exaggerated) the impact can be deleterious. Aging appears to be an instance when microglia display heightened activation in response to an immune stimulus. For example, researchers have consistently shown that aged animals show prolonged proinflammatory cytokine production in the brain following LPS administration. In adults, cytokine levels in the brain return to baseline levels within 24 h, whereas aged animals continue to show increased cytokine levels (30, 50, 74). Some report that in addition to the increase in duration of cytokine release, aged animals show exaggerated cytokine production compared to younger animals a few hours after LPS administration (75, 76). However, this initial enhancement is not always observed, possibility due to a ceiling effect, or may only occur in some areas of the brain (77, 78), indicating that regional differences in cytokine production may develop with aging. Collectively these data highlight that priming of microglia during the aging process sets up the brain to initiate an exaggerated and prolonged immune response in an environment that may be less able to terminate the response.

Not surprisingly, the age-related change in the neuroinflammatory response prolongs the expression of sickness-associated behaviors that are mediated by proinflammatory cytokines following immune activation (30, 74, 78, 79). For example, Godbout et al. (30) reported that mice aged 20–24 months showed prolonged reductions in social exploration and locomotor activity following LPS administration in comparison with young mice. More recent work has shown that immune activation similarly extends the duration of depression-like behavior in aged mice, as only aged mice show increased immobility in the forced swim and tail suspension test 72 h after LPS administration whereas young mice have recovered (79). Evidence that these exaggerated behavioral deficits are mediated by cytokine activity comes from studies that have found inhibiting IL-1β prevents the prolonged sickness behavior in aged animals (74). Additionally, administration of minocycline, a tetracycline-derived antibiotic that inhibits microglia activation, facilitates recovery from sickness behaviors in adult mice and attenuates LPS-induced cytokine expression in the hippocampus of aged mice (76). Ultimately, the evidence indicates that aging exacerbates the time course of sickness associated behaviors that normally show a transient expression and these behavioral abnormalities seem to result from increased and prolonged activation of microglia in the brain.

In addition to extending the duration of sickness behaviors, aging increases the sensitivity to cytokine-induced cognitive deficits. In comparison with younger animals, immune activation induces greater deficits in learning and memory processes in aged animals (75, 77, 80, 81). Aged mice show greater impairments in working memory following LPS administration in a matching-to-place test in a radial arm water maze compared to younger mice (75). These deficits were seen in conjunction with increased expression of IL-1β, IL-6, and TNF-α and enhanced staining for microglia in the hippocampus of aged mice. This increased sensitivity to LPS-induced cognitive deficits may occur as early as middle-age, as year-old animals display enhanced learning deficits compared to adults, but only following repeated administration of LPS (82). Several reports have shown that changes in immune activity within the brain can occur as early as middle age (83, 84) and continue to progress as the organism ages, these changes likely contribute to the increased vulnerability to cognitive deficits. Overall the findings indicate that age-related changes in microglia lead to a prolonged neuroinflammatory response to immune signals from the periphery that increases susceptibility to cytokine-induced cognitive deficits.

4.2. The Role of Inflammation in Age-Related Cognitive Decline

Normal aging is often accompanied by a decline in cognitive function. These age-related deficits in cognitive performance are not a global reduction in all aspects of cognitive function, but rather selective processes seem to be vulnerable to aging. For instance aging is associated with a decline in executive processes including working memory deficits (85). Additionally, processing speed is reduced in aged individuals as well as impairments in selective attention. In contrast sustained attention (i.e., ability to maintain attention), semantic memory (i.e., memory of facts), and procedural or implicit memory are typically unaffected by aging (85). Generally, age-related deficits in performance are most commonly observed in tasks that are difficult and/or require shifting from one task to another (85). Individuals that show memory deficits that exceed what is normally associated with aging are diagnosed with mild cognitive impairment (MCI). Often these deficits progress to more severe forms of dementia including Alzheimer's disease.

One distinct possibility is that the age-associated development of mild chronic inflammation within the brain contributes to cognitive decline, and possibly the progression to more severe deficits such as MCI and dementia. As noted, activation of the immune system, through the release of proinflammatory cytokines, is known to disrupt cognitive performance (10, 60, 61, 63). A major source of inflammatory molecules within the brain is microglial cells, which as previously described acquire an inflammatory profile in aged subjects. Currently, it is unknown whether increased inflammation is a normal part of the aging process or whether these elevations result from sub-clinical infections. Research conducted with humans has shown that increased plasma levels of proinflammatory cytokines, particularly IL-6, IL-1β, and TNF-α, are associated with cognitive impairments (86–88). For example, a prospective study by Yaffe et al. (87) compared the preservation of cognitive function over a 2-year period in elderly (average age of 74) males with and without a diagnosis of metabolic syndrome, a condition characterized by abdominal obesity, hypertension, hyperglycemia, hypertriglyceridemia, and low high-density lipoprotein.

Participants were assessed for plasma levels of the inflammatory molecules C-reactive protein (CRP) and IL-6. Cognitive function was measured at multiple points in the study by the Teng Modified Mini-Mental State Examination test. Findings revealed that individuals with metabolic syndrome showed a greater decline in cognitive performance 2 years after the baseline assessment. However, this was only true in participants that also showed high serum levels of CRP and IL-6. These findings highlight that expression of inflammatory molecules positively correlate with the progression of cognitive deficits. Additionally, research has shown that individuals suffering from dementia show increased plasma levels of TNF-α and IL-1β (88, 89). Associations between elevated levels of peripheral IL-6 and cognitive impairments are more reliably observed than other cytokines, potentially indicating a special role for IL-6 in mediating age-related cognitive decline.

The relevance of peripheral cytokine measures to levels in the brain is of particular importance for the work conducted with humans, as inflammation must also exist in the brain to mediate the cognitive alterations. Prior work has confirmed that cytokines produced within the periphery can gain access to the brain via active transport across the blood brain barrier (BBB), entering at the circumventricular organs that lack the BBB, or inducing *de novo* cytokine production within the brain, particularly from microglia (90–92). Clearly, changes in peripheral cytokine levels can influence inflammation within the brain, suggesting that increased cytokine levels in the peripherally may elevate cytokines within the brain. Post-mortem analysis of cytokine levels in the brains of Alzheimer's patients has shown a marked increase in levels of IL-β (93) and IL-6 (94). Additionally, TNF-α levels are significantly elevated in the cerebral spinal fluid of Alzheimer's patients relative to controls (95). Furthermore, a recent study found that 50% of elderly patients with MCI had increased microglia activation compared to controls (96). These findings in conjunction with the work that indicates a long-term use of nonsteroidal anti-inflammatory drugs (NSAID) offers protection against the development of Alzheimer's disease (97) support the hypothesis that inflammation mediated by microglia in the brain may contribute to age-related cognitive decline and the development of dementia.

In agreement with the human literature, research on aged animals has shown age-related deficits in performing spatial learning, working memory, and associative learning tasks (83, 84, 98). Research has shown that aged animals show exaggerated cognitive deficits following an immune challenge, but whether basal changes in immune activity in the brain contributes to the cognitive deficits in aged animals has not been established. However, treatments that reduce markers of inflammation within the brain are often associated with improvements in cognitive function in aged animals. Currently the most convincing study was conducted by Gemma et al. (25) who demonstrated that chronic infusion of a capase-1 inhibitor into the lateral ventricles improved memory in a context fear conditioning task. Capase-1 is an enzyme that cleaves the pro-form of IL-1β into the active mature form. Inhibition of capase-1 via an antagonist results in reduced levels of active IL-1β within the brain. Gemma et al. (25) report that reducing levels of IL-1β that were elevated in the hippocampus of aged rats via the caspase-1 inhibitor restored performance in a contextual, but not auditory fear conditioning paradigm to levels similar to young rats. These findings suggest that basal elevations in cytokine levels in aged animals may contribute to selective cognitive impairments, as reducing IL-1β levels only improved memory for the hippocampus-dependent task. The hippocampal specificity offers further validity to these results, as in adult animals activation of the immune system produces deficits only in contextual and not auditory conditioning (63, 64), indicating that inflammation in the aged brain may contribute to selective cognitive deficits that involve the hippocampus.

5. Effects of Inflammation on Neuroplasticity

The current literature suggests that the age-related increase in neuroinflammation may contribute to cognitive decline, but the neuromechanisms are unknown. One possibility is that inflammation could impact the capability for plasticity in the brain. Accompanying age-related cognitive deficits are alterations in measures of neural plasticity. For example, aged subjects show deficiencies in adulthood hippocampal neurogenesis and long-term potentiation (LTP) (54, 55, 99). Elucidating the role of neuroinflammation in altering measures of plasticity may further our understanding of how age-related cognitive deficits develop. We briefly cover two forms of neuroplasticity known to show age-related deficits, with an emphasis on the immune systems involvement in these processes (both beneficial and detrimental roles).

5.1. Hippocampal Neurogenesis

Beyond early development only two regions of the brain, the olfactory bulb and the sub-granular zone (SVZ) of the hippocampus, unarguably retain the capacity to generate new neurons throughout life. New hippocampal granule cells result from proliferation of progenitor cells followed by differentiation into neurons and incorporation into hippocampal circuitry. Cells that are not incorporated usually die. A variety of environmental factors can affect the probability that new cells survive and incorporate, one of which is inflammation. These new neurons are suggested to play a role in certain forms of hippocampus-dependent learning and memory (100–104). For instance, many studies show that interventions (e.g., exercise or environment enrichment) that enhance cognitive function also increase hippocampal neurogenesis (100, 105). Furthermore, pharmacological, genetic, or irradiation-induced reductions in hippocampal neurogenesis lead to deficits in hippocampus dependent learning tasks (101, 103, 104). Aged subjects show decreases in both the proliferation and survival of new hippocampal cells, which may contribute to cognitive decline associated with aging (99).

We are just beginning to understand the complex involvement of the immune system in both supporting and impairing hippocampal neurogenesis. Recent evidence indicates that microglia under quiescent (i.e., resting) conditions support hippocampal neurogenesis. For example, cultured neuropoietic cells from the SVZ will eventually lose their ability to proliferate in culture. However, adding microglia or medium from a microglia culture can restore proliferation of these cells, indicating that microglia release factors that facilitate continued neurogenesis (106). Further work has shown that microglia are involved in directing the migration of new cells and can increase the number of cells that differentiate in neurons (107). Microglia play an important role in clearing new cells that do not get incorporated into the granular cell layer via phagocytosis, thereby helping to maintain the microenvironment (108). In an in vivo model, Ziv et al. (109) report that housing animals under enriched environmental conditions enhances both hippocampal neurogenesis as well as microglia proliferation. Additionally, these new microglia were suggested to show the alterative neuroprotective phenotype as they tended to express IGF that is known to promote neurogenesis. Similar effects of microglia were observed in adrenalectomized animals, as the reduction in glucocorticoids significantly increased neurogenesis and activated microglia (110). Following adrenalectomy, microglia showed increased expression of the neuroprotective phenotype and increased expression of the anti-inflammatory cytokine TGF-β (110) that has been found to increase hippocampal neurogenesis if over expressed (111). Collectively, the data indicate that microglia participate in the induction and differentiation of new cells produced in the hippocampus primarily by releasing anti-inflammatory and neuroprotective factors.

In contrast to their supportive role, activation of microglia following an immune challenge is known to inhibit hippocampal neurogenesis via the release of pro-inflammatory cytokines. Classic inflammatory microglia activation is negatively correlated with hippocampal neurogenesis. For example, Ekdahl et al. (112) report that administration of the endotoxin LPS significantly reduced the number of new neurons in the granular cell layer and that this effect was mediated by microglia, as administration of the microglia inhibitor minocycline blocked the reduction in neurogenesis. In agreement, irradiation or LPS-induced reductions in hippocampal neurogenesis can be attenuated by administration of an NSAID (113). Clearly, induction of an inflammatory response within the brain, particularly if prolonged, can impair the ability of the hippocampus to produce new neurons that may have detrimental consequences for cognitive function.

Aged mice show reduced proliferation and survival of new neurons compared to adult mice (99, 114). One mechanism that might contribute to the age-associated deficits in hippocampal neurogenesis could be increased inflammatory signaling in the brain. The age-related reduction in hippocampal neurogenesis is correlated with increased microglia activation and elevated levels of the proinflammatory cytokine IL-1β in the brain (115). Moreover, central administration of a capase-1 inhibitor, that prevents the caspase-1 enzyme from cleaving IL-β into its active form, increased the production of new cells in the hippocampus in aged rats, but not young rats (116). Additionally, inhibiting caspase-1 reduced microglia activation and levels of IL-1β in the hippocampus, indicating that IL-1β likely produced by microglia contributes to the reduction in neurogenesis in the normal aged brain. Additionally, administration of the anti-inflammatory chemokine fractalkine (i.e., CX3CL1 or neurotactin) that helps maintain microglia in a resting state was found to increase hippocampal neurogenesis in aged but not young animals (52). As noted, aged animals show reduced levels of fractalkine, but restoring levels in aged animals reduced microglia activation and subsequently increased neurogenesis. Taken together, the data support the contention that the age-related priming of microglia toward their inflammatory phenotype, possibly through deficiencies in regulatory mechanisms, contributes to the age-associated reduction in hippocampal neurogenesis that may relate to cognitive decline.

5.2. Long-Term Potentiation

Bliss and Lomo (117) demonstrated that stimulating hippocampal fibers with a brief high-frequency stimulus produced an enduring increase in the synaptic strength between the pre- and post-synaptic neurons, a phenomenon termed LTP. After the induction of LTP a fixed stimulus will produce a heightened post-synaptic potential compared to the initial response to the same stimulus. The development of LTP is a calcium-dependent process, thought to be mediated by calcium influx through a sub-type of the glutamate receptor, *N*-methyl d-aspartate (NMDAR). Though an NMDAR-independent form of LTP also exists in which calcium influx occurs through voltage-dependent calcium channels (VDCC). This experience-dependent synaptic modification has been proposed to be a neurobiological correlate of memory formation, as inhibition of LTP impairs performance in a variety of cognitive behavioral tasks (118). Aging is associated with a reduction in the capacity to sustain LTP and may underlie some of the cognitive deficits that develop with normal aging (54, 55, 119, 120).

Induction of microglia activation and proinflammatory cytokines consistently produce impairments in the development of LTP. Chronic infusion of the endotoxin LPS into the fourth ventricle is reported to disrupt both the NMDAR-dependent and NMDAR-independent forms of LTP as well as impair spatial learning ability in the water maze (121). Similarly, systemic bacterial infection with *E.coli* has been reported to reduce LTP in adult rats compared to controls (122). The impairments in LTP following immune activation are likely mediated by the release of proinflammatory cytokines from microglial cells, as elevated levels of IL-1β, TNF-α, and IL-6 inhibit LTP (123, 124). The role of IL-1β is slightly more complex as low levels of IL-1β appear to be necessary to induce LTP, as knockout mice lacking the IL-1 receptor show a complete absence of LTP in the dentate gyrus (73). Additionally, administration of an IL-1 receptor antagonist impairs the maintenance of LTP (125). Taken together, the data indicate that cytokines, particularly IL-1β, participate in synaptic modifications important for cognitive function, but that increases in proinflammatory cytokines following an immune challenge disrupt the induction and maintenance of LTP.

Animal studies provide convincing evidence that the age-related priming of microglia and the slight basal increases in cytokine levels in the brain may contribute to deficits in LTP. For example, Maher et al. (55) identified two distinct subgroups of aged rats, those that showed deficits in LTP maintenance and another group of aged rats that did not differ from young rats. Only the aged rats that failed to sustain LTP showed increased levels of IL-1β, whereas the aged rats with no LTP deficits did not show elevated IL-1β levels. Further age-related deficits in LTP are associated with microglia activation, as 15-month-old rats showed increased expression of the microglia activation markers CD86, CD40, and intercellular adhesion molecule (ICAM) (119). Pretreatment with the microglia inhibitor, minocycline, was reported to partially restore LTP (119). A separate study suggests that age-related elevations in IFN-γ may contribute to the deficits in LTP by activating microglia and inducing their release of IL-1β. Reducing IFN-γ levels was reported to decrease microglia activation, IL-1β levels, and restored the ability of aged rats to sustain LTP (54).

Several studies indicate that decreased expression of the anti-inflammatory cytokine IL-4 contributes to the age-related deficits in LTP maintenance (55, 120). For instance, administration of VPO15 (phospholipids microparticles-incorporating phosphatidylserine), a compound that increases IL-4 levels, blocked the deficits in LTP in both aged and LPS-treated young animals. Additionally, aged animals show reduced expression of IGF that has been shown to attenuate the induction of microglia activation by IFN-γ (54). Collectively, these data indicate that the imbalance between the pro- and anti-inflammatory responses in the brain that develops with normal aging can have detrimental effects on synaptic function.

6. Non-drug Based Interventions to Regulate Microglia

As discussed throughout this chapter anti-inflammatory pharmacological treatments have been shown to offer protection against inflammation-associated cognitive deficits and alterations in measures of synaptic plasticity (126). Additionally, chronic use of anti-inflammatory NSAID is reported to offer protection against the development of neurodegenerative diseases such as Alzheimer's and Parkinson's disease (126). As we further our understanding of the complex role microglia play in maintaining normal brain function as well as their influence on disrupting brain function, it is clear that complete inhibition of microglia may not be an ideal therapy. While the use of anti-inflammatory compounds will reduce inflammation, whether such drugs also inhibit the regenerative processes associated with alternative microglia activation is unclear. The ideal is identifying a way to reduce inflammation while maintaining or possibly enhancing the neuroprotective properties of microglia. Future research will certainly identify novel targets for drug development that may increase the efficiency of anti-inflammatory drugs in attenuating age-related changes in neuroinflammation.

Lifestyle interventions may be an effective alternative to drug-based therapies to attenuate age-related increases in neuroinflammation as well as cognitive decline. We focus on two therapies, namely nutrition and aerobic exercise, which have shown promise in regulating immune activity within the brain.

6.1. Caloric Restriction and Diet

Reducing caloric intake is a powerful method to combat the aging process. Caloric restriction has been shown to increase life-span as well as slow aspects of the aging process including cognitive deficits and neurodegeneration (127). Retrospective studies have shown that Alzheimer's patients tended to have a higher caloric intake prior to the disease onset, potentially suggesting that reducing calorie intake may reduce the risk of Alzheimer's disease (127, 128).

The beneficial effects of caloric restriction may, in part, result from its anti-inflammatory properties. Caloric restriction decreases the age-related increase in the expression of the microglia markers MHC II, CD11b, complement receptor 3 (CR3), and CD68 in the corpus callosum (129, 130), indicating that caloric restriction attenuates the age-induced activation of microglia. In contrast, mice fed a diet high in fat and cholesterol show increased expression of CD45, a marker of microglia activation and elevated basal expression of the inflammatory cytokines IL-1β, IL-6, and TNF-α compared to mice fed a standard diet (131). Furthermore, mice fed the high fat and cholesterol diet showed impaired working memory in a radial arm water maze, which correlates with enhanced microglia activation and cytokine expression. Collectively, the data support that consumption of a poor diet that is high in fat and/or cholesterol exacerbates neuroinflammation while maintaining a healthy diet may attenuate the age-associated increase in inflammatory signaling in the brain.

An alternative to reducing caloric intake is to change what we eat. Increasing consumption of key nutritional elements may represent an effective way of combating age-related changes in neuroinflammation. Aging has been associated with reduced plasma levels of vitamin C and E, both of which have antioxidant and anti-inflammatory properties (132). For instance, vitamin E has been shown to reduce microglia activation in culture. Microglia pre-incubated with vitamin E showed diminished production of IL-1α, TNF-α, and nitric oxide following LPS exposure compared to cells only incubated with LPS (132). Additionally, increasing consumption of flavonoids, polyphenolic compounds found in many fruits and vegetables may attenuate age-related changes in inflammation. For instance, chronic administration of the flavonoids apigenin or quercetin was reported to have attenuated cognitive deficits in avoidance learning in aged and LPS-treated animals (133). In culture, exposing microglia to the flavonoid, luteolin, prior to LPS exposure reduced microglia release of IL-1β and neuronal cell death, indicating that luteolin is neuroprotective (134). Moreover, aged mice that consumed luteolin showed improved performance in a spatial working memory task and reduced expression of IL-1β, IL-6, and marker MHC II in the hippocampus, indicating the cognitive improvements were associated with a reduction in microglia activation (134).

6.2. Aerobic Exercise

The beneficial effects of engaging in aerobic exercise are vast, as exercise improves cognitive function, efficiency of the vascular system, measures of neural plasticity, and increases production of growth factors that support brain health (99, 100, 103, 105). Overall, increasing physical activity is associated with improved cardiovascular health and a reduction in the risk of developing several age-related pathologies such as Alzheimer's and Parkinson's diseases, metabolic syndrome, and diabetes (135, 136). Additionally, aged individuals that had a high level of aerobic fitness had a larger hippocampal volume and improved spatial memory compared to aged individuals with a low level of physical fitness (137). Furthermore, engaging in exercise is reported to slow the progression of cognitive decline in Alzheimer's patients and improve the initiation of movement in Parkinson's patients (136). The preventive and regenerative effects of exercise likely result from the broad physiological changes induced by exercise, including increasing production of growth factors and improving cardiovascular function (136). In addition, exercise-induced changes in immune function are suggested to contribute to the beneficial effects of exercise.

A wealth of evidence indicates that increasing physical activity enhances immune function and facilitates recovery from infection (135). These effects are particularly evident in aged individuals, as exercise has been reported to increase anti-inflammatory cytokines and enhance macrophage phagocytic activity in aged subjects (138, 139). Exercise has well-known immunomodulatory effects within the peripheral nervous system. However, the ability of exercise to modulate immune activity within the CNS has not been thoroughly investigated. Prior work found that treadmill running decreases hippocampal levels of IL-1β (140). A recent study reported that 2 weeks of voluntary wheel running attenuated neuron cell death following administration of trimethyltin, a chemical that induces cell death in the granule cell layer of the hippocampus (141). The protective effects of exercise were proposed to be mediated by increased production of IL-6, as knockout mice deficient in IL-6 failed to show the protective effects of exercise. Though IL-6 is classically considered a pro-inflammatory cytokine, it also has anti-inflammatory properties depending on the signaling pathway activated (142). Evidence that IL-6 mediates some of the anti-inflammatory effects of exercise comes from work by Starkie et al. (143) who reported that exercising for 3 h or an intravenous IL-6 infusion equally attenuated endotoxin-induced increases in TNF-α. The exercise-induced changes in the immune system appear to enhance the overall efficiency of the immune system in defending against an infection, as well as offer some protection against neuronal damage induced by inflammation.

Increasing physical activity has direct effects on microglial cell activity. For example, Ang et al. (144) report that 12 weeks of treadmill running decreased the number of microglia in the septum. Additionally, wheel running decreased the number of new born microglia in the amygdala compared to sedentary mice (145). However, these effects may depend on the brain region assessed and the duration of training, as others report that exercise increases microglia proliferation in the cingulate and motor cortex (146). In the transgenic NSE/*htau*23 mouse model of Alzheimer's disease treadmill running is reported to attenuate the age-dependent increase in microglia activation as measured by staining intensity of CD11b. Aged transgenic mice show increased number of CD11b positive cells in the hippocampus, but exercise reduced the number of CD11b positive cells. Converging evidence that exercise modulates microglial cell activity comes from studies evaluating age-related changes in gene expression using microarray technology. Overwhelmingly, studies report that genes related to inflammation show increased expression in the aged brain compared to young mice (30, 84, 147, 148). Wheel running attenuates expression of many of the inflammatory-related genes that increase with age (147, 148). Additionally, work by Ziv et al. (109) indicated that exposure to an enriched environment that contained a running wheel tended to increase microglia expression of IGF, potentially indicating that microglia shifted toward the alternative neuroprotective phenotype. Collectively, the data indicate that aerobic exercise may be an effective way to attenuate neuroinflammation in the aged brain.

7. Conclusions and Perspectives

Normal aging in the absence of disease increases microglia activation, as these cells appear to be primed toward the inflammatory phenotype. The age-related shift in microglia can lead to increased basal cytokine levels in the brain as well as a heightened and prolonged inflammatory response to injury or infection. Although the mechanisms that initiate these changes in microglia in the aged brain are unknown, it appears that an imbalance in pro-inflammatory and anti-inflammatory molecules contributes to maintaining microglia in their primed state. Neurons appear to lose their ability to regulate microglia activation and levels of anti-inflammatory cytokines are reduced in the aged brain. The age-related changes in microglia likely contribute to the increased vulnerability to age-related cognitive decline and neurodegeneration, particularly following an immune challenge. Future work is needed to identify effective interventions to modulate microglia activity in the aged brain. Optimal therapies would attenuate the overactive inflammatory phenotype associated with aging, while maintaining the cells' ability to initiate a normal inflammatory response in the face of an infection or injury and express the neuroprotective phenotype to support brain health.

References

1. Basu A, Lazovic J, Krady JK, Mauger DT, Rothstein RP, Smith MB et al (2005) Interleukin-1 and the interleukin-1 type 1 receptor are essential for the progressive neurodegeneration that ensues subsequent to a mild hypoxic/ischemic injury. J Cereb Blood Flow Metab 25:17–29
2. Lawson LJ, Perry VH, Dri P, Gordon S (1990) Heterogeneity in the distribution and morphology of microglia in the normal adult mouse brain. Neuroscience 39:151–170
3. Benveniste EN (1997) Role of macrophages/microglia in multiple sclerosis and experimental allergic encephalomyelitis. J Mol Med (Berl) 75:165–173
4. Tambuyzer BR, Ponsaerts P, Nouwen EJ (2009) Microglia: gatekeepers of central nervous system immunology. J Leukoc Biol 85: 352–370
5. Kettenmann H, Hanisch UK, Noda M, Verkhratsky A (2011) Physiology of microglia. Physiol Rev 91:461–553
6. Nimmerjahn A, Kirchhoff F, Helmchen F (2005) Resting microglial cells are highly dynamic surveillants of brain parenchyma in vivo. Science 308:1314–1318
7. Ponomarev ED, Maresz K, Tan Y, Dittel BN (2007) CNS-derived interleukin-4 is essential for the regulation of autoimmune inflammation and induces a state of alternative activation in microglial cells. J Neurosci 27:10714–10721
8. Xiang Z, Chen M, Ping J, Dunn P, Lv J, Jiao B et al (2006) Microglial morphology and its transformation after challenge by extracellular ATP in vitro. J Neurosci Res 83:91–101
9. Aloisi F (2001) Immune function of microglia. Glia 36:165–179
10. Dilger RN, Johnson RW (2008) Aging, microglial cell priming, and the discordant central inflammatory response to signals from the peripheral immune system. J Leukoc Biol 84:932–939
11. Jones LL, Banati RB, Graeber MB, Bonfanti L, Raivich G, Kreutzberg GW (1997) Population control of microglia: does apoptosis play a role? J Neurocytol 26:755–770
12. Gehrmann J, Banati RB (1995) Microglial turnover in the injured CNS: activated microglia undergo delayed DNA fragmentation following peripheral nerve injury. J Neuropathol Exp Neurol 54:680–688

13. Colton CA (2009) Heterogeneity of microglial activation in the innate immune response in the brain. J Neuroimmune Pharmacol 4:399–418
14. Kitamura Y, Taniguchi T, Kimura H, Nomura Y, Gebicke-Haerter PJ (2000) Interleukin-4-inhibited mRNA expression in mixed rat glial and in isolated microglial cultures. J Neuroimmunol 106:95–104
15. Butovsky O, Talpalar AE, Ben-Yaakov K, Schwartz M (2005) Activation of microglia by aggregated beta-amyloid or lipopolysaccharide impairs MHC-II expression and renders them cytotoxic whereas IFN-gamma and IL-4 render them protective. Mol Cell Neurosci 29:381–393
16. Raes G, De Baetselier P, Noel W, Beschin A, Brombacher F, Hassanzadeh Gh G (2002) Differential expression of FIZZ1 and Ym1 in alternatively versus classically activated macrophages. J Leukoc Biol 71:597–602
17. Odegaard JI, Ricardo-Gonzalez RR, Goforth MH, Morel CR, Subramanian V, Mukundan L et al (2007) Macrophage-specific PPARgamma controls alternative activation and improves insulin resistance. Nature 447:1116–1120
18. Chang NC, Hung SI, Hwa KY, Kato I, Chen JE, Liu CH et al (2001) A macrophage protein, Ym1, transiently expressed during inflammation is a novel mammalian lectin. J Biol Chem 276:17497–17506
19. Brodie C, Goldreich N, Haiman T, Kazimirsky G (1998) Functional IL-4 receptors on mouse astrocytes: IL-4 inhibits astrocyte activation and induces NGF secretion. J Neuroimmunol 81:20–30
20. Nakajima K, Tohyama Y, Kohsaka S, Kurihara T (2002) Ceramide activates microglia to enhance the production/secretion of brain-derived neurotrophic factor (BDNF) without induction of deleterious factors in vitro. J Neurochem 80:697–705
21. Butovsky O, Koronyo-Hamaoui M, Kunis G, Ophir E, Landa G, Cohen H et al (2006) Glatiramer acetate fights against Alzheimer's disease by inducing dendritic-like microglia expressing insulin-like growth factor 1. Proc Natl Acad Sci U S A 103:11784–11789
22. Jimenez S, Baglietto-Vargas D, Caballero C, Moreno-Gonzalez I, Torres M, Sanchez-Varo R et al (2008) Inflammatory response in the hippocampus of PS1M146L/APP751SL mouse model of Alzheimer's disease: age-dependent switch in the microglial phenotype from alternative to classic. J Neurosci 28:11650–11661
23. Sierra A, Gottfried-Blackmore AC, McEwen BS, Bulloch K (2007) Microglia derived from aging mice exhibit an altered inflammatory profile. Glia 55:412–424
24. Frank MG, Barrientos RM, Biedenkapp JC, Rudy JW, Watkins LR, Maier SF (2006) mRNA up-regulation of MHC II and pivotal pro-inflammatory genes in normal brain aging. Neurobiol Aging 27:717–722
25. Gemma C, Bickford PC (2007) Interleukin-1beta and caspase-1: players in the regulation of age-related cognitive dysfunction. Rev Neurosci 18:137–148
26. Perry VH, Matyszak MK, Fearn S (1993) Altered antigen expression of microglia in the aged rodent CNS. Glia 7:60–67
27. Streit WJ, Sparks DL (1997) Activation of microglia in the brains of humans with heart disease and hypercholesterolemic rabbits. J Mol Med 75:130–138
28. Sheffield LG, Berman NE (1998) Microglial expression of MHC class II increases in normal aging of nonhuman primates. Neurobiol Aging 19:47–55
29. Sloane JA, Hollander W, Moss MB, Rosene DL, Abraham CR (1999) Increased microglial activation and protein nitration in white matter of the aging monkey. Neurobiol Aging 20:395–405
30. Godbout JP, Chen J, Abraham J, Richwine AF, Berg BM, Kelley KW et al (2005) Exaggerated neuroinflammation and sickness behavior in aged mice following activation of the peripheral innate immune system. FASEB J 19:1329–1331
31. Ye SM, Johnson RW (1999) Increased interleukin-6 expression by microglia from brain of aged mice. J Neuroimmunol 93:139–148
32. McLinden KA, Kranjac D, Deodati LE, Kahn M, Chumley MJ, Boehm GW (2012) Age exacerbates sickness behavior following exposure to a viral mimetic. Physiol Behav 105(5):1219–1225
33. Kullberg S, Aldskogius H, Ulfhake B (2001) Microglial activation, emergence of ED1-expressing cells and clusterin upregulation in the aging rat CNS, with special reference to the spinal cord. Brain Res 899:169–186
34. Conde JR, Streit WJ (2006) Microglia in the aging brain. J Neuropathol Exp Neurol 65: 199–203
35. Rozovsky I, Finch CE, Morgan TE (1998) Age-related activation of microglia and astrocytes: in vitro studies show persistent phenotypes of aging, increased proliferation, and resistance to down-regulation. Neurobiol Aging 19:97–103
36. Inman DM, Horner PJ (2007) Reactive nonproliferative gliosis predominates in a chronic mouse model of glaucoma. Glia 55:942–953

37. Conde JR, Streit WJ (2006) Effect of aging on the microglial response to peripheral nerve injury. Neurobiol Aging 27:1451–1461
38. Kohman RA, DeYoung EK, Bhattacharya TK, Peterson LN, Rhodes JS (2012) Wheel running attenuates microglia proliferation and increases expression of a proneurogenic phenotype in the hippocampus of aged mice. Brain Behav Immun 26:803–810
39. Long JM, Kalehua AN, Muth NJ, Calhoun ME, Jucker M, Hengemihle JM et al (1998) Stereological analysis of astrocyte and microglia in aging mouse hippocampus. Neurobiol Aging 19:497–503
40. Mouton PR, Long JM, Lei DL, Howard V, Jucker M, Calhoun ME et al (2002) Age and gender effects on microglia and astrocyte numbers in brains of mice. Brain Res 956:30–35
41. Vaughan DW, Peters A (1974) Neuroglial cells in the cerebral cortex of rats from young adulthood to old age: an electron microscope study. J Neurocytol 3:405–429
42. Peters A, Sethares C (2002) The effects of age on the cells in layer 1 of primate cerebral cortex. Cereb Cortex 12:27–36
43. Peters A, Josephson K, Vincent SL (1991) Effects of aging on the neuroglial cells and pericytes within area 17 of the rhesus monkey cerebral cortex. Anat Rec 229:384–398
44. Cunningham C, Wilcockson DC, Campion S, Lunnon K, Perry VH (2005) Central and systemic endotoxin challenges exacerbate the local inflammatory response and increase neuronal death during chronic neurodegeneration. J Neurosci 25:9275–9284
45. Walker LC, LeVine H (2000) The cerebral proteopathies: neurodegenerative disorders of protein conformation and assembly. Mol Neurobiol 21:83–95
46. Streit WJ, Xue QS (2009) Life and death of microglia. J Neuroimmune Pharmacol 4: 371–379
47. Broderick C, Hoek RM, Forrester JV, Liversidge J, Sedgwick JD, Dick AD (2002) Constitutive retinal CD200 expression regulates resident microglia and activation state of inflammatory cells during experimental autoimmune uveoretinitis. Am J Pathol 161: 1669–1677
48. Hoek RM, Ruuls SR, Murphy CA, Wright GJ, Goddard R, Zurawski SM et al (2000) Down-regulation of the macrophage lineage through interaction with OX2 (CD200). Science 290:1768–1771
49. Deckert M, Sedgwick JD, Fischer E, Schluter D (2006) Regulation of microglial cell responses in murine Toxoplasma encephalitis by CD200/CD200 receptor interaction. Acta Neuropathol 111:548–558
50. Wynne AM, Henry CJ, Huang Y, Cleland A, Godbout JP (2010) Protracted downregulation of CX3CR1 on microglia of aged mice after lipopolysaccharide challenge. Brain Behav Immun 24:1190–1201
51. Harrison JK, Jiang Y, Chen S, Xia Y, Maciejewski D, McNamara RK et al (1998) Role for neuronally derived fractalkine in mediating interactions between neurons and CX3CR1-expressing microglia. Proc Natl Acad Sci U S A 95:10896–10901
52. Bachstetter AD, Morganti JM, Jernberg J, Schlunk A, Mitchell SH, Brewster KW et al (2011) Fractalkine and CX(3)CR1 regulate hippocampal neurogenesis in adult and aged rats. Neurobiol Aging 32(11):2030–2044
53. Lyons A, Lynch AM, Downer EJ, Hanley R, O'Sullivan JB, Smith A et al (2009) Fractalkine-induced activation of the phosphatidylinositol-3 kinase pathway attentuates microglial activation in vivo and in vitro. J Neurochem 110:1547–1556
54. Maher FO, Clarke RM, Kelly A, Nally RE, Lynch MA (2006) Interaction between interferon gamma and insulin-like growth factor-1 in hippocampus impacts on the ability of rats to sustain long-term potentiation. J Neurochem 96:1560–1571
55. Maher FO, Nolan Y, Lynch MA (2005) Downregulation of IL-4-induced signalling in hippocampus contributes to deficits in LTP in the aged rat. Neurobiol Aging 26: 717–728
56. Hart BL (1988) Biological basis of the behavior of sick animals. Neurosci Biobehav Rev 12:123–137
57. Kent S, Bret-Dibat JL, Kelley KW, Dantzer R (1996) Mechanisms of sickness-induced decreases in food-motivated behavior. Neurosci Biobehav Rev 20:171–175
58. Kent S, Bluthe RM, Dantzer R, Hardwick AJ, Kelley KW, Rothwell NJ et al (1992) Different receptor mechanisms mediate the pyrogenic and behavioral effects of interleukin 1. Proc Natl Acad Sci U S A 89:9117–9120
59. Dantzer R (2001) Cytokine-induced sickness behavior: mechanisms and implications. Ann N Y Acad Sci 933:222–234
60. Sparkman NL, Kohman RA, Garcia AK, Boehm GW (2005) Peripheral lipopolysaccharide administration impairs two-way active avoidance conditioning in C57BL/6J mice. Physiol Behav 85:278–288
61. Kohman RA, Tarr AJ, Sparkman NL, Day CE, Paquet A, Akkaraju GR et al (2007)

Alleviation of the effects of endotoxin exposure on behavior and hippocampal IL-1beta by a selective non-peptide antagonist of corticotropin-releasing factor receptors. Brain Behav Immun 21:824–835

62. Sparkman NL, Kohman RA, Scott VJ, Boehm GW (2005) Bacterial endotoxin-induced behavioral alterations in two variations of the Morris water maze. Physiol Behav 86: 244–251
63. Pugh CR, Kumagawa K, Fleshner M, Watkins LR, Maier SF, Rudy JW (1998) Selective effects of peripheral lipopolysaccharide administration on contextual and auditory-cue fear conditioning. Brain Behav Immun 12: 212–229
64. Thomson LM, Sutherland RJ (2005) Systemic administration of lipopolysaccharide and interleukin-1beta have different effects on memory consolidation. Brain Res Bull 67:24–29
65. Reichenberg A, Yirmiya R, Schuld A, Kraus T, Haack M, Morag A et al (2001) Cytokine-associated emotional and cognitive disturbances in humans. Arch Gen Psychiatry 58: 445–452
66. Grigoleit JS, Oberbeck JR, Lichte P, Kobbe P, Wolf OT, Montag T et al (2010) Lipopolysaccharide-induced experimental immune activation does not impair memory functions in humans. Neurobiol Learn Mem 94:561–567
67. Shaw KN, Commins S, O'Mara SM (2001) Lipopolysaccharide causes deficits in spatial learning in the watermaze but not in BDNF expression in the rat dentate gyrus. Behav Brain Res 124:47–54
68. Arai K, Matsuki N, Ikegaya Y, Nishiyama N (2001) Deterioration of spatial learning performances in lipopolysaccharide-treated mice. Jpn J Pharmacol 87:195–201
69. Aubert A, Vega C, Dantzer R, Goodall G (1995) Pyrogens specifically disrupt the acquisition of a task involving cognitive processing in the rat. Brain Behav Immun 9:129–148
70. Barrientos RM, Higgins EA, Sprunger DB, Watkins LR, Rudy JW, Maier SF (2002) Memory for context is impaired by a post context exposure injection of interleukin-1 beta into dorsal hippocampus. Behav Brain Res 134:291–298
71. Goshen I, Kreisel T, Ounallah-Saad H, Renbaum P, Zalzstein Y, Ben-Hur T et al (2007) A dual role for interleukin-1 in hippocampal-dependent memory processes. Psychoneuroendocrinology 32:1106–1115
72. Frank MG, Barrientos RM, Hein AM, Biedenkapp JC, Watkins LR, Maier SF (2010) IL-1RA blocks E. coli-induced suppression of Arc and long-term memory in aged F344xBN F1 rats. Brain Behav Immun 24:254–262
73. Avital A, Goshen I, Kamsler A, Segal M, Iverfeldt K, Richter-Levin G et al (2003) Impaired interleukin-1 signaling is associated with deficits in hippocampal memory processes and neural plasticity. Hippocampus 13: 826–834
74. Abraham J, Johnson RW (2009) Central inhibition of interleukin-1beta ameliorates sickness behavior in aged mice. Brain Behav Immun 23:396–401
75. Chen J, Buchanan JB, Sparkman NL, Godbout JP, Freund GG, Johnson RW (2008) Neuroinflammation and disruption in working memory in aged mice after acute stimulation of the peripheral innate immune system. Brain Behav Immun 22:301–311
76. Henry CJ, Huang Y, Wynne A, Hanke M, Himler J, Bailey MT et al (2008) Minocycline attenuates lipopolysaccharide (LPS)-induced neuroinflammation, sickness behavior, and anhedonia. J Neuroinflammation 5:15
77. Tarr AJ, McLinden KA, Kranjac D, Kohman RA, Amaral W, Boehm GW (2011) The effects of age on lipopolysaccharide-induced cognitive deficits and interleukin-1beta expression. Behav Brain Res 217:481–485
78. Huang Y, Henry CJ, Dantzer R, Johnson RW, Godbout JP (2008) Exaggerated sickness behavior and brain proinflammatory cytokine expression in aged mice in response to intracerebroventricular lipopolysaccharide. Neurobiol Aging 29:1744–1753
79. Godbout JP, Moreau M, Lestage J, Chen J, Sparkman NL, O'Connor J et al (2008) Aging exacerbates depressive-like behavior in mice in response to activation of the peripheral innate immune system. Neuropsychopharmacology 33:2341–2351
80. Abraham J, Johnson RW (2009) Consuming a diet supplemented with resveratrol reduced infection-related neuroinflammation and deficits in working memory in aged mice. Rejuvenation Res 12:445–453
81. Barrientos RM, Higgins EA, Biedenkapp JC, Sprunger DB, Wright-Hardesty KJ, Watkins LR et al (2006) Peripheral infection and aging interact to impair hippocampal memory consolidation. Neurobiol Aging 27:723–732
82. Kohman RA, Tarr AJ, Byler SL, Boehm GW (2007) Age increases vulnerability to bacterial endotoxin-induced behavioral decrements. Physiol Behav 91:561–565
83. Kohman RA, Crowell B, Kusnecov AW (2010) Differential sensitivity to endotoxin exposure in young and middle-age mice. Brain Behav Immun 24:486–492

84. Verbitsky M, Yonan AL, Malleret G, Kandel ER, Gilliam TC, Pavlidis P (2004) Altered hippocampal transcript profile accompanies an age-related spatial memory deficit in mice. Learn Mem 11:253–260
85. Drag LL, Bieliauskas LA (2010) Contemporary review 2009: cognitive aging. J Geriatr Psychiatry Neurol 23:75–93
86. Weaver, J.D., Huang, M.H., Albert, M., Harris, T., Rowe, J.W. and Seeman, T.E. (2002) Interleukin-6 and risk of cognitive decline: MacArthur studies of successful aging. Neurology 59:371–8.
87. Yaffe K, Kanaya A, Lindquist K, Simonsick EM, Harris T, Shorr RI et al (2004) The metabolic syndrome, inflammation, and risk of cognitive decline. JAMA 292:2237–2242
88. Alvarez XA, Franco A, Fernandez-Novoa L, Cacabelos R (1996) Blood levels of histamine, IL-1 beta, and TNF-alpha in patients with mild to moderate Alzheimer disease. Mol Chem Neuropathol 29:237–252
89. Licastro F, Pedrini S, Caputo L, Annoni G, Davis LJ, Ferri C et al (2000) Increased plasma levels of interleukin-1, interleukin-6 and alpha-1-antichymotrypsin in patients with Alzheimer's disease: peripheral inflammation or signals from the brain? J Neuroimmunol 103:97–102
90. Banks WA, Farr SA, La Scola ME, Morley JE (2001) Intravenous human interleukin-1alpha impairs memory processing in mice: dependence on blood–brain barrier transport into posterior division of the septum. J Pharmacol Exp Ther 299:536–541
91. Watkins LR, Goehler LE, Relton JK, Tartaglia N, Silbert L, Martin D et al (1995) Blockade of interleukin-1 induced hyperthermia by subdiaphragmatic vagotomy: evidence for vagal mediation of immune-brain communication. Neurosci Lett 183: 27–31
92. Dantzer R (2004) Cytokine-induced sickness behaviour: a neuroimmune response to activation of innate immunity. Eur J Pharmacol 500:399–411
93. Griffin WS, Stanley LC, Ling C, White L, MacLeod V, Perrot LJ et al (1989) Brain interleukin 1 and S-100 immunoreactivity are elevated in Down syndrome and Alzheimer disease. Proc Natl Acad Sci U S A 86: 7611–7615
94. Bauer J, Strauss S, Schreiter-Gasser U, Ganter U, Schlegel P, Witt I et al (1991) Interleukin-6 and alpha-2-macroglobulin indicate an acute-phase state in Alzheimer's disease cortices. FEBS Lett 285:111–114
95. Tarkowski E, Liljeroth AM, Minthon L, Tarkowski A, Wallin A, Blennow K (2003) Cerebral pattern of pro- and anti-inflammatory cytokines in dementias. Brain Res Bull 61:255–260
96. Okello A, Edison P, Archer HA, Turkheimer FE, Kennedy J, Bullock R et al (2009) Microglial activation and amyloid deposition in mild cognitive impairment: a PET study. Neurology 72:56–62
97. Etminan M, Gill S, Samii A (2003) Effect of non-steroidal anti-inflammatory drugs on risk of Alzheimer's disease: systematic review and meta-analysis of observational studies. BMJ 327:128
98. Rosenzweig ES, Barnes CA (2003) Impact of aging on hippocampal function: plasticity, network dynamics, and cognition. Prog Neurobiol 69:143–179
99. van Praag H, Shubert T, Zhao C, Gage FH (2005) Exercise enhances learning and hippocampal neurogenesis in aged mice. J Neurosci 25:8680–8685
100. van Praag H, Christie BR, Sejnowski TJ, Gage FH (1999) Running enhances neurogenesis, learning, and long-term potentiation in mice. Proc Natl Acad Sci U S A 96:13427–13431
101. Jessberger S, Clark RE, Broadbent NJ, Clemenson GD Jr, Consiglio A, Lie DC et al (2009) Dentate gyrus-specific knockdown of adult neurogenesis impairs spatial and object recognition memory in adult rats. Learn Mem 16:147–154
102. Dupret D, Revest JM, Koehl M, Ichas F, De Giorgi F, Costet P et al (2008) Spatial relational memory requires hippocampal adult neurogenesis. PLoS One 3:e1959
103. Clark PJ, Brzezinska WJ, Thomas MW, Ryzhenko NA, Toshkov SA, Rhodes JS (2008) Intact neurogenesis is required for benefits of exercise on spatial memory but not motor performance or contextual fear conditioning in C57BL/6J mice. Neuroscience 155:1048–1058
104. Shors TJ, Townsend DA, Zhao M, Kozorovitskiy Y, Gould E (2002) Neurogenesis may relate to some but not all types of hippocampal-dependent learning. Hippocampus 12:578–584
105. Clark PJ, Brzezinska WJ, Puchalski EK, Krone DA, Rhodes JS (2009) Functional analysis of neurovascular adaptations to exercise in the dentate gyrus of young adult mice associated with cognitive gain. Hippocampus 19:937–950
106. Walton NM, Sutter BM, Laywell ED, Levkoff LH, Kearns SM, Marshall GP 2nd et al (2006)

Microglia instruct subventricular zone neurogenesis. Glia 54:815–825

107. Aarum J, Sandberg K, Haeberlein SL, Persson MA (2003) Migration and differentiation of neural precursor cells can be directed by microglia. Proc Natl Acad Sci U S A 100: 15983–15988
108. Sierra A, Encinas JM, Deudero JJ, Chancey JH, Enikolopov G, Overstreet-Wadiche LS et al (2010) Microglia shape adult hippocampal neurogenesis through apoptosis-coupled phagocytosis. Cell Stem Cell 7:483–495
109. Ziv Y, Ron N, Butovsky O, Landa G, Sudai E, Greenberg N et al (2006) Immune cells contribute to the maintenance of neurogenesis and spatial learning abilities in adulthood. Nat Neurosci 9:268–275
110. Battista D, Ferrari CC, Gage FH, Pitossi FJ (2006) Neurogenic niche modulation by activated microglia: transforming growth factor beta increases neurogenesis in the adult dentate gyrus. Eur J Neurosci 23:83–93
111. Mathieu P, Piantanida AP, Pitossi F (2010) Chronic expression of transforming growth factor-beta enhances adult neurogenesis. Neuroimmunomodulation 17:200–201
112. Ekdahl CT, Claasen JH, Bonde S, Kokaia Z, Lindvall O (2003) Inflammation is detrimental for neurogenesis in adult brain. Proc Natl Acad Sci U S A 100:13632–13637
113. Monje ML, Toda H, Palmer TD (2003) Inflammatory blockade restores adult hippocampal neurogenesis. Science 302:1760–1765
114. Walter J, Keiner S, Witte OW, Redecker C (2011) Age-related effects on hippocampal precursor cell subpopulations and neurogenesis. Neurobiol Aging 32(10):1906–1914
115. Kuzumaki N, Ikegami D, Imai S, Narita M, Tamura R, Yajima M et al (2010) Enhanced IL-1beta production in response to the activation of hippocampal glial cells impairs neurogenesis in aged mice. Synapse 64:721–728
116. Gemma C, Bachstetter AD, Cole MJ, Fister M, Hudson C, Bickford PC (2007) Blockade of caspase-1 increases neurogenesis in the aged hippocampus. Eur J Neurosci 26: 2795–2803
117. Bliss TV, Lomo T (1973) Long-lasting potentiation of synaptic transmission in the dentate area of the anaesthetized rabbit following stimulation of the perforant path. J Physiol 232:331–356
118. Martin SJ, Grimwood PD, Morris RG (2000) Synaptic plasticity and memory: an evaluation of the hypothesis. Annu Rev Neurosci 23:649–711
119. Griffin R, Nally R, Nolan Y, McCartney Y, Linden J, Lynch MA (2006) The age-related attenuation in long-term potentiation is associated with microglial activation. J Neurochem 99:1263–1272
120. Nolan Y, Maher FO, Martin DS, Clarke RM, Brady MT, Bolton AE et al (2005) Role of interleukin-4 in regulation of age-related inflammatory changes in the hippocampus. J Biol Chem 280:9354–9362
121. Min SS, Quan HY, Ma J, Han JS, Jeon BH, Seol GH (2009) Chronic brain inflammation impairs two forms of long-term potentiation in the rat hippocampal CA1 area. Neurosci Lett 456:20–24
122. Chapman TR, Barrientos RM, Ahrendsen JT, Maier SF, Patterson SL (2010) Synaptic correlates of increased cognitive vulnerability with aging: peripheral immune challenge and aging interact to disrupt theta-burst late-phase long-term potentiation in hippocampal area CA1. J Neurosci 30:7598–7603
123. Cunningham AJ, Murray CA, O'Neill LA, Lynch MA, O'Connor JJ (1996) Interleukin-1 beta (IL-1 beta) and tumour necrosis factor (TNF) inhibit long-term potentiation in the rat dentate gyrus in vitro. Neurosci Lett 203:17–20
124. Tancredi V, D'Antuono M, Cafe C, Giovedi S, Bue MC, D'Arcangelo G et al (2000) The inhibitory effects of interleukin-6 on synaptic plasticity in the rat hippocampus are associated with an inhibition of mitogen-activated protein kinase ERK. J Neurochem 75:634–643
125. Schneider H, Pitossi F, Balschun D, Wagner A, del Rey A, Besedovsky HO (1998) A neuromodulatory role of interleukin-1beta in the hippocampus. Proc Natl Acad Sci U S A 95: 7778–7783
126. Gorelick PB (2010) Role of inflammation in cognitive impairment: results of observational epidemiological studies and clinical trials. Ann N Y Acad Sci 1207:155–162
127. Morgan TE, Wong AM, Finch CE (2007) Anti-inflammatory mechanisms of dietary restriction in slowing aging processes. Interdiscip Top Gerontol 35:83–97
128. Luchsinger JA, Tang MX, Shea S, Mayeux R (2002) Caloric intake and the risk of Alzheimer disease. Arch Neurol 59:1258–1263
129. Morgan TE, Xie Z, Goldsmith S, Yoshida T, Lanzrein AS, Stone D et al (1999) The mosaic of brain glial hyperactivity during normal ageing and its attenuation by food restriction. Neuroscience 89:687–699

130. Wong AM, Patel NV, Patel NK, Wei M, Morgan TE, de Beer MC et al (2005) Macrosialin increases during normal brain aging are attenuated by caloric restriction. Neurosci Lett 390:76–80
131. Thirumangalakudi L, Prakasam A, Zhang R, Bimonte-Nelson H, Sambamurti K, Kindy MS et al (2008) High cholesterol-induced neuroinflammation and amyloid precursor protein processing correlate with loss of working memory in mice. J Neurochem 106:475–485
132. Li Y, Liu L, Barger SW, Mrak RE, Griffin WS (2001) Vitamin E suppression of microglial activation is neuroprotective. J Neurosci Res 66:163–170
133. Patil CS, Singh VP, Satyanarayan PS, Jain NK, Singh A, Kulkarni SK (2003) Protective effect of flavonoids against aging- and lipopolysaccharide-induced cognitive impairment in mice. Pharmacology 69:59–67
134. Jang S, Dilger RN, Johnson RW (2010) Luteolin inhibits microglia and alters hippocampal-dependent spatial working memory in aged mice. J Nutr 140:1892–1898
135. Woods JA, Vieira VJ, Keylock KT (2009) Exercise, inflammation, and innate immunity. Immunol Allergy Clin North Am 29:381–393
136. Cotman CW, Berchtold NC, Christie LA (2007) Exercise builds brain health: key roles of growth factor cascades and inflammation. Trends Neurosci 30:464–472
137. Erickson KI, Prakash RS, Voss MW, Chaddock L, Hu L, Morris KS et al (2009) Aerobic fitness is associated with hippocampal volume in elderly humans. Hippocampus 19: 1030–1039
138. Jankord R, Jemiolo B (2004) Influence of physical activity on serum IL-6 and IL-10 levels in healthy older men. Med Sci Sports Exerc 36:960–964
139. Ferrandez MD, De la Fuente M (1999) Effects of age, sex and physical exercise on the phagocytic process of murine peritoneal macrophages. Acta Physiol Scand 166:47–53
140. Chennaoui M, Drogou C, Gomez-Merino D (2008) Effects of physical training on IL-1beta, IL-6 and IL-1ra concentrations in various brain areas of the rat. Eur Cytokine Netw 19:8–14
141. Funk JA, Gohlke J, Kraft AD, McPherson CA, Collins JB, Jean Harry G (2011) Voluntary exercise protects hippocampal neurons from trimethyltin injury: Possible role of interleukin-6 to modulate tumor necrosis factor receptor-mediated neurotoxicity. Brain Behav Immun 25(6):1063–1077
142. Scheller J, Chalaris A, Schmidt-Arras D, Rose-John S (2011) The pro- and anti-inflammatory properties of the cytokine interleukin-6. Biochim Biophys Acta 1813: 878–888
143. Starkie R, Ostrowski SR, Jauffred S, Febbraio M, Pedersen BK (2003) Exercise and IL-6 infusion inhibit endotoxin-induced TNF-alpha production in humans. FASEB J 17: 884–886
144. Ang ET, Wong PT, Moochhala S, Ng YK (2004) Cytokine changes in the horizontal diagonal band of Broca in the septum after running and stroke: a correlation to glial activation. Neuroscience 129:337–347
145. Ehninger D, Wang LP, Klempin F, Romer B, Kettenmann H, Kempermann G (2011) Enriched environment and physical activity reduce microglia and influence the fate of NG2 cells in the amygdala of adult mice. Cell Tissue Res 345:69–86
146. Ehninger D, Kempermann G (2003) Regional effects of wheel running and environmental enrichment on cell genesis and microglia proliferation in the adult murine neocortex. Cereb Cortex 13:845–851
147. Stranahan AM, Lee K, Becker KG, Zhang Y, Maudsley S, Martin B et al (2010) Hippocampal gene expression patterns underlying the enhancement of memory by running in aged mice. Neurobiol Aging 31:1937–1949
148. Kohman RA, Rodriguez-Zas SL, Southey BR, Kelley KW, Dantzer R, Rhodes JS (2011) Voluntary wheel running reverses age-induced changes in hippocampal gene expression. PLoS One 6(8):e22654

Chapter 12

Autism Spectrum Disorders: From Immunity to Behavior

Milo Careaga and Paul Ashwood

Abstract

Autism spectrum disorders (ASD) are complex and heterogeneous with a spectrum of diverse symptoms. Mounting evidence from a number of disciplines suggests a link between immune function and ASD. Although the causes of ASD have yet to be identified, genetic studies have uncovered a host of candidate genes relating to immune regulation that are altered in ASD, while epidemiological studies have shown a relationship with maternal immune disturbances during pregnancy and ASD. Moreover, decades of research have identified numerous systemic and cellular immune abnormalities in individuals with ASD and their families. These include changes in immune cell number, differences in cytokine and chemokine production, and alterations of cellular function at rest and in response to immunological challenge. Many of these changes in immune responses are associated with increasing impairment in behaviors that are core features of ASD. Despite this evidence, much remains to be understood about the precise mechanism by which the immune system alters neurodevelopment and to what extent it is involved in the pathogenesis of ASD. With estimates of ASD as high as 1% of children, ASD is a major public health issue. Improvements in our understanding of the interactions between the nervous and immune system during early neurodevelopment and how this interaction is different in ASD will have important therapeutic implications with wide ranging benefits.

Key words: Adaptive immune system, Antibodies, Autism spectrum disorders, Autoantibodies, Behavior, Brain, Chemokine, Cytokine, Innate immune system, Immunity

1. Introduction

Autism spectrum disorders (ASD) are neurodevelopment disorders characterized by impairments in verbal and nonverbal communication, social interactions, and the presence of restricted repetitive behaviors, which are typically diagnosed by 3 years of age (1). In the United States, the incident rate among children is estimated to be 1 in 150 (2). Despite the large number of afflicted individuals, the etiology of ASD is not well understood and all evidence pointing to a cause remains speculative, but likely involves a complex interaction of genetic and environmental factors. Adding to the

Qing Yan (ed.), *Psychoneuroimmunology: Methods and Protocols*, Methods in Molecular Biology, vol. 934,
DOI 10.1007/978-1-62703-071-7_12, © Springer Science+Business Media, LLC 2012

confusion, symptoms and the disease course among patients with ASD vary greatly, making both effective research and treatment difficult. A rise in the number of cases in the last few decades has additionally peaked concern; however, it remains to be determined if the rise is merely a result of a broadening of diagnostic criteria and increased awareness, or if other factors are at work (3). Despite extensive research from a host of disciplines, ASD remains an enigmatic disorder, but mounting evidence suggests a role for immune involved in the etiology of ASD.

The etiology(ies) of ASD and the relative contribution from genetic, epigenetic, and environmental factors are currently unknown. However, as early as 1971 Money et al. postulated that there was an immunological contribution to the pathogenesis of ASD and observed a familial link of ASD with polyendocrine autoimmune disorder (4). Numerous small studies and case reports followed throughout the 1970s and 1980s and the theory of immune dysfunction in the pathology of ASD was developed; however, the exact role altered immune responses have on neurodevelopment and ASD has remained controversial both in terms of its existence as well as its role in the etiology of the disorder.

Since the late 1990s a number of epidemiology studies have found that a familial link exists between ASD and immune dysfunction. The scope of these studies has varied greatly, with studies ranging from small cohort studies to large population-based studies, while the methods utilized range from self-reporting to examination of medical records or clinician evaluation. Furthermore, given the limited rates of some immunological disease in the general population, as well as varying rates between ethnic or geographical background, direct comparisons among the various studies are often difficult (5). However, despite these differences a number of significant observations were repeatedly reported including the association of risk for ASD with immunological conditions such as maternal asthma and allergy (6), celiac disease (7, 8), type-1 diabetes (6, 7, 9–11), autoimmune thyroid disease (12, 13), rheumatoid arthritis (7, 8, 11, 14), and rheumatic fever (9, 14). Data from these epidemiology studies show that the familial link for ASD is not confined to maternal immune dysfunction and that paternal immune conditions are also important (7, 9, 12–14). Arguably, since fathers lack the interaction that occurs with the child during fetal development and postnatally through breast milk, the paternal role that altered immune dysfunctions plays is likely a result of heritable factors. Together these studies point to abnormal immune function in first-degree relatives of families of children with ASD and suggests that immune dysfunction is a risk factor for ASD. Furthermore, the increased risk may stem from genetic changes or altered physiological pathways that are shared between immune conditions/diseases and ASD.

2. Gestational Immune Activation

Pregnancy involves a unique and complex dynamic for the maternal immune system: protection of the mother from pathogens/infections, but also support and acceptance of fetal tissue that contains many "nonself" paternal antigens. During pregnancy the uterus and placenta become tightly regulated immune environments, with uterine NK cells (uNK) together with macrophage and dendritic cells establishing a maternal–fetal interface that promotes fetal health and development including early brain development (15). However, because of the complexity of regulating this balance between immune tolerance and protection from pathogens, pregnancy represents a period of vulnerability to immune insult not only for the mother, but for the developing fetus as well. Both epidemiological and animal studies suggest that any disturbances in immune regulation during this vulnerable period can result in altered neurodevelopment.

One such risk factor that can alter the gestational immune profile and impact neurodevelopment is maternal infection. For example, studies examining birth records of bacterial and viral outbreaks show that children born of exposed mothers have highly increased rates for the neurodevelopmental disorder schizophrenia (reviewed in ref. (16)). Similar case reports and small comparative studies have also shown a casual link between maternal infection and ASD (17–19). In a large population-based study using Denmark's medical registry, consisting of data from over a million children during the period of 1980–2005, an increased rate of children with ASD was born from mothers who were hospitalized for viral infections in the first trimester and bacterial infections in the second trimester when compared with mothers with typically developing children (20). Most maternal infections, however, do not result in the development of ASD in offspring, suggesting other factors such as a genetic susceptibility that control how the mothers respond to infections are also involved. In individuals with known genetic disorders that are associated with high rates of ASD, such as tuberous sclerosis (TCS) which has a 25–50% rate of ASD (21), associations are found between the incidence of ASD, season of birth, and whether the peak flu season occurs during the later stages of pregnancy (22).

Animal models support the role of gestational immune activation on neurodevelopment (23). Using both viral and bacterial analogs as instigators of maternal immune activation, altered neurodevelopment and behavioral changes in offspring can be observed (24, 25). These experiments highlight that a generalized host immune response to a pathogen rather than a pathogen-specific response is involved. It is not fully understood how immune activation affects early brain development, but it is believed that activation of the maternal immune system leads to changes either in the placenta or directly in the fetal brain which alter neurodevelopment (26–28). A number of cytokines are induced during maternal immune activation, of which IL-6 appears to be one of the major mediators that can elicit neurodevelopmental changes in the various maternal immune activation models. Using IL-6 knock-out mice or blocking IL-6 with an antibody ameliorates the effect of maternal immune activation (29). Similarly, inhibition of downstream signaling pathways associated with IL-6 signaling such as JAK2/STAT3 resulted in attenuation of social deficits in the offspring following maternal immune activation (30). In addition to IL-6, other cytokines such as IL-2 can also alter neurodevelopment. IL-2 is a potent modulator of dopamine activity in the brain and can increase motor activity when injected in mice; a finding that is attenuated with a D-1 antagonist (31). Models where pregnant dams are injected with IL-2 result in offspring that demonstrate increased open-field activity, grooming, and rearing behavior (32). Therefore, in these animal models the deficits in behaviors exhibited by the offspring of animals exposed during gestation to infections or immune activation are likely the result of complex interactions of a number of molecules produced both by the mother as well as the offspring. Pinpointing the exact mechanisms and molecules may help develop preventive strategies that could be useful in cases of overt gestational immune activation.

Genetic factors may further contribute to the neuropathology in offspring during maternal immune activation. Mice with disruptions to genes associated with altered neurodevelopment, such as DISC1 or TSC1, appear to show a more exaggerated behavioral phenotype with greater impairments in social interaction after maternal immune activation (22, 33). The affects of maternal immune activation are not limited to altered neurodevelopment in offspring and appear to result in ongoing immune dysfunction in the offspring as well (34–37). It is currently unclear whether the immune dysregulation contributes to the behavioral endophenotype seen in offspring, but increased dysregulation of immune cells, as well as altered cytokine and chemokine profiles, has been linked to greater impairments of behaviors in children with ASD (38–43).

2.1. Antifetal Brain Antibodies

The transfer of antibodies from the mother to child during pregnancy is important physiologically and confers protection from a wide range of infectious agents to the fetus. However, alongside antibodies that provide immunoprotection, antibodies that are immunoreactive to fetal proteins also cross the placental barrier and can affect neonatal outcome (44). For example, the transfer to the fetus of maternal anti-Ro/SS-A and anti-La/SS-B antibodies in mothers with systemic lupus erythematosus (SLE) causes neonatal lupus syndrome, often leading to congenital heart block (45–48).

Brain reactive autoantibodies are also transferred and in experimental models can alter brain development, for example, neurotoxic antibodies from patients with SLE when transferred into pregnant mice result in abnormal brain development in the offspring (45). In addition, abnormal thyroid function caused by placental transfer of maternal antithyroid antibodies is often seen in infants born to mothers with Hashimoto's thyroiditis or Graves' disease (49), and some cases of neonatal antiphospholipid syndrome (APS) are thought to occur due to the transfer of maternal autoantibodies from mothers with primary APS (50). The presence of autoantibodies directed against neuronal components of fetal brain extracts in some mothers of children with ASD children suggests a similar mechanism may occur in ASD (51–53). In approximately 12% of mothers with children with ASD, a strong pattern of antibody reactivity to fetal but not adult brain proteins is observed (51). The exact target of these antibodies is not known but they appear to be specific for mothers of children with autism and have so far not been observed in mothers of children who are typically developing or mothers of children who have developmental disorders other than ASD (51).

The ASD-specific nature of these antibodies is exciting and warrants further study. One possibility is that these antibodies bind to their neuronal targets during development, thereby interfering with, or altering neurodevelopment. Although it is hard to recapitulate exactly the core features of ASD in animal models, certain behaviors associated with ASD such as repetitive behaviors, difficulty in learning, and hyperactivity can be replicated (54). In one model the transference of IgG isolated from mothers with children with ASD into Rhesus macaque monkeys during midgestation resulted in increased stereotypical behavior and hyperactivity in the offspring that were not observed in monkeys which received IgG from mothers of typically developing children or monkeys treated with saline (55). Evidence of a potential role for these antibodies and altered neurodevelopment was also observed in a murine model (56). Whether these behavioral changes are directly related to ASD or are themselves distinct phenomena is not clear; however, these models suggest that antibodies isolated from some mothers with children with ASD may alter the course of early neurodevelopment leading to changes in behavior. Given the potential risk these antibodies may present (51), more work is needed to better characterize them both in terms of their cellular targets as well as the behavioral changes they evoke. Despite being present in only a fraction of mothers of children with ASD, these antibodies may lend clues which could lead to a better understanding of the pathology of ASD and may even represent a potential avenue for screening or therapy.

3. Altered Cytokine Production

Complex neuroimmune interactions occur early during development and continue throughout life. Cytokines and their receptors are produced and expressed by neurons and help to shape neuronal differentiation, proliferation, migration, and synaptic plasticity (57). This interaction occurs either directly or through endocrine intermediates (58). The neuroimmune system works by maintaining an intricate balance, and dysregulation in one system often results in dysregulation of the others (reviewed in ref. (59)).

Increased immune activation is associated with a number of neurodegenerative disorders and is speculated to play a role in psychiatric disorders such as schizophrenia (60), obsessive compulsive disorder (61), depression (62), bipolar disorder (63), Gilles de La Tourette syndrome (61), and ASD (64–66). Elevated levels of inflammatory cytokines in the CNS could reflect inflammatory processes that modulate neuronal function. Increased levels of pro-inflammatory cytokines such as IL-6, TNF-α, and MCP-1, in brain specimens and cerebral spinal fluid (CSF) obtained from young and old individuals with ASD (age range 5–44 years), suggest ongoing neuroinflammatory processes in ASD (67, 68). Studies that have assessed cytokine levels in the periphery also show increases in pro-inflammatory cytokines (39, 69–72). Inflammatory processes are kept in check by the release of cytokines that have anti-inflammatory or regulatory properties such as IL-10 and TGFβ1. In ASD, production of IL-10 (69, 73) and circulating levels of TGFβ1 (74, 75) are decreased. These data indicate a shift towards a pro-inflammatory state in ASD. Furthermore, in a recent large population based case–control study increased plasma cytokines levels were associated with late onset of symptoms and greater impairment of communication as well as more aberrant behaviors in ASD (39). These data suggest that immune activation and atypical cytokine levels are directly related to the behavioral symptoms in ASD and potentially represent a novel area for therapeutic intervention.

However, the literature on cytokines and ASD is not always consistent and likely reflects complex patterns of immune activation among different subgroups of individuals with ASD. The data is further complicated by the use of siblings of children with ASD as controls as these siblings are themselves often on a broader autism phenotype spectrum (76). In addition to behavioral similarities in siblings of children with ASD, researchers have demonstrated that unaffected sibling often have immune profiles more similar to children with ASD than controls (77), i.e. the siblings are on a broader behavioral and immune autism phenotype.

4. Innate Immune Abnormalities

The immune system is generally described as having two arms: the innate immune system which uses genetically encoded receptors and nonspecific mechanisms to defend the host, and the adaptive immune system which responds to a particular threat and develops memory for future insults. These two systems work together to protect the host and maintain proper homeostasis.

The innate immune system develops early during fetal development and appears to initially play more of a housekeeping role than one of host defense. The earliest cells of this system derive from primitive cells of the yolk sac (78–80). These cells migrate from the yolk sac and eventually become the progenitors for both the hematopoietic cells of the peripheral immune system as well as the initial population of the CNS microglia. It was recently reported that abnormalities in these innate CNS immune cells can directly contribute to abnormal behaviors such as pathological grooming in mice (81). In mice homozygous for a loss-of-function mutation in Hoxb8 that reduces the number of peripherally derived microglia cells compulsive grooming and hair removal is observed, but symptoms are improved upon bone marrow transplant from mice without the associate gene mutation (81). In addition, in immune deficient mice, cognitive impairments have been observed, but can be improved when mice receive alternatively activated macrophages, suggesting that epigenetic as well as genetic alternations in innate immune cells can contribute to behavioral alterations (82). Notably, many of the cytokines produced by innate immune cells such as TNF-α, IL-1β, and IL-6 mediate direct affect on neuronal activity and are elevated in ASD (39).

These cytokines have multiple functions in the CNS which vary with both dose and timing. TNF-α can induce neuronal cell death and is thought to play an important role in synaptic pruning (83, 84). However, depending on the local environment, dose, and timing, TNF-α can also induce proliferation (85). This opposing function is also apparent in the actions of IL-1β and IL-6 which have varied effects on neuronal survival and proliferation as well as synapse formation, migration, and differentiation resulting in altered or reduced neurogenesis (86–91).

Given the role of the innate immune system in both appropriate neuronal development and function, it is of great interest that a numbers of studies have demonstrated abnormalities in innate immune function in ASD. Significant findings include alterations in natural killer (NK) cell activity (92). NK cells play an important role in viral defense, tumor surveillance, and help maintain the uterine environment during pregnancy. Early observations showed that NK cell-mediated killing of the target cell K562 was lower in some individuals with ASD (93). Similar results were found in a larger multisite study, with nearly half of the individuals with ASD being having low NK cell cytotoxicity activity against the target cell (94). A more in-depth investigation into NK cell function in ASD demonstrated that under resting conditions NK cells from young children with ASD were more activated, potentially reflecting their in vivo status, but when these cells were challenged in vitro in cultures with K562 cells, they fail to kill the target cells or produce cytokines (92). In circulation, the numbers of NK cells are 40% higher in children with ASD compared with controls, again reflecting potential increases in the in vivo status of NK cells (95). This feature has also been described in several autoimmune diseases and suggests that the immune cells may be maximally stimulated in vivo but cannot respond further once challenged. In addition to NK cells, several studies have reported differences in monocytes and macrophages in ASD.

Alterations in the function of cells of the myeloid lineage, namely monocytes and macrophages, have been directly and indirectly reported in a number of studies in children with ASD. Monocytes and macrophages share many similarities to their CNS localized counterparts, the microglia, and may even contribute to the microglial population (96, 97). Prominent microglia cell activation and infiltration of monocytes and macrophages is observed in brain specimens of individuals with ASD (67). Moreover, powerful transcriptome network mapping techniques highlight the presence of gene networks suggestive for microglial dysregulation in the brains of subjects with ASD, a dysregulation that also appears to be present in peripheral monocytes and macrophages (98). Sweeten et al. reported increased number of circulating monocytes in subjects with ASD (99). Moreover, plasma cytokine levels in children with ASD show higher levels of the "monokines" IL-1β, IL-6, and IL-12, which are produced predominantly by cells of the myeloid lineage, i.e. monocytes and dendritic cells (39). Jyonouchi et al. found that peripheral blood mononuclear cells (PBMC) when stimulated with the innate immune activating TLR-4 agonist LPS released more IL-1β in ASD compared to similarly treated cultures from control subjects (100). In a subset of ASD patients with recurrent infections, altered responses to a number of TLR ligands were also demonstrated (101). These studies, however, used mixed cultures of peripheral cells and it is unclear if the altered response was from monocytes alone or from a more complex interaction between monocytes and other cells including adaptive immune cells. By using only isolated monocytes, Enstrom et al. attempted to better elucidate innate immune findings in ASD and found that IL-1β, IL-6, and TNF-α responses were elevated following TLR-2 stimulation and IL-1β production was higher following TLR-4 stimulation in children with ASD but not typically developing controls (41). These increases in cytokines also correlated with impairments in ASD-specific behaviors as measured by gold-standard assessments. How this inappropriate immune response to pathogen contributes to symptomology of ASD may be through direct interactions between immune messengers and neuronal or neuroendocrine targets, or more circuitously by modulating the adaptive immune response. However, monocytes isolated from subjects with ASD showed a reduced production of IL-1β, IL-6, GM-CSF, and TNF-α following challenge with TLR-9 ligands (41). This differential innate immune response might explain the increased rate of early childhood (first 30 days) infections seen in children with ASD compared with typically developing controls (102). During this early postnatal period, the adaptive immune system is being educated and the body is most reliant on the innate immune system for host defense.

5. Adaptive Immune Abnormalities

The second arm of the immune system develops later in development and does not fully mature until early childhood. Unlike the innate immune system that is genetically coded to recognize and respond to conserved pathogen markers, the adaptive immune system is more dynamic and is educated to respond to pathogens and toxins upon exposure. Similar to the innate immune system, however, the adaptive immune system can also affect both neuronal development and function (reviewed in ref. (103)).

Rodent models have provided much of the evidence that the adaptive immune can alter neuronal development and function. In mice strains lacking an adaptive immune system, or specific elements of it, cognitive deficits have been observed (104). This has also been demonstrated in mice strains with typical immune system where T-cells are depleted (105). The exact mechanism by which T-cells modulate neuronal function is not fully understood; however, in neuronal injury models, CD4+ T-cells have been shown to mediate neuronal survival in an IL-4/STAT6-dependent manner (106, 107). IL-4 has recently been shown to regulate learning and memory by modulating the innate immune system, demonstrating the importance of cross-talk between both arms of the immune system in maintaining neuronal homeostasis (108, 109).

Cellular studies in ASD have demonstrated functional alterations in the adaptive immune response. Early work by Stubbs was the first to suggest irregularities in cellular immune function in ASD; however, this early study was small and poorly controlled (110). Further work was performed by Warren et al., who found T-cell abnormalities, including skewed CD4:CD8 T-cell numbers and altered antigen recall responses (111). More recent work has shown the same decreases in T-cell numbers but only in children with ASD that also have gastrointestinal issues (112) and may reflect the efflux of T-cells from the periphery into the mucosa in this subset of ASD individuals. Cellular markers show that there is an altered T-cell activation in children with ASD, suggesting an incomplete or altered activation profile (40, 73, 113). A skewing towards a T_H2 cytokine profile has been hypothesized for ASD (114). However, as is true for most human research the pattern of cytokines produced in T-cells in ASD is complex and do not easily fit into the traditional T_H2 classification. In a recent study, dynamic T-cell function following stimulation with PHA was assessed in 63 children with ASD and 73 age-matched typically developing controls. After stimulation, levels of GM-CSF, TNF-α, and IL-13 were increased and IL-12 (p40) was decreased in subjects with ASD compared with controls. Furthermore, the induced cytokine production was found to be associated with altered behaviors in children with ASD, such that increased pro-inflammatory or T_H1 cytokine production was associated with greater impairments in core features of ASD as well as aberrant behaviors (39). In contrast, production of GM-CSF and T_H2 cytokines was associated with better cognitive and adaptive function (40). Taken together, these findings suggest that altered T-cell activation and function are present in ASD and likely play a role in the ongoing pathophysiological process.

Currently no studies exist that have directly studied B-cell function in ASD; however, there are several lines of indirect evidence that suggest altered B-cell dysfunction is present in individuals with ASD. The primary role of B-cells is the production of immunoglobins against pathogens. In order to best protect the host, B-cells produce a variety of immunoglobins, each with a dedicated role and in some cases specificity to a particular tissue. IgA is present mainly in mucosal tissue where it serves as a sentinel against pathogens. Deficiencies in IgA are associated with increased infections (115). In ASD, lower circulating levels of IgA have previously been reported (116); however, more recent studies have not validated this finding (42, 117, 118). Instead, reduced production of the IgM and IgG classes of immunoglobins has been reported, with lower levels found to correlate with more aberrant behaviors (42). Further evidence of imbalance of antibody levels was reported in a recent study that looked at IgG levels in neonatal blood. At this developmental age, most IgG present in the neonate will be maternal derived via placenta transfer. IgG levels were found to be lower in children who went on to develop ASD (119). Analysis of specific IgG subclasses in children with ASD found that although total levels for IgG are low, the less abundant IgG2 subtype (118) and IgG4 subtype (117, 118) are elevated in ASD compared with controls. Interestingly, IgG2 is important for immune responses to carbohydrate antigens, and increases in this subtype of IgG might suggest increased exposure to specific pathogens. IgG4 functions as a blocking antibody and is associated with chronic infection. It has also been shown to function as a pathogenic antibody in certain autoimmune disorders (120). Differences in Ig levels in plasma or sera could reflect differences in absolute B-cells numbers, as children with ASD have been reported to have 20% more B-cells on average when compared with controls (95) but that immature $CD5^{+}$ B-cells predominate. In addition to altered immunoglobulin levels, a number of autoantibodies reactive to brain and CNS tissue have been identified in ASD.

6. Autoantibodies in ASD

The presence of antibodies directed against fetal brain or CNS tissue but not adult brain tissue has been repeatedly reported in children with ASD (reviewed in refs. (65, 121)). Several studies demonstrated that subjects with ASD possess autoantibodies directed against specific neurological targets, including serotonin receptors (122), brain-derived neurotrophic factor (BDNF) (123), myelin basic protein (MBP) (123, 124), neuron-axon acidic protein (NAFP) (125), and glial fibrillary acidic protein (GFAP) (125). However, specificity of these antibodies is not the same across studies and there has been difficulty in replicating studies showing antibodies to specific targets such as MBP or GFAP (126, 127). It is also clear that these antibodies are not present in all individuals with ASD (128).

In addition to specific neuronal targets, a number of unidentified neuronal targets have also been detected and appear to be associated with certain behavioral endophenotype in ASD. Antibodies recognizing a 45 kDa cerebellum protein were found more frequently in children with ASD and were associated with lower adaptive and cognitive function, as well as increases in aberrant behaviors (121, 129). Further evaluation of these neuronal targets has suggested that they are presented on or in GABAergic neurons, although not all GABAergic neurons are targeted by these autoantibodies (130). Although it is unclear if any of these autoantibodies have direct pathogenic relevance, or are secondary to previous cellular damage or inflammatory reactions, these studies provide provocative evidence that specific molecular targets represent a possible means by which these autoantibodies are pathogenic and could reveal a subgroup of children with ASD with distinct immune dysfunction.

7. Mucosal Immunity in Autism

It is now accepted that a significant number of individuals with ASD have frequent gastrointestinal (GI) symptoms. The most commonly described GI symptoms are increases in constipation or diarrhea and food insensitivities/food allergies. The latter finding has led some investigators to focus on immunological responses to dietary proteins such as gluten and casein. Jyonouchi et al. (100) found that PBMC responses to gliadin, cow's milk protein, and soy were increased in children with ASD and GI symptoms compared with control children. However, children with ASD in this study were selected on the basis of having previously seen behavior improvements on a restricted diet, and therefore the adverse responses to dietary peptides may be restricted to a specific endophenotype of ASD. In mucosal tissue obtained during colonoscopy and endoscopy, children with ASD who have GI symptoms show increased pan-enteric infiltration of T-cells, monocytes, NK cells, and eosinophils, a finding that suggests there is mucosal immune activation, leading to increased homing of cells to the mucosa, likely as a result of increased cytokine and chemokine signaling (112, 131–133). Isolation of lamina propria mononuclear cells showed increased frequencies of T-cells that were positive for TNF-α in duodenum, ileum, and colonic tissue specimens from children with ASD compared to noninflamed GI symptom controls, and children with celiac disease or inflammatory bowel diseases (69, 73, 112). Concurrently with increased TNFα production there were demonstrable decreases in lower IL-10 production, indicating a shift to a pro-inflammatory environment. Moreover, antibodies directed against the basal membrane and the basal surface of gut epithelium were also observed in children with ASD (131, 132). These autoantibodies may be representative of an autoimmune response directed at the epithelial barrier, one that could lead to the perturbation of the epithelial barrier and potentially increased permeability. In line with this hypothesis, several groups have shown increased gut permeability in individuals with ASD (134, 135). However, there is still controversy regarding the size of the ASD population that suffers from GI symptoms. A retrospective study examining 589 subjects with idiopathic, familial ASD and 163 of their unaffected sibling controls found a more than twofold rate, 42% compared with 19%, of GI issues in subjects with ASD compared to their sibling. Furthermore, the presence of GI issues correlated with increased severity of behaviors in ASD (136). Whether GI symptoms are representative or GI pathology, and how this is associated with behavioral symptoms is still not known. A few small studies suggest that GI symptoms in ASD are associated with increased aggression and hyperactivity but these studies need further replication (137, 138). Some studies suggest that an abnormal immune response to dietary peptides could contribute to behavioral abnormalities associated with ASD and may represent a fruitful avenue for therapeutic intervention (139).

8. Immunogenetics in ASD

ASD is one of the most heritable psychological disorders, with a 70–80% concordance rates among monozygotic twins and a 30–40% concordance rate among dizygotic twins (140–143). Even among nontwin siblings, there is a 25-fold increased risk of developing ASD when compared to the general population, suggesting a strong genetic component in the pathogenesis of this disorder (144). However, variations in primary symptoms domains are present in twins, with the most variance existing in repetitive behaviors and interests (142). Despite the strong evidence for a genetic component in ASD, studies have failed to pinpoint a single gene responsible for ASD, and instead a number of genes have been implicated. These genes vary widely among individuals and family clusters, but together they appear to be involved in important physiological systems including synapse formation, neuronal migration, and immune function.

Among the genes implicated in ASD, restriction of HLA genes is often reported and is associated with increased risk of developing ASD (145–149). The HLA genes are located within a large genomic region referred to as the major histocompatibility complex (MHC) on chromosome 6. These genes are involved in immune function and are among the strongest predictors of risk for autoimmune conditions, and in addition to ASD have been associated with neurodevelopmental disorders such as schizophrenia (150). Several studies have found that a number of HLA haplotypes, in particular HLA-DR4, occur more often in children with ASD compared to the general population (146–149). However, two studies by Guerini et al. (151, 152) found that there was no apparent HLA linkage, and instead there are several microsatellite linkages within the MHC which are associated with ASD. This suggests that genetic abnormalities in the MHC are not solely confined to HLA genes themselves but that other immune genes in the region may be indicated.

Another gene associated with ASD in the MHC region is the gene coding for the complement protein C4. Complement is an important element of innate immunity and is vital in protecting the host from a number of infectious agents as well as synapse pruning in the CNS. Deficiencies in complement protein C4 have been associated with autoimmune disorders such as SLE (153). In ASD, deficiencies in the C4B allele, as well as its protein product, have been reported (154–157). Furthermore, proteomic analyses of sera samples indicate that several complement proteins are differential produced in ASD (158).

A number of other ASD candidate genes have been identified that are integral to immune function. These include macrophage migration inhibitory factor (MIF) (159), MET tyrosine receptors

(160, 161), serine and threonine kinase C gene PRKCB1 (162), and reelin (163–165). In addition, a number of syndromic disorders with high rates of ASD are defined by alterations in genes with significant roles in immune regulation including tuberous sclerosis complex (either TSC1 or TSC2) (Tuberous Sclerosis) (21), protein phosphatase and tensin homolog (PTEN) (Cowden's Syndrome) (166), calcium channel, L type, alpha-1 polypeptide (CACNA1C) (Timothy Syndrome) (167), methyl CpG binding protein 2 (MeCP2) (Rett's Syndrome) (168). Many of these genes are involved in key cellular pathways such as the mTOR/Akt pathway utilized by both the nervous and immune system. The mTOR/Akt pathway is involved in immune signaling, activation, and survival, and alterations to genes within this pathway may contribute to the immune dysfunction seen in ASD (reviewed in ref. (64)). However, it is currently unclear how dysregulation of these pathways contributes to the development of ASD, or to what degree the immune response is involved.

9. Conclusion

The nervous and immune systems are intimately tied together, and immune cells and their products are capable of directly alerting neuronal architecture and function. A convergence of evidence from a number of disciplines has demonstrated the presence of immune dysregulation in ASD, both in the children and parents. This inappropriate immune function can have devastating effects, and both epidemiological and animal model studies suggest that an inappropriate immune response during early development can lead to neurodevelopmental disorders including ASD. Much remains to be understood about the precise mechanism by which the immune system contributes to the pathology of ASD as well as how genetic and environmental factors contribute to the heterogeneity of core features. Further research is needed to elucidate these questions, but it is clear the immune system offers many avenues for better understanding as well as possible targets for therapies in ASD.

References

1. American Psychiatric Association (1994) Diagnostic and statistical manual of mental disorders, 4th edn. American Psychiatric Association, Washington, DC
2. Fombonne E (2003) Epidemiological surveys of autism and other pervasive developmental disorders: an update. J Autism Dev Disord 33:365–382
3. King M, Bearman P (2009) Diagnostic change and the increased prevalence of autism. Int J Epidemiol 38:1224–1234
4. Money J, Bobrow NA, Clarke FC (1971) Autism and autoimmune disease: a family study. J Autism Child Schizophr 1:146–160
5. Cooper GS, Bynum ML, Somers EC (2009) Recent insights in the epidemiology of

autoimmune diseases: improved prevalence estimates and understanding of clustering of diseases. J Autoimmun 33:197–207

6. Croen LA, Grether JK, Yoshida CK, Odouli R, Van de Water J (2005) Maternal autoimmune diseases, asthma and allergies, and childhood autism spectrum disorders: a case–control study. Arch Pediatr Adolesc Med 159:151–157
7. Atladottir HO, Pedersen MG, Thorsen P, Mortensen PB, Deleuran B, Eaton WW, Parner ET (2009) Association of family history of autoimmune diseases and autism spectrum disorders. Pediatrics 124:687–694
8. Valicenti-McDermott MD, McVicar K, Cohen HJ, Wershil BK, Shinnar S (2008) Gastrointestinal symptoms in children with an autism spectrum disorder and language regression. Pediatr Neurol 39:392–398
9. Keil A, Daniels JL, Forssen U, Hultman C, Cnattingius S, Soderberg KC, Feychting M, Sparen P (2010) Parental autoimmune diseases associated with autism spectrum disorders in offspring. Epidemiology 21:805–808
10. Mouridsen SE, Rich B, Isager T, Nedergaard NJ (2007) Autoimmune diseases in parents of children with infantile autism: a case–control study. Dev Med Child Neurol 49:429–432
11. Mostafa GA, Kitchener N (2009) Serum antinuclear antibodies as a marker of autoimmunity in Egyptian autistic children. Pediatr Neurol 40:107–112
12. Molloy CA, Morrow AL, Meinzen-Derr J, Dawson G, Bernier R, Dunn M, Hyman SL, McMahon WM, Goudie-Nice J, Hepburn S, Minshew N, Rogers S, Sigman M, Spence MA, Tager-Flusberg H, Volkmar FR, Lord C (2006) Familial autoimmune thyroid disease as a risk factor for regression in children with Autism Spectrum Disorder: a CPEA study. J Autism Dev Disord 36:317–324
13. Sweeten TL, Bowyer SL, Posey DJ, Halberstadt GM, McDougle CJ (2003) Increased prevalence of familial autoimmunity in probands with pervasive developmental disorders. Pediatrics 112:e420
14. Comi AM, Zimmerman AW, Frye VH, Law PA, Peeden JN (1999) Familial clustering of autoimmune disorders and evaluation of medical risk factors in autism. J Child Neurol 14:388–394
15. Mor G, Cardenas I (2010) The immune system in pregnancy: a unique complexity. Am J Reprod Immunol 63:425–433
16. Brown AS, Derkits EJ (2010) Prenatal infection and schizophrenia: a review of epidemiologic and translational studies. Am J Psychiatry 167:261–280
17. Chess S (1977) Follow-up report on autism in congenital rubella. J Autism Child Schizophr 7:69–81
18. Libbey JE, Sweeten TL, McMahon WM, Fujinami RS (2005) Autistic disorder and viral infections. J Neurovirol 11:1–10
19. Sweeten TL, Posey DJ, McDougle CJ (2004) Brief report: autistic disorder in three children with cytomegalovirus infection. J Autism Dev Disord 34:583–586
20. Atladottir HO, Thorsen P, Ostergaard L, Schendel DE, Lemcke S, Abdallah M, Parner ET (2010) Maternal infection requiring hospitalization during pregnancy and autism spectrum disorders. J Autism Dev Disord 40:1423–1430
21. Wiznitzer M (2004) Autism and tuberous sclerosis. J Child Neurol 19:675–679
22. Ehninger D, Sano Y, de Vries PJ, Dies K, Franz D, Geschwind DH, Kaur M, Lee YS, Li W, Lowe JK, Nakagawa JA, Sahin M, Smith K, Whittemore V, Silva AJ (2012) Gestational immune activation and Tsc2 haploinsufficiency cooperate to disrupt fetal survival and may perturb social behavior in adult mice. Mol Psychiatry 17(1):62–70
23. Smith SEP, Hsiao E, Patterson PH (2010) Activation of the maternal immune system as a risk factor for neuropsychiatric disorders. In: Zimmerman AW, Connors SL (eds) Maternal influences on fetal neurodevelopment. Springer, New York, pp 97–115
24. Borrell J, Vela JM, Arevalo-Martin A, Molina-Holgado E, Guaza C (2002) Prenatal immune challenge disrupts sensorimotor gating in adult rats. Implications for the etiopathogenesis of schizophrenia. Neuropsychopharmacology 26: 204–215
25. Gilmore JH, Jarskog LF, Vadlamudi S (2005) Maternal poly I:C exposure during pregnancy regulates TNF alpha, BDNF, and NGF expression in neonatal brain and the maternal-fetal unit of the rat. J Neuroimmunol 159:106–112
26. Hsiao EY, Patterson PH (2011) Activation of the maternal immune system induces endocrine changes in the placenta via IL-6. Brain Behav Immun 25(4):604–615
27. Meyer U, Nyffeler M, Yee BK, Knuesel I, Feldon J (2008) Adult brain and behavioral pathological markers of prenatal immune challenge during early/middle and late fetal development in mice. Brain Behav Immun 22:469–486
28. Jonakait GM (2007) The effects of maternal inflammation on neuronal development: possible mechanisms. Int J Dev Neurosci 25:415–425

29. Smith SE, Li J, Garbett K, Mirnics K, Patterson PH (2007) Maternal immune activation alters fetal brain development through interleukin-6. J Neurosci 27:10695–10702
30. Parker-Athill E, Luo D, Bailey A, Giunta B, Tian J, Shytle RD, Murphy T, Legradi G, Tan J (2009) Flavonoids, a prenatal prophylaxis via targeting JAK2/STAT3 signaling to oppose IL-6/MIA associated autism. J Neuroimmunol 217:20–27
31. Zalcman SS (2002) Interleukin-2-induced increases in climbing behavior: inhibition by dopamine D-1 and D-2 receptor antagonists. Brain Res 944:157–164
32. Ponzio NM, Servatius R, Beck K, Marzouk A, Kreider T (2007) Cytokine levels during pregnancy influence immunological profiles and neurobehavioral patterns of the offspring. Ann N Y Acad Sci 1107:118–128
33. Abazyan B, Nomura J, Kannan G, Ishizuka K, Tamashiro KL, Nucifora F, Pogorelov V, Ladenheim B, Yang C, Krasnova IN (2010) Prenatal interaction of mutant DISC1 and immune activation produces adult psychopathology. Biol Psychiatry 68:1172–1181
34. Lasala N, Zhou H (2007) Effects of maternal exposure to LPS on the inflammatory response in the offspring. J Neuroimmunol 189: 95–101
35. Surriga O, Ortega A, Jadeja V, Bellafronte A, Lasala N, Zhou H (2009) Altered hepatic inflammatory response in the offspring following prenatal LPS exposure. Immunol Lett 123:88–95
36. Mandal M, Marzouk AC, Donnelly R, Ponzio NM (2010) Preferential development of Th17 cells in offspring of immunostimulated pregnant mice. J Reprod Immunol 87: 97–100
37. Mandal M, Marzouk AC, Donnelly R, Ponzio NM (2011) Maternal immune stimulation during pregnancy affects adaptive immunity in offspring to promote development of TH17 cells. Brain Behav Immun 25: 863–871
38. Ashwood P, Krakowiak P, Hertz-Picciotto I, Hansen R, Pessah IN, Van de Water J (2011) Associations of impaired behaviors with elevated plasma chemokines in autism spectrum disorders. J Neuroimmunol 232(1–2):196–199
39. Ashwood P, Krakowiak P, Hertz-Picciotto I, Hansen R, Pessah I, Van de Water J (2011) Elevated plasma cytokines in autism spectrum disorders provide evidence of immune dysfunction and are associated with impaired behavioral outcome. Brain Behav Immun 25:40–45
40. Ashwood P, Krakowiak P, Hertz-Picciotto I, Hansen R, Pessah IN, Van de Water J (2011) Altered T cell responses in children with autism. Brain Behav Immun 25(5):840–849
41. Enstrom AM, Onore CE, Van de Water JA, Ashwood P (2010) Differential monocyte responses to TLR ligands in children with autism spectrum disorders. Brain Behav Immun 24:64–71
42. Heuer L, Ashwood P, Schauer J, Goines P, Krakowiak P, Hertz-Picciotto I, Hansen R, Croen LA, Pessah IN, Van de Water J (2008) Reduced levels of immunoglobulin in children with autism correlates with behavioral symptoms. Autism Res 1:275–283
43. Sandler RH, Finegold SM, Bolte ER, Buchanan CP, Maxwell AP, Vaisanen ML, Nelson MN, Wexler HM (2000) Short-term benefit from oral vancomycin treatment of regressive-onset autism. J Child Neurol 15:429–435
44. Tincani A, Rebaioli CB, Frassi M, Taglietti M, Gorla R, Cavazzana I, Faden D, Taddei F, Lojacono A, Motta M, Trepidi L, Meroni P, Cimaz R, Ghirardello A, Doria A, Pisoni MP, Muscara M, Brucato A (2005) Pregnancy and autoimmunity: maternal treatment and maternal disease influence on pregnancy outcome. Autoimmun Rev 4:423–428
45. Lee JY, Huerta PT, Zhang J, Kowal C, Bertini E, Volpe BT, Diamond B (2009) Neurotoxic autoantibodies mediate congenital cortical impairment of offspring in maternal lupus. Nat Med 15:91–96
46. Neri F, Chimini L, Bonomi F, Filippini E, Motta M, Faden D, Lojacono A, Rebaioli CB, Frassi M, Danieli E, Tincani A (2004) Neuropsychological development of children born to patients with systemic lupus erythematosus. Lupus 13:805–811
47. McAllister DL, Kaplan BJ, Edworthy SM, Martin L, Crawford SG, Ramsey-Goldman R, Manzi S, Fries JF, Sibley J (1997) The influence of systemic lupus erythematosus on fetal development: cognitive, behavioral, and health trends. J Int Neuropsychol Soc 3:370–376
48. Tincani A, Danieli E, Nuzzo M, Scarsil M, Motta M, Cimaz R, Lojacono A, Nacinovich R, Taddei F, Doria A, Brucato A, Meroni P (2006) Impact of in utero environment on the offspring of lupus patients. Lupus 15:801–807
49. Fu J, Jiang Y, Liang L, Zhu H (2005) Risk factors of primary thyroid dysfunction in early infants born to mothers with autoimmune thyroid disease. Acta Paediatr 94:1043–1048

50. Rolim A, Castro M, Santiago M (2006) Neonatal antiphospholipid syndrome. Lupus 15:301
51. Braunschweig D, Ashwood P, Krakowiak P, Hertz-Picciotto I, Hansen R, Croen LA, Pessah IN, Van de Water J (2008) Autism: maternally derived antibodies specific for fetal brain proteins. Neurotoxicology 29:226–231
52. Silva SC, Correia C, Fesel C, Barreto M, Coutinho AM, Marques C, Miguel TS, Ataide A, Bento C, Borges L, Oliveira G, Vicente AM (2004) Autoantibody repertoires to brain tissue in autism nuclear families. J Neuroimmunol 152:176–182
53. Zimmerman AW, Connors SL, Matteson KJ, Lee LC, Singer HS, Castaneda JA, Pearce DA (2007) Maternal antibrain antibodies in autism. Brain Behav Immun 21:351–357
54. Klauck SM, Poustka A (2006) Animal models of autism. Drug Discov Today Dis Models 3:313–318
55. Martin LA, Ashwood P, Braunschweig D, Cabanlit M, Van de Water J, Amaral DG (2008) Stereotypies and hyperactivity in rhesus monkeys exposed to IgG from mothers of children with autism. Brain Behav Immun 22:806–816
56. Singer HS, Morris C, Gause C, Pollard M, Zimmerman AW, Pletnikov M (2009) Prenatal exposure to antibodies from mothers of children with autism produces neurobehavioral alterations: a pregnant dam mouse model. J Neuroimmunol 211:39–48
57. Deverman BE, Patterson PH (2009) Cytokines and CNS development. Neuron 64:61–78
58. Silverman MN, Pearce BD, Biron CA, Miller AH (2005) Immune modulation of the hypothalamic-pituitary-adrenal (HPA) axis during viral infection. Viral Immunol 18:41–78
59. Schwartz M, Kipnis J (2011) A conceptual revolution in the relationships between the brain and immunity. Brain Behav Immun 25(5):817–819
60. Strous RD, Shoenfeld Y (2006) Schizophrenia, autoimmunity and immune system dysregulation: a comprehensive model updated and revisited. J Autoimmun 27:71–80
61. Murphy TK, Kurlan R, Leckman J (2010) The immunobiology of Tourette's disorder, pediatric autoimmune neuropsychiatric disorders associated with Streptococcus, and related disorders: a way forward. J Child Adolesc Psychopharmacol 20:317–331
62. Dantzer R, O'Connor JC, Freund GG, Johnson RW, Kelley KW (2008) From inflammation to sickness and depression: when the immune system subjugates the brain. Nat Rev Neurosci 9:46–56
63. Eaton WW, Pedersen MG, Nielsen PR, Mortensen PB (2010) Autoimmune diseases, bipolar disorder, and non-affective psychosis. Bipolar Disord 12:638–646
64. Careaga M, Van de Water J, Ashwood P (2010) Immune dysfunction in autism: a pathway to treatment. Neurotherapeutics 7:283–292
65. Enstrom AM, Van de Water JA, Ashwood P (2009) Autoimmunity in autism. Curr Opin Investig Drugs 10:463–473
66. Goines P, Van de Water J (2010) The immune system's role in the biology of autism. Curr Opin Neurol 23:111–117. doi:110.1097/WCO.1090b1013e3283373514
67. Vargas DL, Nascimbene C, Krishnan C, Zimmerman AW, Pardo CA (2005) Neuroglial activation and neuroinflammation in the brain of patients with autism. Ann Neurol 57:67–81
68. Li X, Chauhan A, Sheikh AM, Patil S, Chauhan V, Li X-M, Ji L, Brown T, Malik M (2009) Elevated immune response in the brain of autistic patients. J Neuroimmunol 207:111–116
69. Ashwood P, Anthony A, Torrente F, Wakefield AJ (2004) Spontaneous mucosal lymphocyte cytokine profiles in children with autism and gastrointestinal symptoms: mucosal immune activation and reduced counter regulatory interleukin-10. J Clin Immunol 24:664–673
70. Jyonouchi H, Sun S, Le H (2001) Proinflammatory and regulatory cytokine production associated with innate and adaptive immune responses in children with autism spectrum disorders and developmental regression. J Neuroimmunol 120:170–179
71. Singh VK, Warren RP, Odell JD, Cole P (1991) Changes of soluble interleukin-2, interleukin-2 receptor, T8 antigen, and interleukin-1 in the serum of autistic children. Clin Immunol Immunopathol 61:448–455
72. Singh VK (1996) Plasma increase of interleukin-12 and interferon-gamma. Pathological significance in autism. J Neuroimmunol 66:143–145
73. Ashwood P, Wakefield AJ (2006) Immune activation of peripheral blood and mucosal CD3+ lymphocyte cytokine profiles in children with autism and gastrointestinal symptoms. J Neuroimmunol 173:126–134
74. Ashwood P, Enstrom A, Krakowiak P, Hertz-Picciotto I, Hansen RL, Croen LA, Ozonoff S, Pessah IN, Van de Water J (2008) Decreased transforming growth factor beta1 in autism: a

potential link between immune dysregulation and impairment in clinical behavioral outcomes. J Neuroimmunol 204:149–153

75. Okada K, Hashimoto K, Iwata Y, Nakamura K, Tsujii M, Tsuchiya KJ, Sekine Y, Suda S, Suzuki K, Sugihara G, Matsuzaki H, Sugiyama T, Kawai M, Minabe Y, Takei N, Mori N (2007) Decreased serum levels of transforming growth factor-beta1 in patients with autism. Prog Neuropsychopharmacol Biol Psychiatry 31:187–190
76. Constantino JN, Zhang Y, Frazier T, Abbacchi AM, Law P (2010) Sibling recurrence and the genetic epidemiology of autism. Am J Psychiatry 167:1349–1356
77. Saresella M, Marventano I, Guerini FR, Mancuso R, Ceresa L, Zanzottera M, Rusconi B, Maggioni E, Tinelli C, Clerici M (2009) An autistic endophenotype results in complex immune dysfunction in healthy siblings of autistic children. Biol Psychiatry 66:978–984
78. Alliot F, Godin I, Pessac B (1999) Microglia derive from progenitors, originating from the yolk sac, and which proliferate in the brain. Brain Res Dev Brain Res 117:145–152
79. Ginhoux F, Greter M, Leboeuf M, Nandi S, See P, Gokhan S, Mehler MF, Conway SJ, Ng LG, Stanley ER, Samokhvalov IM, Merad M (2010) Fate mapping analysis reveals that adult microglia derive from primitive macrophages. Science 330:841–845
80. Palis J, Yoder MC (2001) Yolk-sac hematopoiesis: the first blood cells of mouse and man. Exp Hematol 29:927–936
81. Chen SK, Tvrdik P, Peden E, Cho S, Wu S, Spangrude G, Capecchi MR (2010) Hematopoietic origin of pathological grooming in Hoxb8 mutant mice. Cell 141: 775–785
82. Derecki NC, Quinnies KM, Kipnis J (2011) Alternatively activated myeloid (M2) cells enhance cognitive function in immune compromised mice. Brain Behav Immun 25(3):379–385
83. Cacci E, Claasen JH, Kokaia Z (2005) Microglia-derived tumor necrosis factor-alpha exaggerates death of newborn hippocampal progenitor cells in vitro. J Neurosci Res 80:789–797
84. Stellwagen D, Malenka RC (2006) Synaptic scaling mediated by glial TNF-alpha. Nature 440:1054–1059
85. Widera D, Mikenberg I, Elvers M, Kaltschmidt C, Kaltschmidt B (2006) Tumor necrosis factor alpha triggers proliferation of adult neural stem cells via IKK/NF-kappaB signaling. BMC Neurosci 7:64
86. Banks WA, Farr SA, La Scola ME, Morley JE (2001) Intravenous human interleukin-1 alpha impairs memory processing in mice: dependence on blood–brain barrier transport into posterior division of the septum. J Pharmacol Exp Ther 299:536–541
87. Depino AM, Alonso M, Ferrari C, del Rey A, Anthony D, Besedovsky H, Medina JH, Pitossi F (2004) Learning modulation by endogenous hippocampal IL-1: blockade of endogenous IL-1 facilitates memory formation. Hippocampus 14:526–535
88. Goshen I, Yirmiya R (2009) Interleukin-1 (IL-1): a central regulator of stress responses. Front Neuroendocrinol 30:30–45
89. Schneider H, Pitossi F, Balschun D, Wagner A, del Rey A, Besedovsky HO (1998) A neuromodulatory role of interleukin-1beta in the hippocampus. Proc Natl Acad Sci U S A 95:7778–7783
90. Baier PC, May U, Scheller J, Rose-John S, Schiffelholz T (2009) Impaired hippocampus-dependent and -independent learning in IL-6 deficient mice. Behav Brain Res 200:192–196
91. Harden LM, du Plessis I, Poole S, Laburn HP (2008) Interleukin (IL)-6 and IL-1 beta act synergistically within the brain to induce sickness behavior and fever in rats. Brain Behav Immun 22:838–849
92. Enstrom AM, Lit L, Onore CE, Gregg JP, Hansen RL, Pessah IN, Hertz-Picciotto I, Van de Water JA, Sharp FR, Ashwood P (2009) Altered gene expression and function of peripheral blood natural killer cells in children with autism. Brain Behav Immun 23:124–133
93. Warren RP, Foster A, Margaretten NC (1987) Reduced natural killer cell activity in autism. J Am Acad Child Adolesc Psychiatry 26: 333–335
94. Vojdani A, Mumper E, Granpeesheh D, Mielke L, Traver D, Bock K, Hirani K, Neubrander J, Woeller KN, O'Hara N, Usman A, Schneider C, Hebroni F, Berookhim J, McCandless J (2008) Low natural killer cell cytotoxic activity in autism: the role of glutathione, IL-2 and IL-15. J Neuroimmunol 205:148–154
95. Ashwood P, Corbett BA, Kantor A, Schulman H, Van de Water J, Amaral DG (2011) In search of cellular immunophenotypes in the blood of children with autism. PLoS One 6:e19299
96. Wilson EH, Weninger W, Hunter CA (2010) Trafficking of immune cells in the central nervous system. J Clin Invest 120:1368–1379

97. Lima FRS, da Fonseca ACC, Faria GP, Dubois LGF, Alves TR, Faria J, Neto VM (2010) The origin of microglia and the development of the brain. In: Ulrich H (ed) Perspectives of stem cells. Springer, Netherlands, pp 171–189
98. Voineagu I, Wang X, Johnston P, Lowe JK, Tian Y, Horvath S, Mill J, Cantor RM, Blencowe BJ, Geschwind DH (2011) Transcriptomic analysis of autistic brain reveals convergent molecular pathology. Nature 474:380–384
99. Sweeten TL, Posey DJ, McDougle CJ (2003) High blood monocyte counts and neopterin levels in children with autistic disorder. Am J Psychiatry 160:1691–1693
100. Jyonouchi H, Sun S, Itokazu N (2002) Innate immunity associated with inflammatory responses and cytokine production against common dietary proteins in patients with autism spectrum disorder. Neuropsychobiology 46:76–84
101. Jyonouchi H, Geng L, Cushing-Ruby A, Quraishi H (2008) Impact of innate immunity in a subset of children with autism spectrum disorders: a case control study. J Neuroinflammation 5:52
102. Rosen NJ, Yoshida CK, Croen LA (2007) Infection in the first 2 years of life and autism spectrum disorders. Pediatrics 119:e61–e69
103. Moynihan JA, Santiago FM (2007) Brain behavior and immunity: twenty years of T cells. Brain Behav Immun 21:872–880
104. Ziv Y, Ron N, Butovsky O, Landa G, Sudai E, Greenberg N, Cohen H, Kipnis J, Schwartz M (2006) Immune cells contribute to the maintenance of neurogenesis and spatial learning abilities in adulthood. Nat Neurosci 9:268–275
105. Kipnis J, Cohen H, Cardon M, Ziv Y, Schwartz M (2004) T cell deficiency leads to cognitive dysfunction: implications for therapeutic vaccination for schizophrenia and other psychiatric conditions. Proc Natl Acad Sci U S A 101:8180–8185
106. Serpe CJ, Coers S, Sanders VM, Jones KJ (2003) CD4+ T, but not CD8+ or B, lymphocytes mediate facial motoneuron survival after facial nerve transection. Brain Behav Immun 17:393–402
107. Deboy CA, Xin J, Byram SC, Serpe CJ, Sanders VM, Jones KJ (2006) Immune-mediated neuroprotection of axotomized mouse facial motoneurons is dependent on the IL-4/STAT6 signaling pathway in CD4(+) T cells. Exp Neurol 201:212–224
108. Derecki NC, Cardani AN, Yang CH, Quinnies KM, Crihfield A, Lynch KR, Kipnis J (2010) Regulation of learning and memory by meningeal immunity: a key role for IL-4. J Exp Med 207:1067–1080
109. Fairweather D, Cihakova D (2009) Alternatively activated macrophages in infection and autoimmunity. J Autoimmun 33: 222–230
110. Stubbs EG (1976) Autistic children exhibit undetectable hemagglutination-inhibition antibody titers despite previous rubella vaccination. J Autism Child Schizophr 6:269–274
111. Warren RP, Margaretten NC, Pace NC, Foster A (1986) Immune abnormalities in patients with autism. J Autism Dev Disord 16:189–197
112. Ashwood P, Anthony A, Pellicer AA, Torrente F, Walker-Smith JA, Wakefield AJ (2003) Intestinal lymphocyte populations in children with regressive autism: evidence for extensive mucosal immunopathology. J Clin Immunol 23:504–517
113. Plioplys AV, Greaves A, Kazemi K, Silverman E (1994) Lymphocyte function in autism and Rett syndrome. Neuropsychobiology 29: 12–16
114. Gupta S, Aggarwal S, Rashanravan B, Lee T (1998) Th1- and Th2-like cytokines in CD4+ and CD8+ T cells in autism. J Neuroimmunol 85:106–109
115. Aghamohammadi A, Cheraghi T, Gharagozlou M, Movahedi M, Rezaei N, Yeganeh M, Parvaneh N, Abolhassani H, Pourpak Z, Moin M (2009) IgA deficiency: correlation between clinical and immunological phenotypes. J Clin Immunol 29:130–136
116. Warren RP, Odell JD, Warren WL, Burger RA, Maciulis A, Daniels WW, Torres AR (1997) Brief report: immunoglobulin A deficiency in a subset of autistic subjects. J Autism Dev Disord 27:187–192
117. Enstrom A, Krakowiak P, Onore C, Pessah IN, Hertz-Picciotto I, Hansen RL, Van de Water JA, Ashwood P (2009) Increased IgG4 levels in children with autism disorder. Brain Behav Immun 23:389–395
118. Croonenberghs J, Wauters A, Devreese K, Verkerk R, Scharpe S, Bosmans E, Egyed B, Deboutte D, Maes M (2002) Increased serum albumin, gamma globulin, immunoglobulin IgG, and IgG2 and IgG4 in autism. Psychol Med 32:1457–1463
119. Grether JK, Croen LA, Anderson MC, Nelson KB, Yolken RH (2010) Neonatally measured immunoglobulins and risk of autism. Autism Res 3:323–332

120. Qaqish BF, Prisayanh P, Qian Y, Andraca E, Li N, Aoki V, Hans-Filho G, dos Santos V, Rivitti EA, Diaz LA (2009) Development of an IgG4-based predictor of endemic pemphigus foliaceus (fogo selvagem). J Invest Dermatol 129:110–118
121. Wills S, Cabanlit M, Bennett J, Ashwood P, Amaral D, Van de Water J (2007) Autoantibodies in autism spectrum disorders (ASD). Ann N Y Acad Sci 1107:79–91
122. Todd RD, Ciaranello RD (1985) Demonstration of inter- and intraspecies differences in serotonin binding sites by antibodies from an autistic child. Proc Natl Acad Sci U S A 82:612–616
123. Connolly AM, Chez M, Streif EM, Keeling RM, Golumbek PT, Kwon JM, Riviello JJ, Robinson RG, Neuman RJ, Deuel RM (2006) Brain-derived neurotrophic factor and autoantibodies to neural antigens in sera of children with autistic spectrum disorders, Landau-Kleffner syndrome, and epilepsy. Biol Psychiatry 59:354–363
124. Singh VK, Warren RP, Odell JD, Warren WL, Cole P (1993) Antibodies to myelin basic protein in children with autistic behavior. Brain Behav Immun 7:97–103
125. Singh VK, Warren R, Averett R, Ghaziuddin M (1997) Circulating autoantibodies to neuronal and glial filament proteins in autism. Pediatr Neurol 17:88–90
126. Libbey JE, Coon HH, Kirkman NJ, Sweeten TL, Miller JN, Stevenson EK, Lainhart JE, McMahon WM, Fujinami RS (2008) Are there enhanced MBP autoantibodies in autism? J Autism Dev Disord 38:324–332
127. Kirkman NJ, Libbey JE, Sweeten TL, Coon HH, Miller JN, Stevenson EK, Lainhart JE, McMahon WM, Fujinami RS (2008) How relevant are GFAP autoantibodies in autism and Tourette syndrome? J Autism Dev Disord 38:333–341
128. Morris CM, Zimmerman AW, Singer HS (2009) Childhood serum anti-fetal brain antibodies do not predict autism. Pediatr Neurol 41:288–290
129. Goines P, Haapanen L, Boyce R, Duncanson P, Braunschweig D, Delwiche L, Hansen R, Hertz-Picciotto I, Ashwood P, Van de Water J (2011) Autoantibodies to cerebellum in children with autism associate with behavior. Brain Behav Immun 25(3):514–523
130. Wills S, Rossi CC, Bennett J, Cerdeno VM, Ashwood P, Amaral DG, Van de Water J (2011) Further characterization of autoantibodies to GABAergic neurons in the central nervous system produced by a subset of children with autism. Mol Autism 2:5
131. Torrente F, Anthony A, Heuschkel RB, Thomson MA, Ashwood P, Murch SH (2004) Focal-enhanced gastritis in regressive autism with features distinct from Crohn's and Helicobacter pylori gastritis. Am J Gastroenterol 99:598–605
132. Torrente F, Ashwood P, Day R, Machado N, Furlano RI, Anthony A, Davies SE, Wakefield AJ, Thomson MA, Walker-Smith JA, Murch SH (2002) Small intestinal enteropathy with epithelial IgG and complement deposition in children with regressive autism. Mol Psychiatry 7(375–382):334
133. Furlano RI, Anthony A, Day R, Brown A, McGarvey L, Thomson MA, Davies SE, Berelowitz M, Forbes A, Wakefield AJ, Walker-Smith JA, Murch SH (2001) Colonic CD8 and gamma delta T-cell infiltration with epithelial damage in children with autism. J Pediatr 138:366–372
134. de Magistris L, Familiari V, Pascotto A, Sapone A, Frolli A, Iardino P, Carteni M, De Rosa M, Francavilla R, Riegler G, Militerni R, Bravaccio C (2010) Alterations of the intestinal barrier in patients with autism spectrum disorders and in their first-degree relatives. J Pediatr Gastroenterol Nutr 51:418–424
135. D'Eufemia P, Celli M, Finocchiaro R, Pacifico L, Viozzi L, Zaccagnini M, Cardi E, Giardini O (1996) Abnormal intestinal permeability in children with autism. Acta Paediatr 85:1076–1079
136. Wang LW, Tancredi DJ, Thomas DW (2011) The prevalence of gastrointestinal problems in children across the United States with autism spectrum disorders from families with multiple affected members. J Dev Behav Pediatr 32:351–360
137. Buie T, Campbell DB, Fuchs GJ III, Furuta GT, Levy J, Vandewater J, Whitaker AH, Atkins D, Bauman ML, Beaudet AL, Carr EG, Gershon MD, Hyman SL, Jirapinyo P, Jyonouchi H, Kooros K, Kushak R, Levitt P, Levy SE, Lewis JD, Murray KF, Natowicz MR, Sabra A, Wershil BK, Weston SC, Zeltzer L, Winter H (2010) Evaluation, diagnosis, and treatment of gastrointestinal disorders in individuals with ASDs: a consensus report. Pediatrics 125(suppl 1):S1–S18
138. Adams JB, Johansen LJ, Powell LD, Quig D, Rubin RA (2011) Gastrointestinal flora and gastrointestinal status in children with autism–comparisons to typical children and correlation with autism severity. BMC Gastroenterol 11:22
139. Genuis SJ, Bouchard TP (2010) Celiac disease presenting as autism. J Child Neurol 25(1):114–119

140. Constantino JN, Todd RD (2000) Genetic structure of reciprocal social behavior. Am J Psychiatry 157:2043–2045
141. Ronald A, Happe F, Bolton P, Butcher LM, Price TS, Wheelwright S, Baron-Cohen S, Plomin R (2006) Genetic heterogeneity between the three components of the autism spectrum: a twin study. J Am Acad Child Adolesc Psychiatry 45:691–699
142. Kolevzon A, Smith CJ, Schmeidler J, Buxbaum JD, Silverman JM (2004) Familial symptom domains in monozygotic siblings with autism. Am J Med Genet B Neuropsychiatr Genet 129B:76–81
143. Kates WR, Burnette CP, Eliez S, Strunge LA, Kaplan D, Landa R, Reiss AL, Pearlson GD (2004) Neuroanatomic variation in monozygotic twin pairs discordant for the narrow phenotype for autism. Am J Psychiatry 161:539–546
144. Jorde LB, Hasstedt SJ, Ritvo ER, Mason-Brothers A, Freeman BJ, Pingree C, McMahon WM, Petersen B, Jenson WR, Mo A (1991) Complex segregation analysis of autism. Am J Hum Genet 49:932–938
145. Stubbs EG, Magenis RE (1980) HLA and autism. J Autism Dev Disord 10:15–19
146. Daniels WW, Warren RP, Odell JD, Maciulis A, Burger RA, Warren WL, Torres AR (1995) Increased frequency of the extended or ancestral haplotype B44-SC30-DR4 in autism. Neuropsychobiology 32:120–123
147. Lee LC, Zachary AA, Leffell MS, Newschaffer CJ, Matteson KJ, Tyler JD, Zimmerman AW (2006) HLA-DR4 in families with autism. Pediatr Neurol 35:303–307
148. Torres AR, Maciulis A, Stubbs EG, Cutler A, Odell D (2002) The transmission disequilibrium test suggests that HLA-DR4 and DR13 are linked to autism spectrum disorder. Hum Immunol 63:311–316
149. Warren RP, Singh VK, Cole P, Odell JD, Pingree CB, Warren WL, DeWitt CW, McCullough M (1992) Possible association of the extended MHC haplotype B44-SC30-DR4 with autism. Immunogenetics 36:203–207
150. Fernando MM, Stevens CR, Walsh EC, De Jager PL, Goyette P, Plenge RM, Vyse TJ, Rioux JD (2008) Defining the role of the MHC in autoimmunity: a review and pooled analysis. PLoS Genet 4:e1000024
151. Guerini FR, Bolognesi E, Manca S, Sotgiu S, Zanzottera M, Agliardi C, Usai S, Clerici M (2009) Family-based transmission analysis of HLA genetic markers in Sardinian children with autistic spectrum disorders. Hum Immunol 70:184–190
152. Guerini FR, Bolognesi E, Chiappedi M, De Silvestri A, Ghezzo A, Zanette M, Rusconi B, Manca S, Sotgiu S, Agliardi C, Clerici M (2011) HLA polymorphisms in Italian children with autism spectrum disorders: results of a family based linkage study. J Neuroimmunol 230:135–142
153. Mascart-Lemone F, Hauptmann G, Goetz J, Duchateau J, Delespesse G, Vray B, Dab I (1983) Genetic deficiency of C4 presenting with recurrent infections and a SLE-like disease. Genetic and immunologic studies. Am J Med 75:295–304
154. Odell D, Maciulis A, Cutler A, Warren L, McMahon WM, Coon H, Stubbs G, Henley K, Torres A (2005) Confirmation of the association of the C4B null allele in autism. Hum Immunol 66:140–145
155. Warren RP, Burger RA, Odell D, Torres AR, Warren WL (1994) Decreased plasma concentrations of the C4B complement protein in autism. Arch Pediatr Adolesc Med 148:180–183
156. Warren RP, Yonk J, Burger RW, Odell D, Warren WL (1995) DR-positive T cells in autism: association with decreased plasma levels of the complement C4B protein. Neuropsychobiology 31:53–57
157. Mostafa GA, Shehab AA (2010) The link of C4B null allele to autism and to a family history of autoimmunity in Egyptian autistic children. J Neuroimmunol 223:115–119
158. Corbett BA, Kantor AB, Schulman H, Walker WL, Lit L, Ashwood P, Rocke DM, Sharp FR (2007) A proteomic study of serum from children with autism showing differential expression of apolipoproteins and complement proteins. Mol Psychiatry 12: 292–306
159. Grigorenko EL, Han SS, Yrigollen CM, Leng L, Mizue Y, Anderson GM, Mulder EJ, de Bildt A, Minderaa RB, Volkmar FR, Chang JT, Bucala R (2008) Macrophage migration inhibitory factor and autism spectrum disorders. Pediatrics 122:e438–e445
160. Correll PH, Morrison AC, Lutz MA (2004) Receptor tyrosine kinases and the regulation of macrophage activation. J Leukoc Biol 75:731–737
161. Campbell DB, Sutcliffe JS, Ebert PJ, Militerni R, Bravaccio C, Trillo S, Elia M, Schneider C, Melmed R, Sacco R, Persico AM, Levitt P (2006) A genetic variant that disrupts MET transcription is associated with autism. Proc Natl Acad Sci U S A 103:16834–16839
162. Lintas C, Sacco R, Garbett K, Mirnics K, Militerni R, Bravaccio C, Curatolo P, Manzi B, Schneider C, Melmed R, Elia M, Pascucci

T, Puglisi-Allegra S, Reichelt KL, Persico AM (2009) Involvement of the PRKCB1 gene in autistic disorder: significant genetic association and reduced neocortical gene expression. Mol Psychiatry 14:705–718

163. Serajee FJ, Zhong H, Mahbubul Huq AH (2006) Association of Reelin gene polymorphisms with autism. Genomics 87:75–83

164. Zhang H, Liu X, Zhang C, Mundo E, Macciardi F, Grayson DR, Guidotti AR, Holden JJ (2002) Reelin gene alleles and susceptibility to autism spectrum disorders. Mol Psychiatry 7:1012–1017

165. Skaar DA, Shao Y, Haines JL, Stenger JE, Jaworski J, Martin ER, DeLong GR, Moore JH, McCauley JL, Sutcliffe JS, Ashley-Koch AE, Cuccaro ML, Folstein SE, Gilbert JR, Pericak-Vance MA (2005) Analysis of the RELN gene as a genetic risk factor for autism. Mol Psychiatry 10:563–571

166. Herman GE, Butter E, Enrile B, Pastore M, Prior TW, Sommer A (2007) Increasing knowledge of PTEN germline mutations: two additional patients with autism and macrocephaly. Am J Med Genet A 143:589–593

167. Splawski I, Timothy KW, Priori SG, Napolitano C, Bloise R (1993) Timothy syndrome. In: Pagon RA, Bird TD, Dolan CR, Stephens K (eds) GeneReviews. University of Washington, Seattle, WA

168. Nagarajan RP, Patzel KA, Martin M, Yasui DH, Swanberg SE, Hertz-Picciotto I, Hansen RL, Van de Water J, Pessah IN, Jiang R, Robinson WP, LaSalle JM (2008) MECP2 promoter methylation and X chromosome inactivation in autism. Autism Res 1:169–178

Part III

Technologies and Models in Psychoneuroimmunology Studies

Chapter 13

Mouse Testing Methods in Psychoneuroimmunology: An Overview of How to Measure Sickness, Depressive/ Anxietal, Cognitive, and Physical Activity Behaviors

Jason M. York, Neil A. Blevins, Tracy Baynard, and Gregory G. Freund

Abstract

The field of psychoneuroimmunology (PNI) aims to uncover the processes and consequences of nervous, immune, and endocrine system relationships. Behavior is a consequence of such interactions and manifests from a complex interweave of factors including immune-to-neural and neural-to-immune communication. Often the signaling molecules involved during a particular episode of neuroimmune activation are not known but behavioral response provides evidence that bioactives such as neurotransmitters and cytokines are perturbed. Immunobehavioral phenotyping is a first-line approach when examining the neuroimmune system and its reaction to immune stimulation or suppression. Behavioral response is significantly more sensitive than direct measurement of a single specific bioactive and can quickly and efficiently rule in or out relevance of a particular immune challenge or therapeutic to neuroimmunity. Classically, immunobehavioral research was focused on sickness symptoms related to bacterial infection but neuroimmune activation is now a recognized complication of diseases and disorders ranging from cancer to diabesity. Immunobehaviors include lethargy, loss of appetite, and disinterest in social activity and the surrounding environment. In addition, neuroimmune activation can precipitate feelings of depression and anxiety while negatively impacting cognitive function and physical activity. Provided is a detailed overview of behavioral tests frequently used to examine neuroimmune activation in mice with a special emphasis on preexperimental conditions that can confound or prevent successful immunobehavioral experimentation.

Key words: Mouse, Maze, Exploration, Brain based, Biobehaviors, Memory, Motor activity, Anhedonia

1. Introduction

Since its inception as an interdisciplinary field of science in the 1970s, behavior has been an integral part of psychoneuroimmunology (PNI). Indeed, PNI is generally defined as the study of the interactions between behavior, neural, immune, and endocrine

Qing Yan (ed.), *Psychoneuroimmunology: Methods and Protocols*, Methods in Molecular Biology, vol. 934, DOI 10.1007/978-1-62703-071-7_13, © Springer Science+Business Media, LLC 2012

system functions (1, 2). Behavior can be, and is largely, used to assess whether a particular stimuli or experimental treatment has the potential to activate the neuroimmune system (1, 2). An important concept to recognize in PNI is the bidirectionality that exists between the nervous system and the immune system (2). This is to say that both neural-to-immune and immune-to-neural signaling can and do occur. Shared pathways exist between the nervous and immune systems that use a repertoire of signaling molecules such as cytokines and neurotransmitters (3) that are capable of interacting with both immune and nervous system cells. These bioactives can convey the state of peripheral immunity to the neuroimmune system, communicate the status of neuroimmunity to the peripheral immune system (3–5), and provide immunoactivating and deactivating signals to immune cells throughout the body (6).

Observation of innate immune-mediated behavioral change (immunobehaviors) is largely used as a method of measuring neuroimmune activation in response to pathogenic insult of infectious (6) or noninfectious (7) etiology. Sickness behavior, in a classical sense, is a set of coordinated behavioral changes in response to immune stimulation aimed at conserving and redirecting body energy stores toward combating illness and promoting recovery (4, 8). Immunobehaviors are best known for their manifestation in association with bacterial infection (8), but materialize in spectrum of conditions and diseases including cancer (8), autoimmune disorders (9), wounding (10), depression (11), and obesity (12). In any circumstance in which the innate immune system is activated, peripheral inflammatory mediators can impact the brain, altering normal function and causing symptoms of illness/loss of well-being (4, 8). Typical sickness behavior symptoms include reduction in food intake, lethargy, malaise, loss of interest in social and/or environmental surroundings, changes in sleep patterns, and impaired cognition (4, 8, 11). Furthermore, continued or dysregulated activation of the neuroimmune system can progress beyond acute sickness symptoms and transition to behaviors observed in the anxious or depressed (11). Fatigue is often a lingering complication of neuroimmune activation (6) and can present as purely mental or physical or (most commonly) in a combinational form (13). In rodents, exercise behaviors like spontaneous wheel running (SWR) (14) are helping to unravel the complex biology of physical fatigue while tests examining memory formation (learning) and memory recall are being used to explore mental fatigue (15).

Finally, immunobehaviors are a powerful indicator of neuroimmune status offering insight into the pro-inflammatory milieu of the brain. Altered behavior manifests prior to detectable changes in brain-based bioactives and lingers past their resolution. Such conditions indicate that the brain is very sensitive to small perturbations and that traditional chemical bioassays are often not sensitive enough or appropriately targeted to detect brain-based dysfunction at the molecular level. Hence, use of behavioral testing provides highly sensitive and phenomenologically relevant information in regard to brain function but lacks significant specificity from a mechanistic standpoint. This is either due to an evolution-derived paucity of immunobehavioral phenotypes or a current knowledge/ technical deficiency in the ability to parse such behaviors into a multitude of biologically relevant subsets. In this review, methods for measuring sickness, depressive/anxietal, cognitive and physical activity behaviors in mice are described. The tests were chosen based on common usage and validated outcomes.

2. Preexperimental Considerations

Behavior is a valuable tool for gauging the presence, severity, and duration of innate immune activation. Prior to behavioral experimentation, preparatory procedures are required so that meaningful and repeatable results can be obtained. Mice, like most animals used for laboratory research, are responsive to the environment. Consistency and reproducibility of results as in any field of science is dependent on the decisions made and precautions taken before initiation of testing. While the following does not account for every possible preexperimental housing and husbandry scenario, it does seek to articulate and define significant areas of preexperimental bias. Every animal facility, like every laboratory, is unique with differences obvious and subtle. Standardizing and controlling for clear confounds related to mouse strain, gender, and scientific model; maintaining housing and husbandry practices that support animal behavioral well-being and physical health are key. In addition, the following is not intended to be an absolute guide for "correct" mouse immunobehavioral experimentation, for it is critical that the investigator identify, develop, and hone best practice related to the particular area of study with a firm eye on federal laboratory animal regulations and local institutional rules and guidelines.

2.1. Model and Strain Choice

A first consideration should be the animal model and strain chosen. The vast majority of PNI behavioral testing utilizes rats and mice. Porcine models have been used (16), as have other types of rodents, especially prairie voles (17). Mice are especially useful in neuroimmune and immunobehavioral research due to their ability to reproduce and mature rapidly and the relative ease to which genetic modification can be applied through mutational, transgenic, and knockout approaches (18). Different behavioral phenotypes exist between strains. Therefore, it is important to be aware of and control for potential inter-strain and inter-substrain variances (18), as well as intra-strain variation between mice raised/housed by disparate commercial venders and institutional facilities. Furthermore, genetically altered/modified mice are especially prone to immunobehavioral alteration and should be selected with such in mind. With genetically altered/modified mice, diligent baseline testing in comparison to wild-type animals is essential to ensure the behavior noted is causative (i.e., due to knockout of a specific target gene) and not a result of an unexpected consequence (e.g., saccharin preference anomalies in leptin unresponsive mice (*db/db* and *ob/ob*) related to the importance of leptin to sweet taste and not due to a type 2 diabetes phenotype (19)).

2.2. Gender

Depending on strain, genetic alteration/modification, and behavioral test, male and female mice will perform differently. For example, in the elevated plus maze (EPM) females exhibit less general activity (20). When female mice are compared to male mice in a freely explorable open field arena, female mice are less active, are less willing to leave their home cage to enter the open field, and are less likely to explore the open field (21). Female mice generally run for shorter distances in a voluntary wheel running paradigm than male mice (22) and will run different distances depending on their current state in the estrous cycle (23). Thus, regardless of identical housing and husbandry practices, care must be taken in mixing genders during behavioral testing. Such care can be especially frustrating when using genetically altered/modified animals due to in-house breeding deficiencies and difficulty in acquiring adequate numbers of similarly aged animals from commercial suppliers.

2.3. Age

Natural aging effects decreases in immune functioning with individual variation in severity depending on factors such as lifelong physiological stressor exposure (24). It comes with little surprise then that neuroimmune-based behavior can also be affected by age. While sickness behavior appears beneficial to young mice, it may be maladaptive in older mice (25). Age can also negatively impact physical activity where aged mice run less (26). Young mice present difficulty in running analyses as well due to progressive increases in distance traveled (27). Investigators should be aware of potential differences arising from non-age-matched experimental mice and older mice reared under disparate conditions.

2.4. Transportation

Environmental factors play a significant role in how mice behave and respond to neuroimmune stimuli and immunobehavioral treatments. Mice should be allowed a transition phase to acclimatize to a new environment. Whether this is the procedure experimentation room itself (28, 29), or the housing room following arrival from a commercial supplier or other outside source (28, 30). Biochemically, transportation stress increases plasma corticosterone levels in mice regardless of transport duration, and up to 48 h of acclimation is required for corticosterone to return to pretransportation values (29). Behavioral change in response to transport has been shown to persist for 4 days (29), and body weight reduction returns to pretransport levels within 4 days (28, 30). Therefore, a period of 5 days of acclimatization is generally required as a minimum for mice undergoing behavioral testing following off-site transportation (30). A minimum of 24 h of acclimatization time following on-site transportation (i.e., between housing and experimental rooms) should also be utilized (30). These are minimum time recommendations for acclimatization. Longer times may be necessary depending on the type of mice used, the duration of transport, and the breadth of difference between initial and relocated environmental conditions (28, 30). As with any laboratory test, validation studies are recommended to confirm preexperimental choice decisions.

2.5. Light Cycle

Alteration of light cycle has been shown to affect natural murine behavioral patterns (30), as well as neuroimmune behavior (e.g., anxiety) (31). Mice are under control of a genetically driven circadian clock that serves to regulate physiological and behavioral processes in a diurnal fashion (32). Therefore, it is important to ensure that experimental rooms have a similar light cycle to the housing room. In addition, it is advisable to initiate behavioral experiments at the same time of "day" especially when performing repeat testing. Mice are active at night, and, for the majority of testing, should be tested during the dark cycle. Reverse light cycle housing is beneficial so as not to put undue burden on personnel performing the behavioral tests. Mice also are crepuscular (33), with heightened activity during the early (dusk) and late (dawn) components of the light cycle dark phase and should be tested during these peak activity times. Methods for determining the timing of these active periods are described in Subheading 3.2.

2.6. Temperature/Humidity

Temperature should be largely similar across animal housing facilities, as it is federally regulated by the Office of Laboratory Animal Welfare (OLAW) in the United States (34). According to the Guide for the Care and Use of Laboratory Animals, mice should be housed in a room/environment with temperatures ranging from 68 to 79 °F (20–26 °C) (34). Mice show neuroimmune and behavioral sensitivity to both heat- (35) and cold-stress (36) indicating the potential for altered behaviors with temperature fluctuations. Relative humidity should also be maintained at similar levels across animal housing facilities, and the Guide for the Care and Use of Laboratory Animals indicates a range of 30–70%. Cage style, construction, bedding, and enrichment materials as well as housing density affect temperature and humidity within the cage microenvironment (34). It is therefore important to recognize that room temperature and humidity may not necessarily reflect intracage temperature and humidity, depending on housing factors.

2.7. Noise

Noise also has the potential to activate neuroimmune signaling pathways and alter behavior, as bell ringing (37) and noise produced by vacuuming (38) have been shown to stress laboratory mice as evidenced by activation of the hypothalamic-pituitary-adrenal (HPA) axis (39, 40). White noise generators that create a constant background have been shown to reduce behavioral response to sudden loud noise (41).

2.8. Odors

Mice use odors for communication, marking territory, and in individual and group recognition signaling (30). In addition to using patterns of urine deposition for communication, mice also produce specialized odors via several glandular secretions (30). There is also evidence that neuroimmune activation can alter odor production and that odors can induce behavioral change. When mice are administered the classical neuroimmune activator lipopolysaccharide (LPS) they generate olfactory cues to indicate that they may have a transmissible pathogen causing healthy cage mates to socially withdraw from the sick mouse (42). This phenomenon is also seen in healthy mice housed with tumor-bearing cage mates (43). Finally, exposure to foreign/strange odors (e.g., human associated odors) can result in stress responses (30). Unfortunately, no specific research has been performed examining the duration of olfactory stress responses in mice, nor is there an identified acclimation or exhaustion time for evocative scents. It should also go without mention that eliminating as many olfactory cues within rooms, cages, and on experimental apparatuses (e.g., through use of 70% v/v ethanol) is best practice. Mouse handler odors (i.e., perfumes and predator scents (e.g., feline)) should be minimized and/or eliminated.

2.9. Handling

Physical handling of mice is a well-studied modifier of mouse physiology and behavior (44). Therefore, it is advisable to handle mice at least daily so as to acclimate them to their human researchers and to physical contact. With this, mice will be more likely to appropriately and consistently respond to experimental treatment and have a reduced opportunity to succumb to handling stress which can elevate blood corticosterone (45). The handling method used, however, appears important. Mice respond to handling more readily when removed from their cage passively, such as with a tube or cupped hands, as opposed to the more traditional removal by grasping the base of the tail with the thumb and forefinger or soft forceps (46). Hurst and West noted that mice develop a consistent response (measured as voluntary interaction with handlers) by the ninth day of single 60 s handling sessions, regardless whether the mice were picked up by grasping the tail base or allowed to enter a tube or cupped hands before handling (46). Of note, mice picked up by the base of the tail had a lower level of voluntary interaction, compared to tube and cupping methods (46). Furthermore, when investigators acclimated mice by removing mice from their cages with tubes or cupped hands, the mice were not aversive to scruff restraint, whereas those removed via tail base grasping showed increased distress when scruffed (46). As such, a period of at least 9–10 days of daily handling appears sufficient to ensure a consistent and nonaversive response in mice. If injections are a necessary component of a behavioral experiment, a passive method of mouse cage removal appears best.

2.10. Housing Method/Environmental Enrichment

Mice are social animals and should be housed as often as possible with other mice (34). Several studies have investigated the impact that individual housing/social isolation has on neuroimmunity and immunobehaviors, and social isolation induces aggression in male mice (47). Individually housed male mice also appear more prone to developing anxiety- and depressive-like behaviors following exposure to unpredictable chronic mild stress (48) despite their increased propensity to explore (21, 29). Group housed mice order themselves into a social hierarchy, with 1–2 dominant mice and several subordinate mice. Subordinates as well as dominant mice show similar exploratory levels in an open field context (21) but this seems dependent on the relatedness of the group-housed mice, for an introduced nonsibling dominant intruder mouse evokes social stress and immune cell glucocorticoid resistance in the group-housed mice (49). Therefore, housing mice in groups at a density of one 25–30 g mouse per 77.4–96.7 cm^2 of cage floor area by 12.7 cm of cage ceiling height appears advantageous (34).

Interestingly, a clean cage environment (30, 50) and novel cage construction materials can reduce mouse welfare and induce aberrant behaviors (30, 34). Introduction to a clean/novel cage has been shown to increase plasma corticosterone in mice and to increase physical activity within the first 24 h of exposure. Metal cages, as opposed to more commonly used plastic cages (34), are colder to the touch, more conducive to noise generation, and less permeable to light (30, 34). Additionally, the use of solid flooring with absorbent bedding is recommended by most institutional care and use committees, as well as federal regulatory bodies, because wire mesh flooring can lead to paw injury (34) that can confound behavioral experiments involving the innate immune system (6).

Environmental enrichment is thought to enhance mouse well-being by providing motor and sensory stimulation. Environmental enrichment may include nesting material, structures, and/or shelters within the cage (34). Lack of environmental enrichment dampens mouse reactivity and alertness in many behavioral tests (51). Environmental enrichment is, however, somewhat strain dependent because the loss of reactivity and alertness noted earlier was observed in BALB/c mice but not seen in C57BL/6 mice. In fact, Van de Weerd et al. concluded that male BALB/c mice housed in enriched environments were anxious (51). Olsson and Dahlborn noted simply changing the barren cage environment by placing objects within it does not necessarily lead to "enrichment" (52). Instead, it is important to observe what, how, and when behavioral and physiological changes occur in the animal, and if these changes result in long-term improved health and well-being of the animal. Some "environmental enrichers" are felt to result in increased stress and anxiety (51, 52). Thus, the environment within the cage may be as important as the environment in which the cage is housed in when establishing appropriate preexperimental procedures.

3. Sickness Behaviors

Sickness behavior is classically defined as the nonspecific set of symptoms associated with the body's response to innate immune challenge (6). Symptoms of sickness behavior include anorexia, fatigue, malaise, reduced locomotor activity, loss of interest in environmental and social surroundings, and disappearance of body-care activity (6, 53). These changes occur in response to brain-based increases in the proinflammatory cytokines interleukin-1β (IL-1β) and tumor necrosis factor-α (TNF-α), resulting in changes in the motivational state of an organism (6, 11). Sick individuals also experience psychological symptoms such as anxiety and depression, and cognitive deficits such as learning and memory loss (discussed in later sections). Frequently used methods for quantifying sickness behavior include social exploratory activity (54), locomotor activity (4, 55), food disappearance (4, 55), and rotarod testing (56, 57).

3.1. Social Exploration of a Novel Juvenile

The paradigm of social exploration appears to have evolved from work done by Thor and Holloway showing that adult laboratory rats actively investigate and form social memories of conspecifics (58), principally via ano-genital sniffing, nosing, mutual grooming, and close following (59). Rodents also do not show behavioral habituation during social investigation provided the conspecific juvenile is novel at each presentation into the home cage of the adult (60). Furthermore, adult male rats do not exhibit aggression towards prepubertal male juveniles but do toward unrelated post-pubertal males, which is a function of androgen-related odors from the postpubertal rat eliciting aggressive attacks from the adult due to infamiliarity (58). It is this basis in social recognition that first allowed Dantzer et al. to show that social memory could be modulated by neurohypophyseal peptides (54). This is likely the first experiment that used social exploration as a tool to measure the effects of neuroactive compounds. Social exploratory behavior was adapted from social memory testing by using a different juvenile at each observation time point (61), and due to the advantage of the lack of habituation when using a novel juvenile, social exploration has been routinely used as a sensitive test of immunobehavioral perturbation. Bluthé et al. adapted the rat-based Dantzer procedure to mice, and since the test has remained largely unchanged (59).

3.1.1. Procedure

All observations should be made during the dark/active cycle of the mice. Mice should be housed individually at least 24 h prior to the initial measurement and be allowed to acclimatize to the procedure room (if procedure room differs from housing room) for the time period in which they are individually housed. In some studies, infrared light is used with the aid of infrared- or nightvision-capable cameras (59, 61), but use of red-tinted lighting is also acceptable, as mice only have limited ability to detect light from the red portion of the visible spectra (34). All observations of adult–juvenile interaction are video recorded during social exploration testing for later analysis. Within each observation/recording session, each adult mouse to be experimentally observed (subject mouse) is only exposed to a juvenile (challenge mouse) once. Social exploration is initially measured immediately prior to any experimental treatments so as to serve as a baseline of social exploratory activity for each subject mouse. Social exploration is subsequently measured at specific times following experimental treatment, usually every 2 h for the first 12 h posttreatment, and then every 12 thereafter until recovery is reached (59, 61). A test session/observation time point consists of introducing a novel challenge mouse (conspecific juvenile mouse of the same sex) into the home cage of the subject mouse for 5 min before returning the juvenile to its own home cage (59, 61, 62). In some instances, the juvenile challenge mouse is housed in a clean 7.62 cm × 7.62 cm × 7.62 cm wire mesh enclosure (baby cage) when introduced into the home cage of the subject mouse (63) to avoid undesired aggressiveness seen with certain mouse strains like C57BL/6 mice. If a baby cage is used, it is best to acclimate subject mice to the wire mesh enclosure by including it in their home cage during single housing. Once the experiment is completed, the duration (in s) of exploration or investigation of the challenge mouse by the subject mouse is recorded from analysis of the video record (59, 61, 63). Preferably, analysis of the video record should utilize automated video tracking software (64) such as that developed by Noldus Information Technology (Leesburg, VA). In general, tracking software eliminates observer bias and provides more consistent results. When using tracking software, care must be given as to mouse color vs. background color so that the animal is easily distinguished. If tracking software is not available, a trained observer blinded to the treatment groups (blinded trained observer) can manually quantify social exploration without significant prejudice (59, 61). Observer training for all video review behavior testing is best accomplished by having personnel new to scoring a behavioral test evaluate previously analyzed videos that have been scored and validated (proficiency testing). When the scoring skills of the trainee observer are within plus/minus 10% of a novel validated video in three consecutive evaluations of novel validated videos, the observer trainee is deemed proficient. This same training should be followed when educating personnel to the use of automated tracking software. During manual video review the blinded trained observer uses a stopwatch to record the time of interaction initiated by the subject mouse with the challenge mouse throughout the 5 min designated investigational period. Social exploration is considered to be subject mouse-to-challenge mouse investigation (not the opposite), including ano-genital sniffing, nosing, following, and grooming. With use of a baby cage, nose-to-cage contact is considered exploration. Social exploration is typically shown in graphical display using either raw seconds of exploration at each time point (59) or as percent control or percent baseline (63).

3.2. Locomotor Activity

As lethargy is a core symptom of sickness behavior, locomotion (53) can be used as a technically easy and high-throughput measure of sickness behavior. Spontaneous locomotor activity is advantageous in that it can be assessed without moving mice from their home cage, and automated video tracking software can be easily used for analysis. In addition, wide screen video capture allows for up to eight mice to be observed at once. Alternatively, specifically designed activity chambers (Versamax from AccuScan Instruments, Columbus, OH) with built-in infrared beam detection systems can be used (65) allowing for real-time analysis. Such testing platforms, however, introduce an element of novel environment and need to be thoroughly cleaned between each mouse tested.

3.2.1. Procedure

All observations should be made during the dark/active cycle of the mice. Mice should be housed individually at least 24 h prior to the initial measurement and be allowed to acclimatize to the procedure room (if procedure room differs from the housing room) for the time period in which they are individually housed. As with social exploration, infrared or red lights can be used to provide illumination. At each time point of interest, mouse movement is recorded for 5 min (12), with a camera placed over the center of a single cage or grouping of cages. If multiple mice are being recorded during a given observation point, they should be shielded from one another's view. Movement including total distance traveled, velocity, and time spent moving is best determined from the video record using automated tracking software. However, if tracking software is not available videos can be hand scored by a blinded trained observer. To score manually, a thin-line grid comprised of six equally sized rectangles is affixed to the television or monitor screen directly over the cage and the blinded trained observer counts the number of times the mouse crosses a line (line crossing) throughout the 5 min designated investigational period.

A mouse is only considered to have line crossed if both fore- and hind limbs cross a line (62).

A more powerful method for assessing mouse locomotor activity is through long duration (hours–days) tracking. This is required when detailing mouse crepuscular movement. While video recording can be used for such evaluation, the data collection, storage, and interpretation can be burdensome-to-prohibitive due to video file sizes. Therefore, the use of biotelemetry is the preferred method for this type of testing (66). With this method, a biotelemetric emitter is surgically implanted within the peritoneum of a mouse and a receiver pad linked to a PC running data collection software is placed directly underneath the home cage of the implanted mouse (Mini Mitter, Bend, OR). Mouse movement is tracked and recorded automatically. Specific procedures and training for this method should be provided by the manufacture of the device chosen.

3.3. Food Consumption

Food consumption, (or disappearance, as discussed below), is an indicator of sickness, as individuals experiencing illness often exhibit anorexia. Food consumption gives an indication of whether anorexia is present, which could further be used to indicate if sickness behavior is occurring (4, 55). Food consumption can be measured in at least two different ways, as outlined below. The first uses "food disappearance," which is often interpreted/estimated as food consumption.

3.3.1. Food Disappearance Procedure

Mice should be individually housed as per social exploration at least 24 h prior to experimentation. With single housing, food should be moved from the overhead cage food hopper and placed in an 8 cm diameter × 5 cm stainless steel bowl in the cage. Steel is preferred over ceramic because ceramic containers can absorb water if they are not completely glazed. In addition, steel dishes can be magnetically secured to the cage bottom or side with the use of a strong magnet. This prevents mice from tipping the bowl and spilling food which can easily occur with plastic bowls. After the acclimation period, and just prior to initiation of testing, new food should be added to the steel bowl and the bowl weighed. This process should occur at the very beginning of the dark/active cycle of the mice in order not to disturb mice during their sleep cycle. Food disappearance is measured by weighing the bowl plus food at fixed intervals, such as every 24 h. For longer term experiments, food can be re-added to the bowl and reweighed (55). The term food disappearance is used in place of food consumption because not all food is ingested. Some food inadvertently falls in the cage bedding (67).

3.3.2. Food Consumption Procedure

Mice should be individually housed as per social exploration at least 24 h prior to experimentation. 24 h prior to testing mice should be fasted but allowed full access to water. An empty 8 cm diameter × 5 cm stainless steel food bowl should be present in the cage. One hour prior to testing, mice should be removed to similarly sized cage without bedding but with full water access. Testing is initiated by wiping the bottom of the bedding-less cage clean and placing a preweighed bowl with food in the cage. After 1 h the food bowl is removed and weighed as are any food remnants within the cage. The difference between food bowl food disappearance and food collected from the cage floor is considered food consumed (65).

A more powerful method for assessing food disappearance and/or consumption is through use of automated food and water intake measurement systems where food and/or water intake initiated by the animal is evaluated by computer controlled electronics (BioDAQ, New Brunswick, NJ). Specific procedures and training for this method should be provided by the manufacture of the device chosen.

3.4. Rotarod Testing

Inducers of neuroimmune activation and sickness behavior impair motor coordination and induce physical fatigue (56). The rotarod performance test can measure motor coordination (57) by assessing how well mice avoid falling of a rotating rod (68). Some strains of mice progressively perform better on the rotorod test during repeated trials at the same rotational speed indicating a physical training or memory component to this procedure (69, 70). Rotarod apparatuses are available via commercial vendors such as AccuScan Instruments (Columbus OH), with some variance in features (number of lanes and/or rod diameter, for example). In general, rotarod apparatuses have the same basic design featuring a 3–9 cm diameter rod (57, 69) partitioned by plastic divider discs spaced evenly longitudinally along the rod. The end point measured is latency to fall from the rod (71). Fall detection ranges from pressure-sensitive pads located under the rod to infrared beams that automatically stop an integrated timer when hit or blocked, respectively. Rotarod performance can, however, be assessed manually from a video record (71) by a blinded trained observer or by automated tracking software.

3.4.1. Procedure

Single housing prior to testing is not required but, like with social exploration, mice require at least 24 h of acclimation to the procedure room. Use of preexperimentation acclimation to the rotarod is not agreed upon. Some have exposed (trained) mice to the rotating rod, by placing mice on the rod at a low speed (4 rpm (56) and 18 rpm (57)), while others have not (69). Preexperimentation exposure to the rod has been done 1 week in advance of testing (57) and immediately prior to testing (56). Finally, the test itself can be performed in 1 of 2 ways. The rotarod performance test measures the duration of time a mouse can remain on the rotating rod at a single or several fixed speeds (71). The accelerating rotarod performance test measures the maximum speed of rotation the mouse can tolerate before it falls from the rod in a fixed amount of time (69, 71). All pretest conditioning and testing should be made during the dark/active cycle of the mice (56), although testing has been performed during the light/inactive cycle as well (57).

3.4.2. Rotarod Performance Test

Rotarods should be calibrated such they rotate at a constant speed, and should be kept clean and as odor free as possible between trials, as urine and feces on the rod can affect performance (71). Testing is initiated by placing mice on the rotating rotarod which rotates at a fixed speed. Mice are allowed to maintain themselves on the rod as long as they can and the test session continues until they fall or a designated time point is achieved such as 1–5 min on the rod. At such time the latency to fall is recorded. Fixed speed trials are best used after significant validation testing on the strain of mouse chosen and are best used on mice with significant loss of coordination because small losses of coordination may not manifest at the speed or time chosen. Some testing protocols investigate several different speeds increasing with each trial. An example of increasing speeds used is 5, 8, 15, 20, 24, 31, 33, and 44 rpm (71). Mouse rest time between increasing speed trials ranges from 10 to 60 min (69, 71).

3.4.3. Accelerating Rotarod Performance Test

Preconditions are similar as for nonaccelerating rotarod testing. This test differs in that the rod accelerates at a constant rate through some specified range of speed (4–40 rpm) over a fixed amount of time (5 min). Mice remain on the rod for as long as they can and speed of the rod at the time of falling is the recorded end point (69).

For both methods of rotarod testing, motor learning can be assessed by performing daily repeated trials to determine if mouse time spent on the rod (fixed rod speed) or rod speed endured (accelerating rod speed) improves from trial to trial (69).

4. Depressive/Anxiety-Like Behaviors

Depression and anxiety are well-known consequences of neuroimmune activation (11, 65, 72). However, the difficulty in assessing and distinguishing depressive/anxiety-like responses to conditions or experimental treatments lies in the fact that sickness behavior symptoms can overlap with depressive/anxiety-like behaviors. Sickness-induced reduced locomotion is a key confound in that most tests designed to measure depressive/anxiety-like behaviors require mouse movement (11). For this reason, behavioral testing for depressive/anxiety-like behaviors following exogenous activation of the neuroimmune system should be performed only after overt physical symptoms of sickness have subsided and spontaneous locomotion has returned to pretreatment levels. Importantly, the presence of depressive/anxiety-like behaviors should be confirmed using antidepressive and/or anxiolytic therapies to improve/resolve the identified depressed or anxious behavior (11). Tests for depressive/anxiety-like behaviors include burrowing (12, 73), the EPM (74), the open field test (OFT) (75, 76), the zero maze test (69), the tail suspension test (TST) (11), sucrose/saccharin preference test (11), and the forced swim (aka Porsolt) test (11). The forced swim test (FST) is the test best validated for depression due to its responsiveness to antidepressives (77). However, investigators should refrain from using any one single test to definitively measure depressive/anxiety-like behaviors. Such behaviors are best examined using a battery of tests. Unfortunately, there is no ideal combination of tests because confounds are mouse strain/model/gender and experimental treatment specific. As an example, sucrose/saccharin preference testing should not be used in mouse testing where serum leptin is affected due to the impact of leptin levels on sweet taste detection by the mouse tongue (19).

4.1. Burrowing

Rodents are well known burrowers (73). This behavior is related to tunnel maintenance and possibly defense. Defensive burying is a known indicator of anxiety and can, itself, be measured (73). Burrowing appears to be largely hippocampal driven but mouse strain differences exist with C57BL/6 mice burrowing more than 129S2/Sv mice (73). Burrowing is associated with depressive/anxiety-like behavior where reduced burrowing reflects an increased depressive/anxiety-like state (12). As burrowing utilizes relatively simple equipment and minimal labor, it is a simple and inexpensive method for evaluating immunobehaviors (12, 73).

4.1.1. Procedure

All observations should be made during the dark/active cycle of the mice. Mice should be individually housed as per social exploration at least 24 h prior to experimentation and, with single housing, a clean empty burrowing tube should be placed in the cage. Burrowing tubes can be constructed from standard white 6.8 cm diameter PVC piping cut to 20 cm in length (73). The open end of the burrowing tube is elevated 3 cm by bolting two 50 mm machine screws 1 cm from the open end, and spaced so that the tube entrance is elevated. This elevation keeps burrowing substrate from spilling out of the open end. The closed end is sealed with a standard PVC end cap (12). Testing should begin 3 h prior to the onset of the dark/active phase of the light cycle and is initiated with addition of burrowing substrate to the tube (12). The burrowing substrate used needs to be suitable to the mouse strain and experimental treatment. Pelleted mouse chow, gravel, or sand are common materials used for burrowing (73). The burrowing tube can be completely filled (73) or filled with a fixed amount of substrate (12) if ceiling effects are not a concern. Ceiling effects arise with vigorous borrowers. These mice will remove all substrate from a tube in a rapid time frame obscuring any difference in burrowing activity relative to time. After substrate is placed in the burrow, the burrow plus substrate is weighed and returned to the cage. If mouse chow is used as a substrate, food from the cage food hopper should be removed for the duration of the burrowing test (73). Depending on anticipated mouse burrowing activity, experimental observation time points can range from 1 to 24 h. Amount burrowed (in grams) is calculated from the pre- and postburrowing weight of the tube plus substrate. Following a measurement, the burrowing tube can be refilled, reweighed, and returned to the cage for additional testing (73). Alternatively, a single measurement of burrowing can be utilized (12). Occasionally, with poorly burrowing mice, one or several training sessions may be necessary, and a practice run with the mice to be used in the experiment can, and has been shown to, improve burrowing activity and reduce variability between animals (73).

4.2. Elevated Plus Maze

The EPM is a simple method to measure anxiety-like behavior in mice. Anxiety is assessed by comparing the time spent in the open (exposed) vs. closed (walled) arms of a 4-arm radial maze (74). The advantage to the EPM is that it eschews use of noxious stimuli like foot shock, food/water deprivation, and/or loud noise. Instead, it relies on the predilection of mice to favor dark enclosed spaces over open and obviously elevated environments (74). Accommodation and/or learning can occur with repeated exposures to the maze. Therefore, EPM is generally administered as a single exposure with control mice for comparison (74).

4.2.1. Procedure

All observations should be made during the dark/active cycle of the mice. Single housing prior to testing is not required but, like with social exploration, mice need at least 24 h of acclimation to the procedure room. The maze can be made of a variety of materials but those that can be easily wiped clean between each mouse tested like stainless steel or plastic are recommended. Maze shape is that of a plus sign where the four arms are spaced 90° apart, radiating from an open central 5 cm × 5 cm platform. Arm length and width are 25 cm × 5 cm, respectively. Maze elevation should be at least 40 cm from the floor (74, 79). Arm wall height is 15 cm in the "closed" arms and there are no side walls in the "open" arms. The central 5 cm × 5 cm platform has no walls. The open arms are at 180° from each other, likewise with the closed arms. Unlike the tests described earlier, EPM should be well lit by overhead white light. Significant arm wall-generated shadows, especially those confined to a single arm, should be avoided. Testing is initiated by placing the mouse in the open central 5 cm × 5 cm platform. Each subject mouse needs to be introduced to the maze in a similar fashion and placed on the maze in the same spot with analogous orientation (74). Mouse exploration is video recorded for 5 min (74) to 10 min (78). Time spent in open and closed arms, the number of entries between arms (defined as all four paws of the mouse crossing the threshold of an arm), frequency of head-dips (downward movement of the mouse head toward the floor from an open arm), rears and stretch-attend postures (74) are best determined from the video record using automated tracking software (62). If tracking software is not available videos can be hand scored by a blinded trained observer (74).

4.3. Open Field Test

The OFT can be used to measure movement (76) and anxiety-like behavior (75, 76). OFT apparatuses are walled arenas that vary in shape (square, rectangle, circle) and size (250–2,500 cm^2) (76). OFT testing should not be used as a surrogate test for spontaneous locomotor activity because the OFT uses a novel environment (76). Anxiety-like behavior in the OFT is evaluated by examining mouse movement throughout the arena with a special focus on the amount of time the mouse spends/moves next to walls of the OFT apparatus (thigmotaxis). The novelty, size, and white light illumination of the OFT contribute to anxiogenesis (76). Procedures vary considerably but the open field arena is usually brightly lit in studies investigating anxiety (75).

4.3.1. Procedure

All observations should be made during the dark/active cycle of the mice. Single housing prior to testing is not required but, like with social exploration, mice need at least 24 h of acclimation to the procedure room. For testing of anxiety-like behaviors the arena should be larger than 1,600 cm^2 (76). Arena wall height should be at least 35 cm so as to limit the ability of the mouse to see over/above the arena. The arena can be made of a variety of materials but those that can be easily wiped clean between each mouse tested, like stainless steel or plastic, are recommended. Testing is initiated by placing the mouse in the center of the arena, and each subject mouse needs to be introduced to the arena in a similar fashion and placed in the same spot with analogous orientation. Movement through the arena is video recorded for 5–10 min and analysis of movement is best documented with automated tracking software because thigmotaxis is easily appreciated with this method. Path tracing is a key aid in that overall patterns of movement can be evaluated. Such patterns supplement the usual measurements of time spent adjacent to the arena walls, wall preferences, time spent not adjacent to the arena walls, overall distance traveled, velocity and time spent moving. Videos can be manually examined using a line-crossing scoring approach (similar to that described for spontaneous locomotor activity) but this method should be carefully validated due to the complex grid pattern needed to ascertain time spent close to the arena walls. Due to this intricacy, some have used the end point of total distance moved plus time spent in the central

25% of the arena (79). Finally, OFT has been used as a repeated measure to determine if therapeutics improve performance over time (80).

4.4. Zero Maze

Like the EPM, the zero maze measures anxiety-like behaviors in mice (69) by using elevation and open and closed areas. Therefore, time spent in the open indicates a reduced level of fear/anxiety as demonstrated by use of anxiolytic agents and their ability to increase time spent in the open area of the zero maze (69). The advantage of the zero maze over the EPM is the elimination of the central platform of EPMs, which can complicate analysis of open/closed arm comparisons (81).

4.4.1. Procedure

All observations should be made during the dark/active cycle of the mice. Single housing prior to testing is not required but, like with social exploration, mice need at least 24 h of acclimation to the procedure room. Maze design varies but in general is comprised of a circular track 30–45 cm in diameter that is 3–5 cm wide. Maze elevation should be at least 40 cm from the floor (69, 82). The track should be divided into four quadrants with two quadrants having no side walls and two quadrants having side walls at least 15 cm in height. These open and closed areas should alternate. As with all maze constructions, materials that are easily wiped clean between each mouse tested are recommended (69, 81, 82). Ample but dim (40–60 lux) white lighting should be used to achieve similar illumination of both the open and closed quadrants (81). Testing is initiated by introducing the subject mouse to the middle of a closed quadrant (designated as the starting quadrant). Each subject mouse needs to be introduced to the maze in a similar fashion and placed on the maze in the same place and orientation. Mouse exploration is video recorded for 5 min (81). Time spent in open and walled arms, the number of transitions between open and walled quadrants, number of rears, number of head-dips (the actual dipping of the head over the edge of the track in an open quadrant), time spent grooming, the number of stretch attend postures, and number of fecal boli in each type of quadrant are best determined by using a combination of automated tracking software and direct observation after testing (fecal boli) (69, 81). If tracking software is not available videos can be hand scored by a blinded trained observer. Entry into a quadrant occurs when all four paws cross the threshold of an open or walled area (81).

4.5. Tail Suspension Test

The TST is a commonly used behavioral test for assessing depressive-like behavior in mice. It is thought to induce an escape response (83). With increased depressive-like behavior the mouse fails to extricate itself from the apparatus and becomes immobile. Increased immobility indicates a greater degree of depressive symptoms (84). Importantly, antidepressants shorten immobility offering a degree of validation to the test's usefulness in measuring depressive-like behaviors (83). The TST can be automated through use of commercially available apparatuses that utilize computer-linked linear load cells and load cell filters to determine mouse movement/struggle (Med Associates, St. Albans, VT). As with any commercially purchased device, specific procedures and training should be provided by the manufacture of the device chosen. However, certain basic procedures should be followed and considered with use of the TST including the difficulty in examining young (especially C57BL/6) mice due to their robust tail climbing behavior and penchant for extracting themselves from the device.

4.5.1. Procedure

Unlike all the previous behavioral tests described the TST should be administered during the light/inactive cycle of the mice. Single housing prior to testing is not required but, like with social exploration, mice need at least 24 h of acclimation to the procedure room. Testing is initiated by affixing the mouse to the apparatus "hook" with adhesive tape wrapped around the tail at three quarters of its length from base. Hook the mouse to the apparatus through the tape as close to the tail as possible. The tail should remain straight so as not to injure the mouse. Mice should be suspended as uniformly as possible, and if multimouse devices are used the mice should be shielded from each other's view (84). Immobility verse movement/struggle should be measured for 6 min. Nonautomated devices can be constructed, which are essentially chambers with hooks. Mouse behavior can be video recorded and immobility determined from the video record by automated tracking software (85) or a blinded trained observer (86). With any of the aforementioned analysis techniques, time of immobility is compared between control and experimental groups of mice (84).

4.6. Forced Swim Test

The FST, also called the Porsolt test for the investigator who developed the test in rodents, like the TST, is a tool for assessing depressive-like behavior in mice. The FST is relatively easy to administer (87) and felt to be the best validated test for depression by the pharmaceutical industry (88). This test evolved from the observation that rats will develop an immobile posture after an initial attempt to escape from an inescapable cylinder filled with water. FST-induced immobility is thought to represent behavioral despair (failure of persistent escape behavior) or a development of passive behavior that causes the animal to stop actively coping with a stressor (87). The FST has several disadvantages when compared to the TST. The FST appears to be more stressful for mice and carries a risk of hypothermia (84). Mice of varying fatness are also difficult to assess due to inherent buoyancy differences.

4.6.1. Procedure

Like the TST, the FST should be administered during the light/inactive cycle of the mice (88). Single housing prior to testing is not required but, like with social exploration, mice need at least

24 h of acclimation to the procedure room. As with most device requiring tests, equipment design varies. A simple setup is to use clean white or black cylindrical PVC containers 16 cm in diameter and 31 cm in height (essentially 2 gallon open head pails) containing 20 cm of water maintained at 25 ± 1 °C (89). The FST should be performed under 30 lux white light (90). Testing is initiated by introducing the subject mouse to the water-filled container. Mouse swimming is video recorded for 6 min (89). Immobility is determined from the video record from the last 5 min of the FST using either automated tracking software (91) or a blinded trained observer (89). Immobility scoring should not include movements necessary for the mouse to maintain its head above water (84). Like the TST, time of immobility is compared between control and experimental groups of mice.

4.7. Sucrose/Saccharin Preference

Anhedonia, or the inability to gain pleasure from otherwise enjoyable experiences, is one of the features of depression (92, 93). In mice, their preference for sweetened solutions has been exploited to measure anhedonia. The decreased consumption of a sweet-tasting solution is indicative of anhedonic behavior and can be reversed with antidepressives (93). Sucrose (93) and saccharin (12) solutions are commonly used opposite normal tap water in a 2-choice test. For investigators concerned with mouse caloric intake, saccharin is the recommended sweetener (12). Advantages to the sucrose/saccharin preference test are that it can be run continuously for many days without significant concern of adaptation or learning.

4.7.1. Procedure

Three days prior to testing mice should be singly housed in standard cages adapted for 2-bottle water access (adaptation phase). If the experimental design requires mice to be challenged with a neuroimmune activator, each bottle should contain either saccharin as a 0.4% sodium saccharin solution (1% for sucrose can substituted for saccharin) or water. If the experimental design does not require exogenous challenge as with a comparison of mice of different strains or genders, the adaptation phase should consist of both bottles being filled with water. The adaption phase is especially important to experiments using endogenous immune activators so as not to elicit the behavior of conditioned aversion where the mouse associates a newly introduced substance like saccharin/sucrose with the cause of their loss of well-being (94). After the adaptation phase, mice are usually administered a challenge at the beginning of their dark/active cycle and then returned to the cage in which they were adapted in the presence of both water and saccharin (testing phase). Fluid consumption is recorded every 24 h. Fluid consumption is determined by bottle weight (12). In order to control for the development of bottle bias, bottle position of water vs. sweetened solution should be switched on a regular but defined basis such as halfway through the experiment or every 24 h.

Bottle switching should also be practiced during the adaptation phase usually at 24 h intervals. Sweetened solution preference is generally reported as a percentage of sweetened solution consumption/disappearance to total fluid consumption/disappearance (93). A 50/50 consumption of sweetened solution to water equates to anhedonia but a ratio in which water consumption/disappearance exceeds sweetened solution consumption/disappearance is indicative of aversion and should trigger concerns as to the applicability of the results to the measurement of depressive-like behaviors (12).

5. Cognitive Behaviors

Neuroimmune activation can dramatically impact cognitive function (9) causing learning and memory deficits. Most mouse-based behavioral tests for cognitive function make use of memory and focus either on the ability of the mouse to form new memories (memory formation) or recall old memories (memory retention). Memories involving location (spatial memory) are especially utilized (9). A cornucopia of cognitive function tests exist. Some of these tests have been specifically designed to identify specialized aspects of learning and memory such as olfactory memory (95). Given that peripheral innate immune driven neuroimmune activation is relatively brain-region nonspecific, cognitive tests that cover more global aspects of brain function are favored by PNI investigators.

5.1. Novel Object Recognition

Novel object recognition is a test of working memory in mice. The test exploits the innate tendency of mice to investigate a new entity (96). Novel object testing is one of the simplest of cognition tests, but test variations are described that add significant complexity through mixing of objects, object placement (novel location testing), and testing arena conditions (12, 96–98). The setup for novel object recognition typically depends on what sort of memory function a researcher desires to investigate (96). An advantage of novel object testing over other seemingly more powerful maze-based memory tests is its adaptability to repeated measure testing (96). In essence, as long as the mouse is well adapted to the familiar object, changing out the novel object after each exposure allows for a new round of testing. This feature is very useful when looking at recovery from a neuroimmune challenge.

5.1.1. Memory Recall Procedure

All observations should be made during the dark/active cycle of the mice. Mice should be housed individually at least 24 h prior to the initial measurement. The 24 h training phase is initiated by introducing two identical objects into the home cage (standard shoe-box cage size; 28 cm in length; 17 cm in width; 12.5 cm in height) of the singly housed mouse. The objects are placed 10 cm apart at the short-side wall end, 5 cm from the short side wall and 3.5 cm from the long-side wall. Tall (3–5 cm in height) complex objects are preferred because when a tall complex object is introduced during the testing phase it provokes significantly more exploration time. Tall complex objects can be constructed from Lego® blocks (Enfield, CT). Magnets can be used to secure the structures to the cage floor. All structures should be taken apart and cleaned prior to reuse. After the 24 h training phase, the mouse is subjected to the chosen neuroimmune activator. At relevant times after the applied immunobehavioral challenge, the memory recall testing phase is initiated by placing the mouse in a home-cage like arena (including bedding) which contains a similar object setup as in the training phase where one of the familiar objects has been replaced by a novel tall complex object. The mouse should be introduced at the cage end opposite the objects. No spatial clues should be present in the testing/training area. Object exploratory behavior is video recorded for 5 min and object investigation is determined from the video record by either automated tracking software or by a blinded trained observer. Object exploration is considered as contact by mouth, nose, or paw. Accidental contact such as bumping into an object while passing should not be considered (97). Mice with a memory recall deficit should examine both the familiar and novel objects equally (99). Once recovered from neuroimmune activation, mice should explore the novel object over the familiar object. This test cannot be performed as a repeated measure and, thus, requires separate groups of mice to determine at what time after neuroimmune activation cognitive recovery occurs.

5.1.2. Memory Formation Procedure

All observations should be made during the dark/active cycle of the mice. Single housing prior to testing is not required but, like with social exploration, mice need at least 24 h of acclimation to the procedure room. Memory formation testing differs from recall testing in that training occurs after endogenous activation of the neuroimmune system instead of before (96). The procedure is identical to the above except at relevant times after the applied immunobehavioral challenge mice are trained for 1 h with the two familiar objects in the shoebox-sized testing arena then returned to the home cage. After 1 h in the home cage, testing is initiated by placing the mouse back in the testing arena where one of the familiar objects has been replaced by a novel object. Recording time and scoring are identical to the above. Mice with a formation deficit should examine both the familiar and novel objects equally. Once recovered from neuroimmune activation, mice should explore the novel object over the familiar object. This test can be performed as a repeated measure as long as the novel object is always new.

5.2. Fear Conditioned Learning

Fear conditioned learning is a form of classical (Pavlovian) conditioning where an association between a stimuli and its aversive consequence(s) is made (100). Fear conditioning is a highly conserved behavior that occurs in mice both in the laboratory and in the wild. In PNI research, it is a useful tool for evaluating emotional memory formation and recall (100). Fear conditioned learning is generally a one-trial learning procedure and is unique from other cognitive tests in that the investigator regulates the parameters of the stimulus. Factors that impact mouse hearing, like age, are important to consider prior to use of fear conditioned learning, as auditory sensory decline will negatively affect sound-based contextual cues (100). Like novel object testing, fear conditioned learning can be used to test memory formation and memory recall. For memory formation testing, the training phase (see below) is conducted after neuroimmune stimulation. For memory recall testing, the training phase is conducted prior to neuroimmune stimulation.

5.2.1. Cued Fear Conditioning Procedure

All observations should be made during the dark/active cycle of the mice. Mice should be single housed for this behavioral procedure and, like with social exploration, mice need at least 24 h of acclimation to the procedure room. Automated commercially available fear conditioning apparatuses (San Diego Instruments, San Diego, CA) are the easiest way to adapt this testing paradigm. General apparatus parameters are fairly uniform. There is a shock generator and scrambler that delivers a 0.1–1.0 mA foot shock through a wire grid floor in concert with a sound generator that produces auditory cues, all contained in a shoebox cage-sized chamber (100). It is recommended that sound meters and voltmeters are used to verify and record stimulus intensities (100). Prior to testing mice require training. In the initial training session, mice are placed in the fear conditioning apparatus for 120 s (phase A) before the presentation of a 30 s sound cue (phase B). A 2 s foot shock is delivered immediately after the sound cue (phase C). Mice are returned to their home cages 30 s after the shock ends. Repeat training can be utilized to reinforce the memory. As noted earlier, training relative to neuroimmune stimulation determines whether memory formation or recall is being tested. Testing is usually initiated 24 h posttraining and consists of re-introducing the mouse to the fear conditioning apparatus and representing the sound cue. The sound cue now lasts for 180 s. Mouse behavior during this 180 s period is recorded with a side-mounted video camera. However, apparatuses with a beam detection grid system linked to a PC can automate analysis. With video recording, freezing and nonfreezing behavior is scored by a blinded trained observer at 10 s intervals. Freezing is considered a complete lack of mouse movement (100). Fear conditioning is presented as number of freezing episodes. With an automated detection system, actual time spent frozen can be determined.

5.2.2. Contextual Fear Conditioned Procedure

Contextual fear conditioning uses the same preexperimental and scoring procedures as for cued fear conditioning. However, in contextual fear conditioning, no sound cues are delivered. The mouse is expected to associate the apparatus with the foot shock. Testing time is 180 s. Complexity can be added by using an alterable microenvironment within the fear conditioning apparatus (altered contextual fear conditioning). A variety of cues from visual to olfactory can then be utilized (100).

5.3. Spontaneous Alternation

Spontaneous alternation is the simplest spatial memory test to perform in mice. Increases and decreases in spontaneous or perfect alternations reflect improvements and impairments, respectively, in spatial memory function (12, 101). Spontaneous alternation can be performed in a variety of maze types including radial arm, T and Y (12, 102). Subforms of spontaneous alternation testing have also been described including forced-trial alternation, where one arm of the maze is closed off, forcing the mouse to enter the open arm without choice. In a subsequent testing, the closed arm is then made available (102). Interestingly, certain mouse strains have been shown to be biased in their turning direction (102), and this should be considered and controlled for. Like novel object testing, spontaneous alternation can be used to test memory formation and memory recall. For memory formation testing, spontaneous alternation test is conducted after neuroimmune stimulation. For memory recall testing, the mouse is tested in the Y-maze (which serves as a training period), exposed to a neuroimmune activator and then re-tested in the Y-maze. In addition, spontaneous alternation can be performed as a repeated measure and maze performance usually increases with repetition. Repeated measure testing is generally preferred because a "one and done" testing strategy is more indicative of locomotor activity and less dependent on spatial memory (102).

5.3.1. Procedure

All observations should be made during the dark/active cycle of the mice. Single housing prior to testing is not required but, like with social exploration, mice need at least 24 h of acclimation to the procedure room. As with all mazes described previously, the Y-maze used for spontaneous alternation should be made of a material that can be easily wiped clean between each mouse tested. Clear Plexiglas is preferred so that a different black-colored design (lines, circles, or triangles) can be affixed to the outside wall of each arm to provide intra-maze visual cues. The maze base is an opaque blue. Maze shape is three equally spaced arms 120° from each other (radial Y). Arm length is 40 cm, arm width is 9 cm, and arm wall height is 16 cm (12). Testing is initiated by placing the mouse into the distal end of a randomly chosen arm (as assigned by a random number generator). Each subject mouse needs to be introduced to the maze in a similar fashion and placed on the maze with analogous orientation.

Mouse exploration is recorded for 5 min (3 and 15 min have also been used (103)). If the experimental design allows, mice should be tested every 24 h for 4 consecutive days. Perfect alternations are determined from the video record by a blinded trained observer. A perfect alternation is defined as exploration of two different arms of the maze sequentially before a return to the starting arm (e.g., beginning in arm "C," moving to arm "A," then to arm "B," before returning to arm "C" again) (12). Number of "regular" alternations should also be scored. Regular alternations are defined as entering all three arms within a sequence of four arm entries (e.g., ACAB is considered an alternation, whereas ACAC is not) (102). Arm entries occur when all four paws of the mouse pass the threshold of the arm entrance (12). Results are represented as total alternations or perfect alternations divided into the total possible alternations or perfect alternations, respectively (102). Perfect alternation scoring is considered more rigorous.

5.4. Barnes Maze

The Barnes maze, like spontaneous alternation, is a test of spatial memory. This test combines several aspects of the previously mentioned mazes including elevation, open/exposed illuminated space, and a dark enclosed area (104). Use of the Barnes maze was popularized as an alternative to the Morris water maze (MWM) (described in the next section) because swimming may produce anxiety (105). Removal of water also allows for more balanced testing of mice of different fat density due to elimination of the buoyancy effect. Importantly, the Barnes maze appears to rely on the same hippocampal-dependent memory function as the MWM (104). As with any maze designed to test spatial memory, extra- and intra-maze cues serve as location reference points and without these cues mice perform less well (104). Like spontaneous alternation, the Barnes maze can be used to test memory formation and recall depending on when neuroimmune activation is triggered relative to the training period. However, recall is significantly simpler to measure when using transient memory impairment paradigms.

5.4.1. Procedure

All observations should be made during the dark/active cycle of the mice. Single housing prior to testing is not required but, like with social exploration, mice need at least 24 h of acclimation to the procedure room. As with all mazes, construction materials should be easily cleanable. A typical Barnes maze is a 90 cm diameter white acrylic disc with 12 equally spaced through-and-through holes arranged 5 cm from the outer edge of the disc. Hole diameter is 5 cm and the maze is situated 56 cm off the floor (104). A tunnel-like extension attached to an enclosed sealable $8 \times 8 \times 8$ cm chamber (escape chamber) needs to be freely fittable to one of the holes from underneath the maze. Thus, for the mouse to escape the maze, it must enter a hole. Extra maze cues, such as different geometric shapes are placed around the maze and on the walls of the room (105). Prior to testing multiday training is required. Training occurs four times per day (during the dark/active cycle of the mouse) for a 5-day period. In each session, the mouse is introduced to the maze (lit at 1,200 lux) via a nontransparent holding chamber placed in the center of the maze. Time spent in the holding chamber is 30 s. After the holding chamber is unsealed, the mouse is allowed to explore the maze freely for 5 min. During each training session, the escape chamber should remain under the same assigned escape hole with all other holes blocked. During the 5 min exploration period, the mouse should find the escape chamber hole. If the mouse fails to find the escape chamber hole, it is picked up and placed near the entrance of the escape chamber hole and allowed to enter. Once the mouse enters the escape chamber the mouse is removed from the maze and the training session is ended (104). One hour after the final training session a probe trial is conducted in which all of the holes are blocked (preventing any escape) and the mouse is allowed to explore the maze for 5 min. Successfully trained mice with functional spatial memory should actively search for the remembered escape chamber hole in the appropriate location. Mouse introduction to the maze during the probe trail uses the holding chamber technique as performed during training. After immunobehavioral stimulation, testing is initiated re-performing a single 5 min training procedure. Mouse behavior is video recorded and maze performance evaluated from the video record using a combination of automated tracking software and observation. The mouse should use the extra-maze visual cues to locate the remembered escape chamber (104). Scoring the trials consists of tallying the frequency of errors committed before entering the escape chamber (examination of the incorrect hole), timing the latency to find/enter the escape chamber, and determining the path length to the escape chamber. Different variations of the Barnes maze exist and include a hidden-target fixed-location modification in which the extra-maze cues were always in the same location, but the maze was rotated (104).

5.5. Morris Water Maze

The MWM is used for assessing spatial or place learning. Advantages of the MWM include no requirement for pretraining, high reliability across different tank designs, and proved validity in measuring hippocampal-dependent spatial and reference memory. Learning impairments in the MWM are independent of locomotor deficits, as locomotor reductions do not seem to affect swim speed (106). The MWM is an open circular pool filled with water. Mice must swim and search for a small, hidden platform just below the surface of the water in a fixed location utilizing extra-maze cues. The maze is constructed of a circular, stainless steel tank 122 cm in diameter, with 51 cm high walls, with nonreflective inner surfaces. Contrasting colors between the inside of the tank and the mouse allow easy integration of automated tracking software for the analysis of swim path, duration, and location. As the purpose of the MWM test is to induce the mouse to use distal cues, any seams or recognizable patterns on the inside of the pool are not recommended. The platform (made of a plastic or PVC conduit shaft with a plastic or acrylic platform on top) is typically square or circular in shape and is clear or matching in color to the inside of the swim tank. The platform is positioned just below the water level (0.5–1 cm). Water temperature should range between 24 and 26 °C (107). The room in which the MWM test takes place in should allow for ample distal visual cues like for the Barnes maze. Studies have shown that lack of cues can negatively affect MWM performance (106). The investigator should be aware that their presence in the procedure room during MWM testing may make them a distal visual cue. All variations of the MWM procedure should take place in an illuminated, albeit indirectly lit room (to avoid reflections or glare on the water surface, which can make scoring with automated tracking software difficult) (106). The maze is divided into four, equally sized quadrants with the platform positioned in the center of one of these quadrants (106). The procedures for spatial acquisition and reversal learning are described below but a variety of modifications exist. A key concern in MWM spatial memory testing is that the probe trial should be spaced temporally from the last training session to effectively and reliably measure reference memory formation (106).

5.5.1. Spatial Acquisition Procedure

All testing should take place during the dark/active cycle of the mice. Single housing prior to testing is not required but, like with social exploration, mice need at least 24 h of acclimation to the procedure room. The mouse is placed (not dropped) at the selected start position in the maze, facing the tank wall. A timer or video tracking should be started immediately at the placement of the mouse in the maze. The timer remains on until the mouse reaches (comes in contact with) the platform. Standard trial limits of 1–2 min per trial are usually used, and mice that have not reached the platform should be placed on or guided to it by the investigator (106). The animal should remain on the platform for 15 s. This step helps mice orient their position in space relative to the extra-maze cues (106). Following the inter-trial interval, the mouse is again placed in the maze, this time in a different but predetermined location (most protocols start the mice from one of four positions—south (the investigators position), north (opposite the investigators position), east (to the right of the investigators position), and west (to the left of the investigators position)). Trials are repeated four times per day for 5 days. Following training, the experimental treatment is administered and time is allowed for the treatment to take effect, or in the case of neuroimmune activators, for sickness behavior to resolve so as not to confound the results (11). The probe trial is run, during which the platform is removed from the maze. The probe trial is video recorded and lasts 60 s, after which the mouse is removed. The objective of the probe trial is to determine whether or not the mouse can recall memories of where the platform was during training sessions based on the distal visual cues (106). End points measured in spatial acquisition include the number of platform site crossovers, time and distance swam in the target quadrant relative to the other quadrants, time in a predefined radius around the original platform position (larger than the original platform itself), average distance swam to target site, and latency to first target site crossover. For investigators without automated tracking capabilities, blinded trained observers should use a timer to calculate the time spent in the aforementioned areas, as distance traveled is not feasible to measure with trained observers. Percent time spent in the target quadrant or percent of distance swam in the target quadrant is the most common reported end points in MWM spatial acquisition testing (106).

5.5.2. Spatial Reversal Testing Procedure

Spatial reversal testing determines the ability of the mouse to extinguish a particular memory in favor of forming a new one (106). In this paradigm, training procedures are the same as they were for spatial acquisition, but the probe trial differs. During the reversal training probe trial, the platform is moved, typically to the opposite side of the maze, but cues remain in their same position as during training trials (107). Mice are placed first on the platform for 30 s to allow them to gain some spatial cues as to where the new platform location is. Mice are then given 1–3 trials to reach the platform, starting from different locations if necessary (107). The same end points are used in spatial reversal training as with spatial acquisition (106). Since the platform remains in the maze, latency to reach the platform, swim speed, and total distance swam are also used as end points (107). Some variations of the MWM include repeated learning, latent learning, and cued learning (106).

6. Physical Activities

An acute reduction in physical activity is a sign/symptom of sickness and is associated with fatigue (11). Chronic low-grade inflammation is also linked to altered patterns of physical exertion and fatigue (11). Physical activity and fatigability can be measured with techniques adopted from exercise research and include voluntary running wheel and exhaustive/forced running. These tests are more powerful than spontaneous and long duration locomotion testing described earlier in that they can tease out more subtle activity differences. Animals that engage in more spontaneous physical activity generally have less fatigue, higher fitness levels, and better performance in forced exercise testing (108). Important behavioral differences appear to exist with spontaneous and forced exercise. Wheel running is spontaneous and thought to be under central nervous system control. The concept of motivation is critical to this behavior and sickness-associated fatigue appears to be a modulating factor (109, 110). In contrast, exhaustive exercise, such as forced treadmill running (FTR), is generally controlled by muscle and/or cardiovascular limitations (111). The rapidity with which an animal discontinues an exhaustive exercise test may also be governed by immunobehavioral fatigue (111). PNI investigators most often use SWR (26) and FTR (109) to probe the impact of immunobehaviors on physical activity. SWR is preferred for the high-throughput testing in that it can be remotely monitored with little demand on personnel. FTR is much more labor intensive but allows for considerable customization including alterability of duration, frequency, and intensity. FTR is also considerably more stressful to mice.

6.1. Spontaneous Wheel Running

A key advantage of SWR is that it can be assessed without moving mice from their home cage and the length of examination time can be very long. A disadvantage is that mice need to be singly housed. Specialized caging is needed to accommodate the running wheel and bedding must be correctly adjusted and monitored so as not to interfere with the wheel. A basic running wheel may measure only revolutions of the wheel and may need manual resetting at each data collection point. Advanced running wheel systems (Mini Mitter, Bend, OR) can obtain hourly, daily, or weekly distances run. Regardless of the running wheel sophistication, wheels need to be clean and well lubricated. Running wheel size and structure should also accommodate the size of mouse used. In long duration studies, cage cleaning and contact with animal facility and/or investigative personnel can result in an acute reductions in running. For the below procedure, an automated, multichannel running wheel system (Mini Mitter, Bend, OR) is utilized. Specific procedures and training for any given wheel should be provided by the manufacture of the device chosen.

6.1.1. Procedure

Mice need to be individually housed for experiments with running wheels and need to acclimate to the procedure room for at least 24 h prior to experimentation. Groups of mice in cages with locked running wheels and in cages with no wheel present should be included for proper experimental controls. Prior to experimentation (such as neuroimmune activation), a baseline measurement is recorded in case post hoc normalization of distance run is required. After immunobehavioral stimulation, mice are immediately returned to their cage and allowed access to the wheel (rotating, locked) or cage environment (no wheel). A 10-day course of wheel running is recommended. With automated running wheel systems, total distance run is reported. With manual wheels, wheel revolutions are recorded and distance traveled calculated by multiplying the wheel circumference by the number of revolutions. A limitation in SWR is the absence of a running intensity marker. However, some sophisticated wheel systems can record revolutions/min providing some insight into intensity.

6.2. Forced Treadmill Running

FTR better measures mouse fatigue (111). Like running wheel systems, mouse treadmills vary in sophistication with some allowing both uphill and downhill running (IITC Inc. Life Science, Woodland Hills, CA). Treadmills coupled to oxygen consumption systems can be used to determine mouse "fitness." Nonrodent treadmills (Jog-A-Dog, Ottawa Lake, MI) divided into lanes with Plexiglas dividers allow for high-throughput studies of up to 20 mice. Treadmills should contain a protective end (foam) to prevent mice from being thrown from the device and to provide an impetus to move forward should the mouse reduce its speed or stop running. Mice will respond to the contact of the tail/hind portion with the protective end. A ventilated cover is also recommended. Intra-experimental prodding can be used if a mouse or mice appear to predominantly "ride" the treadmill but this encouragement can lead to bias due to the difficulty of applying prodding evenly to every subject mouse.

6.2.1. Procedure

All observations should be made during the dark/active cycle of the mice. Mice do not need to be single housed prior to this procedure but should be allowed to acclimate for at least 24 h to the procedure room. Prior to experimentation, mice should be trained daily for 3 days at speeds of 14–20 m/min (speed depends on mouse age and strain). Mice that cannot learn the treadmill task should not be included in experimental studies. Training sessions should last until mouse exhaustion (1–2 h). Immunobehavioral stimulation is delivered 24 h after the final training session. Testing is initiated by conducting a treadmill run to exhaustion. Exhaustion is considered as a cease in running that is not motivated by protective end contact. Time to exhaustion is the measured end point. Distance to exhaustion can be calculated from the time run and velocity of the treadmill.

7. Conclusion

Behavioral testing is a fundamental element of PNI research and mice provide a powerful tool for exploring the origins and relevance of sickness symptoms. Like with any experimental procedure, uniform agreement on exact technique between scientists has not been achieved. Therefore, the above should be considered an overview of how to measure sickness, depressive/anxietal, cognitive, and physical activity behaviors. As important as appropriate procedures are to successful behavioral testing, preexperiment considerations are likely the greatest determinate to relevance and reproducibility. It is essential that mice be housed in environments devoid of negative stressors and be well adapted to any change. Variation in the equipment and experimental design is usually irrelevant when compared to unexpected and unpredictable housing conditions. In fact, wet cages, noise, and unfamiliar odors are often used as elicitors of adverse biobehaviors. Thus, consistency, concern, and care in handling mice afford the best foundation for success. Finally, keen observation is an additional reward, and making sure to note unanticipated or unusual behaviors during testing may lead to innovative discoveries toward the creation of new behavioral tests and immunobehavioral paradigms.

Support

This research was supported by the National Institutes of Health (DK064862, NS058525 and AA019357 to G.G.F.), USDA National Institute of Food and Agriculture, Hatch project #ILLU-971-32.

References

1. Ader R (2000) On the development of psychoneuroimmunology. Eur J Pharmacol 405(1–3):167–176
2. Maier SF, Watkins LR, Fleshner M (1994) Psychoneuroimmunology—the interface between behavior, brain and immunity. Am Psychol 49(12):1004–1017
3. Kerschensteiner M, Meinl E, Hohlfeld R (2009) Neuro-immune crosstalk in CNS diseases. Neuroscience 158:1122–1132
4. Kelley KW et al (2003) Cytokine-induced sickness behavior. Brain Behav Immun 17: S112–S118
5. Irwin MR (2008) Human psychoneuroimmunology: 20 years of discovery. Brain Behav Immun 22:129–139
6. Dantzer R (2004) Cytokine-induced sickness behavior: a neuroimmune response to activation of innate immunity. Eur J Pharmacol 500:399–411
7. Johnson DR et al (2007) Acute hypoxia activates the neuroimmune system, which diabetes exacerbates. J Neurosci 27(5):1161–1166
8. Dantzer R (2001) Cytokine-induced sickness behavior: mechanisms and implications. Ann N Y Acad Sci 933:222–234
9. Gibertini M (1998) Cytokines and cognitive behavior. Neuroimmunomodulation 5: 160–165
10. Wingfield JC et al (2006) Contexts and ethology of vertebrate aggression: implications for the evolution of hormone-behavior interactions. In: Nelson RJ (ed) Biology of aggression. Oxford University Press, New York
11. Dantzer R et al (2008) From inflammation to sickness and depression: when the immune system subjugates the brain. Nat Rev Neurosci 9:46–56
12. Lavin DN et al (2011) Fasting induces an anti-inflammatory effect on the neuroimmune system which a high-fat diet prevents. Obesity 19(8):1586–1594
13. Paul RH et al (2000) Fatigue and its impact on patients with Myasthenia Gravis. Muscle Nerve 23(9):1402–1406
14. Carmichael MD et al (2006) Role of brain IL-1β on fatigue after exercise-induced muscle damage. Am J Physiol Regul Integr Comp Physiol 291:R1344–R1348
15. Rönnbäck L, Hansson E (2004) On the potential role of glutamate transport in mental fatigue. J Neuroinflammation 1:22

16. Warren EJ et al (1997) Coincidental changes in behavior and plasma cortisol in unrestrained pigs after intracerebroventricular injection of tumor necrosis factor-α. Endocrinology 138(6):2365–2371
17. Grippo AJ (2009) Mechanisms underlying altered mood and cardiovascular dysfunction: the value of neurobiological and behavioral research in animal models. Neurosci Biobehav Rev 33(2):171–180
18. Crawley JN (2003) Behavioral phenotyping of rodents. Comp Med 53(2):140–146
19. Shigemura N et al (2004) Leptin modulates behavioral responses to sweet substances by influencing peripheral taste structures. Endocrinology 145(2):839–847
20. Rodgers RJ, Cole JC (1993) Influence of social isolation, gender, strain and prior novelty on plus-maze behaviour in mice. Physiol Behav 54(4):729–736
21. Palanza P, Gioiosa L, Parmigiani S (2001) Social stress in mice: gender differences and effects of estrous cycle and social dominance. Physiol Behav 73:411–420
22. Lightfoot JT et al (2004) Genetic influence on daily wheel running activity level. Physiol Genomics 19:270–276
23. Basterfield L, Lumley LK, Mathers JC (2009) Wheel running in female C57BL/6J mice: impact of oestrus and dietary fat and effects on sleep and body mass. Int J Obes 33: 212–218
24. Hawkley LC, Cacioppo JT (2004) Stress and the aging immune system. Brain Behav Immun 18(2):114–119
25. Dilger RN, Johnson RW (2008) Aging, microglial cell priming, and the discordant central inflammatory response to signals from the peripheral immune system. J Leukoc Biol 84(4):932–939
26. Martin SA et al (2011) Voluntary-wheel exercise training attenuates the visceral adipose, but not central, inflammatory response to LPS in aged C57BL/6J mice. Brain Behav Immun 25(S2), S217–S218 (Abstract)
27. Ma H et al (2010) Effects of diet-induced obesity and voluntary wheel running on bone properties in young male C57BL/6J mice. Calcif Tissue Int 86:411–419
28. Obernier JA, Baldwin RL (2006) Establishing an appropriate period of acclimatization following transportation of laboratory animals. ILAR J 47(4):364–369
29. Tuli JS, Smith JA, Morton DB (1995) Stress measurements in mice after transportation. Lab Anim 29:132–138
30. Jennings M et al (1998) Refining rodent husbandry: the mouse. Report of the Rodent Refinement Working Party. Lab Anim 32(3): 233–259
31. Clénet F et al (2006) Light/dark cycle manipulation influences mice behavior in the elevated plus maze. Behav Brain Res 166(1): 140–149
32. Ciarleglio CM et al (2009) Population encoding by circadian clock neurons organizes circadian behavior. J Neurosci 29(6):1670–1676
33. Goulding EH et al (2008) A robust automated system elucidates mouse home cage behavioral structure. Proc Natl Acad Sci U S A 105(52):20575–20582
34. National Research Council of the National Academies (2011) Guide for the care and use of laboratory animals. National Academy of Sciences, Washington, DC
35. Buchanan JB et al (2008) Cognitive and neuroinflammatory consequences of mild repeated stress are exacerbated in aged mice. Psychoneuroendocrinology 33(6):755–765
36. Ajarem JS, Safar E, Ahmad M (2011) Effect of ethanol and thermal stresses on the social behavior of male mice. Asian J Biol Sci 4: 362–368
37. Goshen I et al (2003) The role of endogenous interleukin-1 in stress-induced adrenal activation and adrenalectomy-induced adrenocorticotropic hormone hypersecretion. Endocrinology 144:4453–4458
38. Naff KA et al (2007) Noise produced by vacuuming exceeds the hearing thresholds of C57BL/6 and CD1 mice. J Am Assoc Lab Anim Sci 46(1):52–57
39. Turnbull AV, Rivier C (1995) Regulation of the HPA axis by cytokines. Brain Behav Immun 9(4):253–275
40. Beishuizen A, Thijs LG (2003) Review: endotoxin and the hypothalamo-pituitary-adrenal (HPA) axis. Innate Immun 9(1):3–24
41. Pfaff J (1974) Noise as an environmental problem in the animal house. Lab Anim 8:347–354
42. Arakawa H, Cruz S, Deak T (2011) From models to mechanisms: odorant communication as a key determinant of social behavior in rodents during illness-associated states. Neurosci Biobehav Rev 35(9):1916–1928
43. Alves GJ et al (2010) Odor cues from tumor-bearing mice induces neuroimmune changes. Behav Brain Res 214:357–367
44. Conour LA, Murray KA, Brown MJ (2006) Preparation of animals for research—issues to consider for rodents and rabbits. ILAR J 47(4):283–293
45. Balcombe JP, Barnard ND, Sandusky C (2004) Laboratory routines cause animal stress. Contemp Top Lab Anim Sci 43(6):42–51

46. Hurst JL, West RS (2010) Taming anxiety in laboratory mice. Nat Methods 7(10):825–826
47. Koike H et al (2009) Behavioral abnormality and pharmacologic response in social isolation-reared mice. Behav Brain Res 202(1):114–121
48. Ma X et al (2011) Social isolation-induced aggression potentiates anxiety and depressive-like behavior in male mice subjected to unpredictable chronic mild stress. PLoS One 6(6): e20955
49. Avitsur R, Stark JL, Sheridan JF (2001) Social stress induces glucocorticoid resistance in subordinate animals. Horm Behav 39(4): 247–257
50. Pardon M et al (2004) Repeated sensory contact with aggressive mice rapidly leads to an anticipatory increase in core body temperature and physical activity that precedes the onset of aversive responding. Eur J Neurosci 20(4):1033–1050
51. Van De Weerd HA et al (1994) Strain specific behavioural response to environmental enrichment in the mouse. J Exp Anim Sci 36: 117–127
52. Olsson AS, Dahlborn K (2001) Improving housing conditions for laboratory mice: a review of 'environmental enrichment'. Lab Anim 36:243–270
53. Kent S et al (1992) Sickness behavior as a new target for drug development. Trends Pharmacol Sci 13:24–28
54. Dantzer R et al (1987) Modulation of social memory in male rats by neurohypophyseal peptides. Psychopharmacology 91:363–368
55. Park SE et al (2011) Central administration of insulin-like growth factor-I decreases depressive-like behavior and brain cytokine expression in mice. J Neuroinflammation 8:12
56. Krzyszton CP et al (2008) Exacerbated fatigue and motor deficits in interleukin-10-deficient mice after peripheral immune stimulation. Am J Physiol Regul Integr Comp Physiol 295(4):R1109–R1114
57. Pecaut MJ et al (2002) Behavioral consequences of radiation exposure to simulated space radiation in the C57BL/6 mouse: open field, rotarod, and acoustic startle. Cogn Affect Behav Neurosci 2(4):329–340
58. Thor DH, Holloway WR (1982) Social memory of the male laboratory rat. J Comp Physiol Psychol 96(6):1000–1006
59. Bluthé RM, Dantzer R, Kelley KW (1991) Interleukin-1 mediates behavioural but not metabolic effects of tumor necrosis factor α in mice. Eur J Pharmacol 209:281–283
60. Bluthé RM, Schoenen J, Dantzer R (1990) Androgen-dependent vasopressinergic neurons are involved in social recognition in rats. Brain Res 519:150–157
61. Dantzer R, Bluthé RM, Kelley KW (1991) Androgen-dependent vasopressinergic neurotransmission attenuates interleukin-1-induced sickness behavior. Brain Res 557: 115–120
62. Abraham J et al (2008) Aging sensitizes mice to behavioral deficits induced by central HIV-1 gp120. Neurobiol Aging 29:614–621
63. Sherry CL et al (2009) Behavioral recovery from acute hypoxia is reliant on leptin. Brain Behav Immun 23(2):169–175
64. Cao JL et al (2010) Mesolimbic dopamine neurons in the brain reward circuit mediate susceptibility to social defeat and antidepressant action. J Neurosci 30(49):16453–16458
65. Basso AM et al (2009) Behavioral profile of $P2X_7$ receptor knockout mice in animal models of depression and anxiety: relevance for neuropsychiatric disorders. Behav Brain Res 198:83–90
66. Buchanan JB, Sparkman NL, Johnson RW (2010) A neurotoxic regimen of methamphetamine exacerbates the febrile and neuroinflammatory response to a subsequent peripheral immune stimulus. J Neuroinflammation 7:82
67. Fanelli MT, Kaplan ML (1978) Effects of high fat and high carbohydrate diets on the body composition and oxygen consumption of ob/ob mice. J Nutr 108(9):1491–1500
68. Jones BJ, Roberts DJ (1968) The quantitative measurement of motor incoordination in naïve mice using and accelerating rotarod. J Pharm Pharmacol 20(4):302–304
69. Tarantino LM, Gould TJ, Druhan JP, Bucan M (2000) Behavior and mutagenesis screens: the importance of baseline analysis of inbred strains. Mamm Genome 11:555–564
70. Dang MT et al (2006) Disrupted motor learning and long-term synaptic plasticity in mice lacking NMDAR1 in the striatum. Proc Natl Acad Sci U S A 103(41):15254–15259
71. Carter RJ, Morton AJ, Dunnett SB (2001) Motor coordination and balance in rodents. Curr Protoc Neurosci Chapter 8:Unit 8.12
72. Loftis JM, Huckans M, Morasco BJ (2010) Neuroimmune mechanisms of cytokine-induced depression: current theories and novel treatment strategies. Neurobiol Dis 37:519–533
73. Deacon RMJ (2006) Burrowing in rodents: a sensitive method for detecting behavioral dysfunction. Nat Protoc 1(1):118–121
74. Walf AA, Frye CA (2007) The use of the elevated plus maze as an assay of anxiety-related

behavior in rodents. Nat Protoc 2(2): 322–328

75. Cryan JF, Holmes A (2005) The ascent of mouse: advances in modeling human depression and anxiety. Nat Rev Drug Discov 4: 775–790
76. Gould TD, Dao DT, Kovacsics CE (2009) The open field test. In: Gould T (ed) Mood and anxiety related phenotypes in mice: characterization using behavioral tests. Humana Press, New York
77. Petit-Demouliere B, Chenu F, Bourin M (2004) Forced swimming test in mice: a review of antidepressant activity. Psychopharmacology 177:245–255
78. Komada M, Takao K, Miyakawa T (2008) Elevated plus maze for mice. J Vis Exp 22: e1088
79. Tonelli LH et al (2009) Allergic rhinitis induces anxiety-like behavior and altered social interaction in rodents. Brain Behav Immun 23:784–793
80. Fromm L et al (2004) Magnesium attenuates post-traumatic depression/anxiety following diffuse traumatic brain injury in rats. J Am Coll Nutr 23(5):529S–533S
81. Shepherd JK et al (1994) Behavioural and pharmacological characterisation of the elevated "zero-maze" as an animal model of anxiety. Psychopharmacology 116:56–64
82. Heisler LK et al (1998) Elevated anxiety and antidepressant-like responses in serotonin 5-HT_{1A} receptor knockout mutant mice. Proc Natl Acad Sci U S A 95:15049–15054
83. Cryan JF, Mombereau C, Vassout A (2005) The tail suspension test as a model for assessing antidepressant activity: review of pharmacological and genetic studies in mice. Neurosci Biobehav Rev 29(4–5):571–625
84. Porsolt RD et al (2001) Rodent models of depression: forced swimming and tail suspension behavioral despair tests in rats and mice. Curr Protoc Neurosci 8.10A.1–8.10A.10
85. Lad HV et al (2007) Quantitative traits for the tail suspension test: automation, optimization, and BXD RI mapping. Mamm Genome 18:482–491
86. Steru L et al (1985) The tail suspension test: a new method for screening antidepressants in mice. Psychopharmacology 85:367–370
87. Cryan JF, Markou A, Lucki I (2002) Assessing antidepressant activity in rodents: recent developments and future needs. Trends Pharmacol Sci 23(5):238–245
88. Cryan JF, Page ME, Lucki I (2005) Differential behavioral effects of the antidepressants reboxetine, fluoxetine, and moclobemide in a modified forced swim test following chronic treatment. Psychopharmacology 182:335–344
89. Moreau M et al (2008) Innoculation of Bacillus Calmette-Guerin to mice induces an acute episode of sickness behavior followed by chronic depressive-like behavior. Brain Behav Immun 22(7):1087–1095
90. Udo H et al (2008) Enhanced adult neurogenesis and angiogenesis and altered affective behaviors in mice overexpressing vascular endothelial growth factor 120. J Neurosci 28(53):14522–14536
91. Hédou G et al (2001) An automated analysis of rat behavior in the forced swim test. Pharmacol Biochem Behav 70(1):65–76
92. DSM-IV (1994) Diagnostic and statistical manual of mental disorders, 4th edn. American Psychological Association, Washington, DC
93. Strekalova T, Steinbusch H (2009) Factors of reproducibility of anhedonia induction in a chronic stress depression model in mice. In: Gould T (ed) Mood and anxiety related phenotypes in mice: characterization using behavioral tests. Humana Press, New York
94. Niemi MB et al (2008) Neuro-immune associative learning. In: Lajtha A, Galoyan A, Besedovski HO (eds) Handbook of neurochemistry and molecular neurobiology. Springer, New York
95. Brennan PA, Keverne EB (1997) Neural mechanisms of mammalian olfactory learning. Prog Neurobiol 51(4):457–481
96. Bryan KJ et al (2009) Chapter 1: transgenic mouse models of Alzheimer's disease: behavioral testing and considerations. In: Buccafusco JJ (ed) Methods of behavior analysis in neuroscience, 2nd edn. CRC Press, Boca Raton, FL
97. Bevins RA, Besheer J (2006) Object recognition in rats and mice: a one-trial non-matching-to-sample learning task to study 'recognition memory'. Nat Protoc 1(3):1306–1311
98. Stefanko DP et al (2009) Modulation of long-term memory for object recognition via HDAC inhibition. Proc Natl Acad Sci U S A 106(23):9447–9452
99. Win-Shwe TT, Fujimaki H (2012) Acute administration of toluene affects memory retention in novel object recognition test and memory function-related gene expression in mice. J Appl Toxicol 32(4):300–304
100. Wehner JM, Radcliffe RA (2004) Cued and contextual fear conditioning in mice. Curr Protoc Neurosci Chapter 8:Unit 8.5C
101. Deacon RMJ, Rawlins JNP (2006) T-maze alternation in the rodent. Nat Protoc 1(1): 7–12

102. Lalonde R (2002) The neurological basis of spontaneous alternation. Neurosci Biobehav Rev 26:91–104
103. Bekker A et al (2006) Isoflurane preserves spatial working memory in adult mice after moderate hypoxia. Anesth Analg 102: 1134–1138
104. Harrison FE et al (2006) Spatial and nonspatial escape strategies in the Barnes maze. Learn Mem 13(6):809–819
105. O'Leary TP, Brown RE (2009) Visuo-spatial learning and memory deficits on the Barnes maze in the 16-month-old APPswe/PS1dE9 mouse model of Alzheimer's disease. Behav Brain Res 201:120–127
106. Vorhees CV, Williams MT (2006) Morris water maze: procedures for assessing spatial and related forms of learning and memory. Nat Protoc 1(2):848–858
107. Rosczyk HA, Sparkman NL, Johnson RW (2008) Neuroinflammation and cognitive function in aged mice following minor surgery. Exp Gerontol 43:840–846
108. Dishman RK et al (2006) Neurobiology of exercise. Obesity 14:345–346
109. Leasure JL, Jones M (2008) Forced a voluntary exercise differentially affect brain and behavior. Neuroscience 156:456–465
110. Garland TH Jr et al (2011) The biological control of voluntary exercise, spontaneous physical activity and daily energy expenditure in relation to obesity: human and rodent perspectives. J Exp Biol 214(pt 2):206–229
111. Noakes TD (2011) Time to move behind a brainless exercise physiology: the evidence for complex regulation of human exercise performance. Appl Physiol Nutr Metab 36: 23–35

Chapter 14

The MRL Model: An Invaluable Tool in Studies of Autoimmunity–Brain Interactions

Boris Sakić

Abstract

The link between systemic autoimmunity, brain pathology, and aberrant behavior is still largely unexplored field of biomedical science. Accumulating evidence points to causal relationships between immune factors, neurodegeneration, and neuropsychiatric manifestations. By documenting autoimmunity-associated neuronal degeneration and cytotoxicity of the cerebrospinal fluid from disease-affected subjects, the murine MRL model had shown high validity in revealing principal pathogenic circuits. In addition, unlike any other autoimmune strain, MRL mice produce antibodies commonly found in patients suffering from lupus and other autoimmune disorders. This review highlights importance of the MRL model as an indispensible preparation in understanding the links between immune system and brain function.

Key words: Autoimmunity, Lupus, Behavioral dysfunction, Neurodegeneration, Immunopsychiatry, Animal model

1. Introduction

1.1. Regulatory Metasystem

The basic principal of life is to adapt to the relentlessly changing environment, thus providing the basis for survival of an individual and continuity of a species. When challenged by external and internal stressors, functional homeostasis in mammals regulates itself through a coordinated network of the Regulatory Metasystem, which comprises of diverse interactions between nervous, endocrine, and immune systems (Fig. 1). While the nervous system is hardwired to endocrine glands and immune organs via autonomic fibers, the immune system communicates with other tissues by secreting various soluble messengers, such as cytokines, chemokines, and proteins of the complement system (1). These mediators can affect brain function by activating the vagal and other nerves (2), the secondary messenger system of endothelial cells in brain vasculature (3), or by diffusing into the brain parenchyma if the blood–brain barrier (BBB)

Qing Yan (ed.), *Psychoneuroimmunology: Methods and Protocols*, Methods in Molecular Biology, vol. 934, DOI 10.1007/978-1-62703-071-7_14, © Springer Science+Business Media, LLC 2012

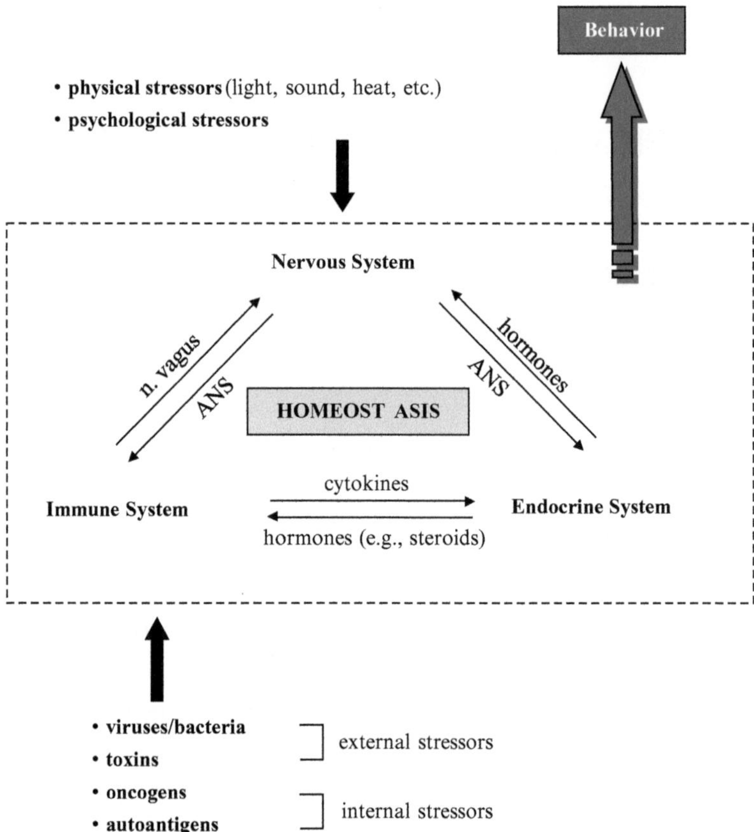

Fig. 1. The principal network of mammal regulatory metasystem. When challenged by various external and internal stressors, functional homeostasis regulates itself through coordinated interactions between neuroendocrine and immune systems, which form the Regulatory Metasystem. While the CNS is hardwired to endocrine glands and immune organs via fibers of the autonomic nervous system, ANS, the immune system communicates with other organs and tissues via release of various soluble messengers that either affect the brain directly via neural pathways (e.g., nervous vagus), or indirectly, by affecting hormonal activity in major endocrine pathways, such as hypothalamic-pituitary-adrenal axis. Imbalanced homeostasis (or allostasis) ultimately results in increased production of steroids and altered behavior, which are part of the adaptive responses to acute and chronic stressors. Acute sickness behavior and cortisol release (corticosterone in animals) are examples of an adaptive mechanism to acute exposure to pathogens. Different forms of mental and neurodegenerative CNS illnesses are proposed to ensue in genetically susceptible organisms when disturbances in their Regulatory Metasystem become severe and chronic. Systemic autoimmune diseases triggered by myriad of autoantigens (such as in SLE) are example of chronic activation in the Regulatory Metasystem.

becomes more permeable. These factors can also alter behavior indirectly by changing hormonal activity in major endocrine pathways, such as the hypothalamic-pituitary-adrenal axis (4). Imbalanced homeostasis (or allostasis) in this Regulatory Metasystem ultimately results in altered behavior, which is an integral part of the adaptive responses to acute and chronic stressors (5).

It is well established that acute and chronic stimuli from the external environment activate neuroendocrine organs and hormones in several stages (6). Similarly, infiltrated pathogens and toxins activate immune cells and organs, which subsequently signal the central neuronal circuits that control diverse aspects of behavior. Sickness behavior is an archetype of an acute interaction between immune response and an adaptive behavioral response (7). Namely, initial activation of the immune system and behavioral changes occur often within several hours or days. However, chronic activation of the immune system in genetically susceptible individuals may result in various forms of brain dysfunction because of sustained allostasis in the Regulatory Metasystem (8–10). Chronic inflammation, allergy, and autoimmune reactions are examples of sustained immune responses that have the potential to irreversibly harm the brain and disturb the Regulatory Metasystem in a prolonged manner. If viewing this homeostatic network more broadly, oncogens and autoantigens can be considered internal stressors which trigger and maintain sustained immune reactions accompanied by diverse immune cells and their products. Given that immunocytes have a unique capacity to inactivate, destroy, and eliminate other cells (including cells of own body), it is conceivable to assume that they have potential to profoundly compromise brain morphology and function. Autoimmune diseases are notorious for their chronicity and severity. As such, they pose a major threat to overall homeostasis and normal brain functioning. Unfortunately, compartmentalization of modern biomedical science into separate disciplines is largely responsible for our ongoing inability to integrate knowledge from different disciplines and gain deeper insight into etiologies of brain disorders accompanied by sustained inflammatory and autoimmune reactions. The sections below summarize a useful animal model that has confirmed its face and construct validity over the past 20 years and has become an indispensable tool in unraveling principal connections between systemic autoimmunity and the neuroendocrine system.

1.2. Involvement of the Nervous System in Systemic Lupus Erythematosus

Systemic lupus erythematosus (SLE) is a chronic autoimmune/inflammatory disorder with a broad spectrum of clinical manifestations. Despite its complexity in presentation and etiology, SLE is a prime example of causal relationships between systemic autoimmunity, brain pathology, and aberrant behavior. Neurologic and psychiatric (NP) manifestations of unknown etiology occur in up to 75 % of patients and are proposed to represent a more severe form of SLE (11). They range from diffuse manifestations (e.g., depression, anxiety, confusion, psychosis) to focal CNS manifestations (i.e., seizures, cerebrovascular disease, chorea, myelopathy, transverse myelitis, demyelinating syndrome, aseptic meningitis). Moreover, disorders of the peripheral nervous system (e.g., polyneuropathies, mononeuropathies, plexopathy, myasthenia gravis) are also common (12).

A significant number of patients experience NP manifestations well before disease onset, at the time of diagnosis, or within the first year after diagnosis is established (13). While a histologically normal brain is a possible finding in NP SLE (or CNS SLE), hypoperfusion (14–17) and regional metabolic abnormalities (18–20) are common neuropathological finding on brain imaging. Brain atrophy, however, is the most frequent observation on CT scans (21–26) and is proposed to reflect widespread and progressive neuronal loss (27, 28).

Apart from complications induced by kidney damage, infections, and steroid therapy, more recent studies confirm autoimmunity as a primary mechanism in the etiology of CNS lupus. Autoantibodies in the serum and cerebrospinal fluid (CSF) of lupus patients have been proposed as a key factor in brain damage (29). Increased intrathecal synthesis (as revealed by an elevated IgG index and oligoclonal banding) in patients with CNS dysfunction (30–32) and antigen-specific autoantibodies in the CSF (33) are shown to be associated with NP manifestations (34). In many cases, however, the correlational nature of clinical data has led to the necessity for animal models. In experimental studies, interactions between autoimmune/inflammatory phenomena and brain function can be examined in a more systematic and direct way. More importantly, due to ethical reasons, cause–effect relationships between specific immune factors and changes in behavior cannot be tested in clinical studies. They can be studied exclusively with well-controlled animal models that have significant face, construct, and predictive validity (35).

2. The MRL Model

2.1. Development

Most commonly studied spontaneous models of SLE include the NZB, (NZB × NZW)F1 hybrid, BXSB, and MRL mouse strains. They are characterized by a wide spectrum of autoimmune manifestations (36) and share common characteristics, such as hypergammaglobulinemia and elevated antinuclear antibodies (ANA), which are serological hallmarks of SLE. Since no animal model is a replica of human brain disease, each of these strains has distinct features that make them less or more useful in studying certain aspects of CNS SLE. Due to profound deficits in behavior of MRL/MpJ-Faslpr/J (MRL/lpr) mice that appear at a high frequency during the onset of spontaneous CNS SLE-like disease, my research over the past 20 years has focused on the nature of behavioral dysfunction during systemic autoimmunity and validity of the MRL model in studies of CNS SLE pathogenesis (37, 38).

There is no doubt that many murine models have made significant contributions to our understanding of SLE in general, and CNS SLE in particular (39). However, the MRL model has several advantages over the other strains. First, MRL mice do not have a high incidence of inherited brain abnormalities (40) that may confound assessment of autoimmunity-induced changes in brain function. They also produce antibodies that are common in SLE patients. Furthermore, MRL mice are convenient for longitudinal studies because they develop autoimmune manifestations early in life (41). Since MRL mice are among the biggest in the mouse kingdom, technically demanding procedures are feasible (e.g., CSF collection from the cisterna magna, retro-orbital bleeding, intra-cerebro-ventricular cannulation). Most importantly, there are two congenic substrains that differ in <0.1 % of their genetic background and disease onset. High levels of circulating cytokines, autoantibodies, and behavioral deficits appear in the MRL/MpJ-Fas^{lpr}/J substrain (MRL/lpr, stock 485 in The Jackson Laboratories) within the first 2 months of life (42). Conversely, the congenic MRL/MpJ ($MRL^{+/+}$) mice (stock 486) develop lupus-like disease much later in life and are asymptomatic at this age, thus representing an adequate control. Indeed, the traits above have helped in establishing the MRL model of CNS SLE, which is largely based on discrepancy in behavior and brain morphology between MRL/lpr and $MRL^{+/+}$ mice (43).

The MRL/MpJ lymphoproliferation wild-type strain was generated at The Jackson Laboratory from a series of crosses with strains C57BL/6J (0.3 %), C3H/HeDi (12.1 %), AKR/J (12.6 %), and LG/J (75 %) (Fig. 2). During development of this strain, the spontaneous mutation Fas^{lpr} was found in MRL/lpr mice at F12. This mutation of a single autosomal recessive gene (designated lymphoproliferative, *lpr* gene) on chromosome 19 results in massive lymphoadenopathy, induced by the accumulation of abnormal T-lymphocytes (44). There is also a spontaneous loss of function associated with the Fas mutation, which leads to a deficit in apoptotic Fas receptor (FasR) expression in MRL/lpr mice (45, 46). Largely due to aberrant apoptosis of self-reactive clones in the thymus (44), these mice develop an accelerated form of SLE-like disease, characterized by skin lesions, alopecia, arthritis, and immune complex glomerulonephrosis. Starting around 3 months of age, levels of circulating immune complexes rise promptly in the MRL/lpr substrain, but not in $MRL^{+/+}$ controls (41). Female MRL/lpr mice die at an average age of 17 weeks of age and males at 22 weeks.

In a series of early studies, we documented brain pathology, CSF cytotoxicity, and deficits in emotional reactivity of both male and female MRL/lpr mice (38). However, we were also aware that the expression of FasR plays an important role in neuronal apoptosis during postnatal development (47). Although the effectiveness of immunosuppressive treatment in preserving normal neuronal morphology pointed to a pathogenic role of autoimmunity (48–51), the possibility that the FasR deficiency in the CNS contributes to aberrant behavior in the MRL/lpr substrain could not be rejected until a new, long-lived stock of MRL/lpr mice was generated.

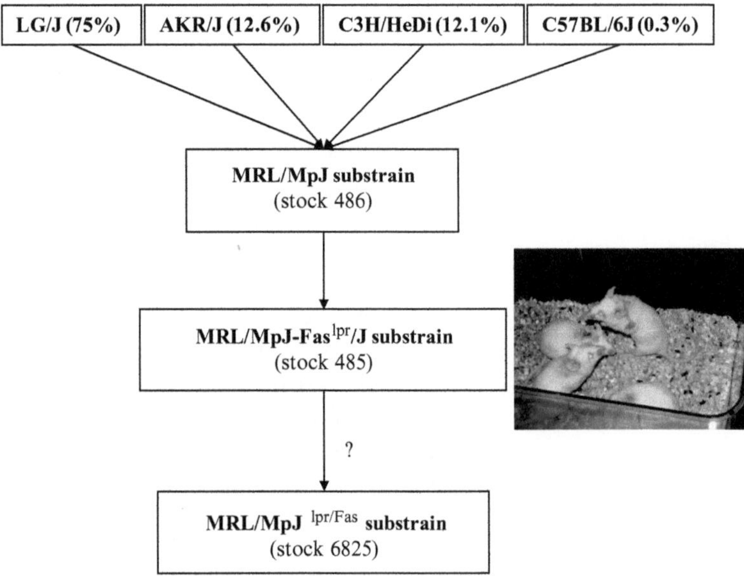

Fig. 2. Genetic background of the MRL mouse strain. Four different strains of mice were used in mid-1970s to produce the lupus-prone MRL strain in The Jackson Laboratories. In comparison to the original stock 486, spontaneous Fas^{lpr} mutation accounted for accelerated disease development in the stock 485 (MRL/lpr mice, shown on the picture). However, unexplained decline in autoimmune phenotype was observed in this stock over the past decade, and the subsequent stock was labeled 6825. As the stock 485, it carries the Fas^{lpr} mutation, thus rendering this group a more adequate control in behavioral studies that test causal links between systemic autoimmunity and brain damage.

Namely, a gradual decline in the autoimmune phenotype was observed in the MRL/lpr colony over the past decade. This phenomenon of unknown origin was also accompanied by a gradual decline in the number and severity of behavioral deficits (52). In 2007, the supplier (Jackson Laboratories, Bar Harbor, ME) publicly announced phenotype loss in the stock 485 and re-assigned it into stock 6825 (MRL/MpJ-Fas^{lpr}/JJ), which still carried the FasR deficiency in their genome (http://jaxmice.jax.org/strain/006825.html). Since embryos of the original stock 485 were cryopreserved in 1993, the original MRL/lpr stock was re-established in the summer of 2008. In brief, stock 485 has been proposed as a model of CNS SLE in reference to control stock 486 (37, 53), while stock 6825 ("mutated" stock 485) emerged as a new, improved control group because it shares FasR deficiency with the stock 485.

2.2. Autoimmunity-Associated Behavioral Syndrome

MRL/lpr and $MRL^{+/+}$ mice are comparable in many respects (e.g., appearance, size, reproductive age), except in the onset of autoimmunity and neurobehavioral dysfunction. Disease progression in MRL/lpr mice parallels emergence of behavioral deficits often seen after exposure to chronic stressors (37). The constellation of behavioral differences between age- and sex-matched MRL/lpr and

$MRL^{+/+}$ mice was operationally termed "autoimmunity-associated behavioral syndrome" (AABS), which has been largely characterized by progressive anxiety- and depressive-like behaviors (38). These constructs were supported by increased thigmotaxis of MRL/lpr mice in large arenas, impaired exploration of novel objects and spaces, performance deficits in the plus-maze and step-down tests, excessive floating in the forced swim test (54–56), reduced responsiveness to palatable stimulation (49, 57), and reduced isolation-induced inter-male fighting (58). Moreover, their "cognitive inflexibility" and poor spatial learning were noted in the Morris water maze (59, 60) and spontaneous alternation test (51). In addition, diseased MRL/lpr animals show lower nocturnal and open-field activity levels, as well as significant deficiencies in neurological (60, 61) and psychomotor tests (62).

2.3. Breached Blood–Brain Barrier

The BBB is formed by endothelial cells that tightly line capillaries and blood vessels of the brain. The BBB has an important role in maintaining a well-regulated CNS micro-environment for reliable neuronal signaling. When its normal function is disrupted, large molecules and cells can infiltrate into the brain and lead to CNS damage. In many CNS SLE patients, the BBB becomes transiently or permanently breached, as evidenced by an increased albumin quotient (63). Increased BBB permeability is an important permissive condition which allows diffusion of cytokines and antineuronal auto-antibodies into CSF and accounts for subsequent CNS manifestations (64).

Similar to patients, a breached BBB has been observed in diseased MRL/lpr mice. This damage occurs at a very early age (7–8 weeks) and is evidenced by perivascular leakage of IgG antibodies and increased albumin levels in the CSF (65, 66). In addition to soluble factors, significant infiltration of macrophages, T cells, B cells, and plasma cells can be demonstrated in the choroid plexus, meninges, and brain parenchyma of MRL/lpr mice (60, 67–69).

2.4. CNS Inflammation

The role of neuroinflammation is emerging as an important component of lupus-like disease. In addition to the previously mentioned infiltration of immunocytes into the brain parenchyma, several other types of inflammation-related pathologies have been observed in brains of MRL/lpr mice. They include upregulation of adhesion molecules (70, 71), the expression of mRNA for pro-inflammatory cytokines (72, 73), and deposition of complement proteins (74) within brains of MRL/lpr mice. Major histocompatibility complex (MHC) upregulation (75) and F4/80 microglia staining provides additional evidence for microglia-induced neuronal excitotoxicity in these animals (76). When assessing the global pattern of neuronal damage in MRL/lpr brains (77), a pattern of degeneration emerges that is typically seen in hydrocephalus, meningoencephalitis, and hypoglycemic encephalopathy

(78–82), all of which result in cerebritis. Supporting this notion, others have reported that MRL/lpr mice have an increased incidence of hydrocephalus (83), meningoencephalitis (67), and altered glucose metabolism (84), with complement activation as a likely precursor to cerebral edema (85).

Congenic MRL$^{+/+}$ animals were found to have greater cell loss and a more aggressive, sustained microglial inflammatory response following mechanical injury and breakdown of the BBB (86). Unlike MRL/lpr animals, which develop spontaneous BBB disruption, MRL$^{+/+}$ mice do not show evidence of CNS damage under normal conditions. However, the MRL strain may have an inherent propensity toward exaggerated CNS inflammatory responses. For example, considering the substantia nigra of mice have more microglia than other areas (87), one may assume that this neuroanatomical trait in lupus mice reflects the region-specific susceptibility to inflammatory and excitotoxic metabolites produced by activated microglia (88).

While neuroinflammation appears to be a contributing factor to disease in MRL/lpr animals, a distinct inflammatory response is not commonly seen in the brains of lupus patients. Some of the most common neuropathological findings in SLE, however, are small vessel cerebral vasculopathy and micro-infarcts. These observed features likely reflect the end result of repeated episodes of acute inflammation in the small brain vessels (89). Elevated levels of soluble adhesion molecules in serum and CSF of patients with CNS involvement (90) also suggests that neuroinflammatory conditions may play an understated role in certain NP manifestations.

2.5. Brain Pathology

Clinical studies clearly demonstrate that NP manifestations are accompanied by cerebral atrophy (91), progressive neuronal loss (19, 27), and parenchymal lesions (92). Similar to CNS SLE patients and effects of chronic stress, MRL/lpr mice show brain atrophy and ventricular enlargement alongside behavioral deficits detected at the onset of SLE-like disease (51, 93, 94).

The MRL strain does not show a high incidence of inherited neuroanatomical abnormalities (40), which minimize the possibility of congenital defects confounding the study of disease-induced neurodegeneration. At the onset of autoimmune symptoms in MRL/lpr mice, reports of reduced complexity of pyramidal neurons, reduced brain weights (94), and selectively neurotoxic CSF (95) provided indirect evidence of neuronal damage in diseased animals. Direct evidence of neuronal death, however, was first confirmed in MRL/lpr brains using the Fluoro Jade B (FJB) cytochemical stain (specific for dying neurons). A small percentage of these neurons were subsequently found to contain TdT-labeled apoptotic nuclei and co-localized with FJB (77) and antineurofilament staining (74). Moreover, while the size of hippocampal fields and neuronal density are not reduced in young Fas-deficient lpr mice

(96), cell densities are reduced within the hippocampus, cortex (51), and midbrain (88) of aged/diseased lupus mice.

In addition to mature neurons, recent findings suggest that progenitor cells also degenerate in MRL/lpr brains. More specifically, the subventricular zone (97), subgranular zone (76, 77), and substantia nigra (88), all of which are known to contain proliferative progenitor cells capable of neurogenesis (98), show signs of damage. CSF from diseased lupus mice is also cytotoxic to neurons and neuronal progenitor cells in vitro (99), thus supporting a link between toxic CSF IgG and neuronal/progenitor cell damage (66). If in vitro findings are predictive of in vivo events, then autoimmune-induced lesions of germinal layers may reduce the developmental and regenerative capacity of MRL/lpr brains. An impairment in this process would likely exacerbate subsequent autoimmune/inflammatory-mediated neuronal death and behavioral deficits. For example, an impaired capacity for hippocampal neurogenesis could account for the cognitive impairments observed in these animals (51). Stress hormones, known to be chronically elevated in lupus mice (100), have also been shown to inhibit cell proliferation and neurogenesis (101). Therefore, one may assume that such mechanisms account for impaired brain growth and regeneration along the progression of autoimmune disease.

Despite parallels between the emergence of behavioral dysfunction and systemic autoimmunity, there is no firm evidence that brain pathology accounts for aberrant behavior in the MRL model. However, significant correlations suggest principal links between structural brain damage and functional/behavioral impairments in MRL/lpr mice. For example, deficits in spatial learning/memory emerge concomitantly with hippocampal damage (51), aberrant performance in the sucrose preference test coincide with lesions of the nucleus accumbens (102), and decreased locomotor activity accompany degeneration in the substantia nigra (88). Although the mechanisms underlying these deficits are not well understood (103), recent pharmacological evidence supports a link between dopaminergic circuit damage and AABS.

2.6. Proposed Neuropathogenic Factors and Mechanisms

The causative role of autoimmunity and inflammation in the pathogenesis of AABS has been supported by studies employing the immunosuppressive drug cyclophosphamide (CY). Sustained treatment with CY from an early age prevents several behavioral deficits and brain pathology in MRL/lpr mice (49–51, 68). More specifically, CY abolishes substrain differences in anxiety- and motivation-related behaviors, as suggested by restored novel object exploration, increased responsiveness to a palatable sucrose solution, and normalized nocturnal activity. Although systemic autoimmunity and inflammation have been proposed as key factors, the possibility that subtle genetic dissimilarities, imbalanced hormonal production, and peripheral tissue involvement contribute to certain aspects of AABS could not be discounted. However, the use of newly developed stock 6825 rejected the possibility that AABS is entirely accounted by FasR mutation in neuronal cells. Namely, the constellation of differences between the lpr stocks 485 and 6825 confirmed the hypothesis that the *lpr* mutation per se does not fully account for the brain pathology and altered behavior in the stock 485 (104). Together with significant correlations between immunological and behavioral measures, this study suggested that soluble immune factors play a key role in CNS pathogenesis. In addition, combined use of immunoprecipitation with homogenates of unaffected brains, 2-dimensional differential in-gel electrophoresis, and mass spectrometry revealed strong binding of CSF IgG antibodies to cytoskeletal antigens in brains of MRL/lpr mice. This finding is consistent with the proposed pathogenic role of brain-reactive autoantibodies (BRA) in the etiology of AABS.

CNS SLE is frequently accompanied by BRA cross-reactive with diverse brain-specific and systemic antigens (11). Most of these autoantibodies have been identified on the basis of their binding to tissues and cells, including neuroblastoma and glioblastoma cell lines (105). There are also autoantibodies against lymphocytes, capable of being adsorbed by brain tissue (106, 107). Some antibodies can react specifically to CNS neurons (108, 109), neuronal cytoplasm (110), and neuronal receptors (111, 112). A current literature review proposes approximately 20 pathogenic BRA (113), including antiribosomal, anticardiolipin, antiphospholipid, and more recently antibodies to an NMDA receptor, or anti-NR2 antibodies (29, 111, 114–119). Consistent with clinical findings in CNS SLE patients (120–123), our recent study with MRL/lpr mice revealed significant reactivity of their CSF and serum IgG molecules to cytoskeletal proteins (104). When the source of BRA is considered, both clinical studies and studies with MRL/lpr mice suggest that BRA from CSF are more pathogenic than BRA from serum (95, 99, 124–126). While the mechanism by which circulating BRAs access the brain is not well understood, aberrant behavioral and emotional manifestations in human and murine forms of lupus suggest that multiple CNS antigens and sites are targeted (111, 117, 118, 127–129). A significant relationship between aberrant behavioral performance and specific BRA has been reported in diseased MRL/lpr mice (130–132). However, certain subsets of BRA might be more important in the induction of permanent neuronal damage, while other subsets might merely affect neuronal functioning in a transient fashion (133). Given these complex modes of action, more direct, invasive studies are required to prove causality between specific classes of pathogenic BRA and certain behavioral deficit/brain pathology.

A dysregulated cytokine network is also hypothesized to play an important role in the etiology of CNS SLE. In general, proinflammatory cytokines are instrumental in expanding peripheral immune reactions to the CNS via endothelial activation (63, 134). Early increases in serum levels of IL-1β, TNF-α, IL-6, and interferon-gamma are principal events facilitating the hyperproduction and maintenance of autoantibodies in the MRL/lpr substrain (57, 135–137). A significant correlation between serum IL-6 levels and responsiveness to a palatable stimulus was documented in MRl/lpr mice (138). Using adeno-vector methodology, a direct cause–effect relationship was shown for both IL-6 and interferon-gamma (139, 140). Similarly, administration of TNF-α enhanced intracellular adhesion molecule (ICAM)-dependent leukocyte–endothelial interactions in MRL/lpr brains (141). Furthermore, these interactions can be prevented by antibody blockade of pro-inflammatory cytokines or ICAM (61, 70). It is important to emphasize that small amounts of pro-inflammatory cytokines can also cross the BBB by specific transport mechanisms (142–144) and activate receptors on endothelial cells of the brain vasculature to release other mediators (e.g., cytokines, nitric oxide, prostaglandins) into the CSF and brain parenchyma (145, 146). However, it remains to be determined whether physiological doses of circulating cytokines can compromise viability of central neurons. On the other hand, it is well documented that pro-inflammatory cytokines have the ability to affect the stress hormone system and alter behavior (147–151). More specifically, these cytokines can regulate corticosteroid levels and autoimmunity through receptors in adrenal gland and pituitary (150, 152–155). Sustained activation of the pituitary-adrenal axis in MRL/lpr mice is evidenced by increased central expression of arginine/vasopressin mRNA (156, 157) and high levels of corticosterone (100). Although an imbalanced neuro-immuno-endocrine network is confirmed to play a key role in the etiology of brain damage, it is still not clear to which extent central neurons are damaged by an inflammation-driven upregulation in corticosterone production vs. direct cytotoxicity of self-reactive immunocytes and their products. Corticosterone-induced atrophy of neurons may be reversible, but it can also be indicative of an early stage of neurodegeneration (158, 159). Indeed, diseased MRL/lpr mice show profound neuronal spine loss (94) which can be further exacerbated with chronic pretreatment with corticosterone. Namely, sustained corticosterone administration attenuated signs of autoimmune disease, but lead to profound dendritic spine deterioration, as revealed by the Golgi method (160). Therefore, based on chronically elevated serum corticosterone levels in MRL/lpr mice (100), one may hypothesize that sustained endogenous immunosuppression is a precursor and necessary factor for neurodegenerative events that occur when autoimmune mechanisms prevail at later stages of the disease (Fig. 3). Indeed, changes in the morphology of neuronal dendrites, cerebral atrophy, and immunoreactive ubiquitin particles (denoting axon terminal degeneration) occur by 14 weeks of age in MRL/lpr brains, but progressive

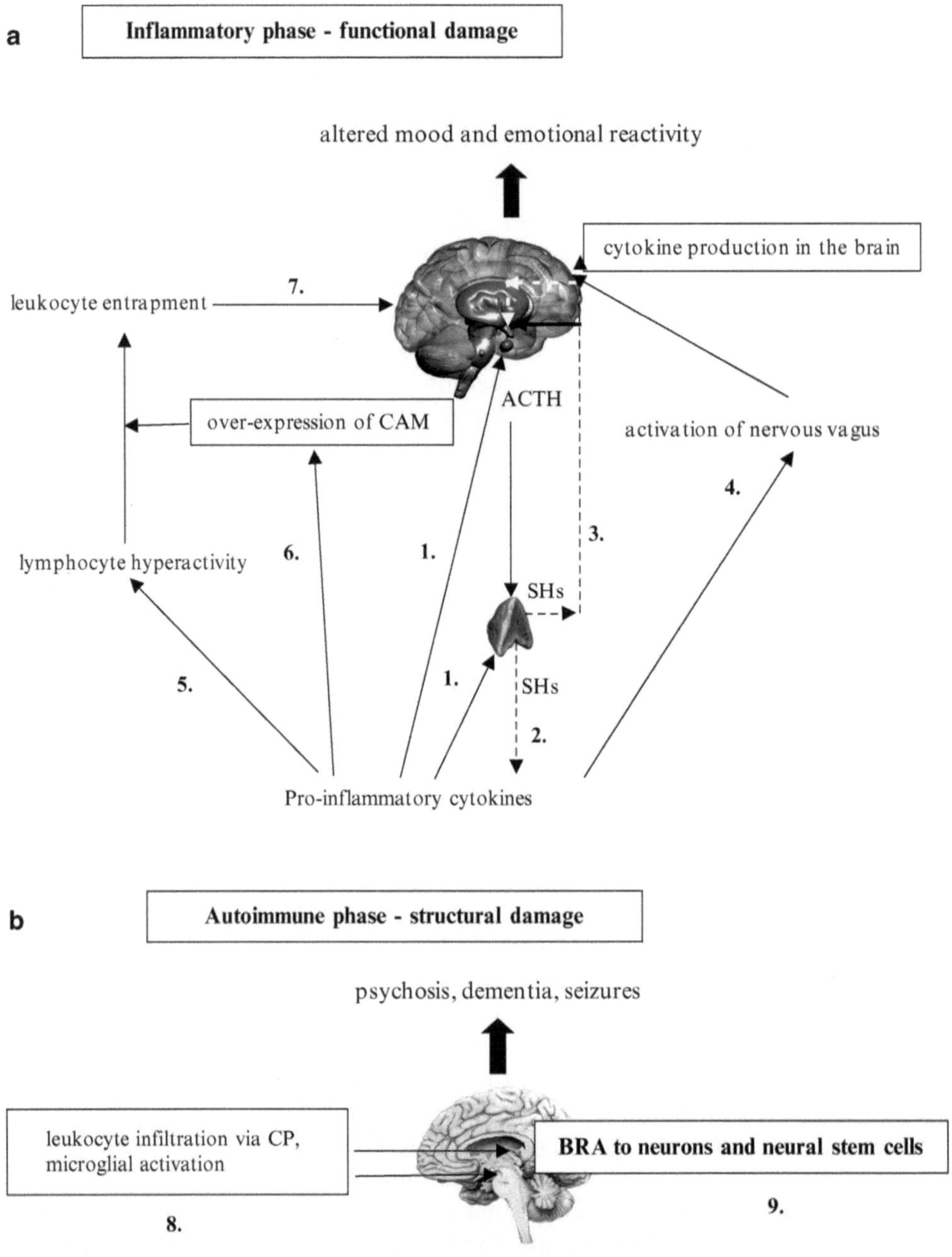

a

Inflammatory phase - functional damage

altered mood and emotional reactivity

cytokine production in the brain

leukocyte entrapment

7.

ACTH

over-expression of CAM

activation of nervous vagus

4.

3.

lymphocyte hyperactivity

6.

1.

SHs

5.

1.

SHs

2.

Pro-inflammatory cytokines

b

Autoimmune phase - structural damage

psychosis, dementia, seizures

leukocyte infiltration via CP,
microglial activation

BRA to neurons and neural stem cells

8.

9.

Fig. 3. Proposed phases and pathways of the CNS damage during systemic autoimmune disease. Behavioral dysfunction and brain damage in lupus-like disease may result from chronic stress-like response induced by sustained autoimmunity and inflammation. In SLE patients and lupus-prone MRL/lpr mice, spontaneous onset of systemic inflammation and autoimmunity are characterized by increased levels of pro-inflammatory cytokines, which may activate pituitary-adrenal axis and promote sustained release of glucocorticoids. In turn, steroid hormones suppress the immune system at multiple levels. Due to chronic nature of the disease, glucocorticoids, cytokines, and other immune components remain elevated, thus compromising the integrity of the blood–brain barrier and neuronal function. (**a**) The inflammatory phase is largely associated with early functional damage of the brain. The upregulation in circulating proinflammatory cytokines (e.g., IL-1β, IL-6, TNF-α, and IFN-γ) is an initial serologic event that disturbs activity of the immune network. These cytokines can also activate the hypothalamic-pituitary-adrenal axis (1), which down-regulates peripheral inflammation via increased production of steroid hormones, SHs (2). However, in addition to the activation of major inhibitory signals from the hippocampus

neurodegeneration and microglial activation do not become pronounced until terminal stages of the disease (~5 months). Few MRL/lpr mice survive beyond 6 months of age (36), which may be attributed to profound CNS damage and brain edema (84). It is viable that such sustained "allostatic load" may ultimately provide the basis for vulnerability of central neurons (161), *bona fide* neurodegeneration, and behavioral dysfunction (51, 77, 94). Future studies examining the effects of cytokines on the endocrine axes and the possibility that adrenalectomy prevents (or delays) central neurodegeneration in MRL/lpr mice are warranted.

Aberrant cytokine production also modulates systemic autoimmunity by sustained activation of B-cells, which later differentiate into pathogenic autoantibody-forming cells. These pathogenic autoantibodies are a prelude to immune complex disease (162), a common feature of lupus. Indeed, deposition of antigen–antibody complexes (immune aggregates) in choroidal blood vessels have been associated with NP manifestations, while vascular deposits within the choroid plexus (CP) are accompanied by histopathological evidence of inflammation (163). Therefore, autoantibodies to endothelial cells, as well as the pathogenic action of circulating-immune complexes (CIC) on microvessels, likely contribute to, if not cause, endothelial cell damage and breakdown of the BBB in lupus patients and MRL/lpr mice (63, 66, 69). Subsequent infiltration of various immunocytes into the brain parenchyma of MRL/lpr mice (68, 69) may merely be another step in a cascade of neuropathogenic events.

There are numerous factors that can induce excitotoxic damage. In an injured or immunologically challenged brain, cytokine-producing microglia appear to play an important role. Microglia readily activate by transforming from a ramified, resting state into amoeboid cells that express MHC molecules (87), as seen in MRL/lpr brains (75). Inflammatory responses are then perpetuated by both cyclooxygenase (COX) and nitric oxide (NO). In MRL/lpr mice, however, abnormalities in prostaglandin production were reported (164), likely rendering COX inhibition ineffective in ameliorating AABS (76). Indirectly, these results suggest that inducible NO synthase and the glutamate system are important

Fig. 3. (continued) to hypothalamic paraventricular nucleus, sustained binding of steroids to receptors in central neurons (3) induces stress-like manifestations (e.g., emotional disturbances, impaired mood, etc.) which are largely under control of the limbic system. This effect on brain function is further amplified by cytokine-induced activation of the nervous vagus and activation of glial cells in the hypothalamus (4). Moreover, activated lymphocytes (5) and cytokine-induced overexpression of cell adhesion molecules on endothelial cells of the BBB and choroid plexus, CP (6) are conducive of immunocyte entrapment (7). (**b**) The autoimmune phase is largely characterized by structural damage, such as neurodegeneration and brain atrophy. Chronic inflammatory responses increase the permeability of the BBB and CP, thus leading to infiltration of immunocytes into perivascular spaces and cerebrospinal fluid (8). Structural brain damage can result from neurotoxic metabolites that accumulate after sustained activation of microglia (9) and chronic binding of brain-reactive antibodies (BRA) to adult and immature neurons (10). Loss of periventricular and cortical mass may underlie psychosis, dementia, and seizures that frequently accompany neuropsychiatric lupus. *Note*: dashed lines represent inhibitory pathways.

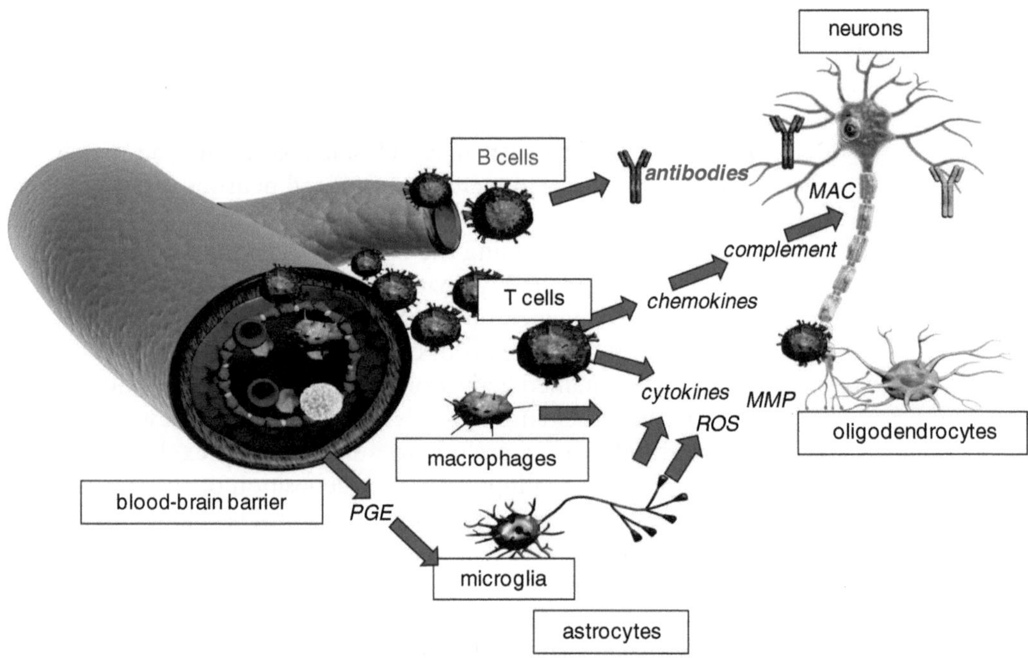

Fig. 4. Summary of putative factors and cellular mechanisms underlying neuronal damage in CNS lupus. When BBB is breached, various immune cells and mediators can compromise the viability of brain cells at different stages of disease progress, age, and genetic deficits in affected individuals. These factors include cytotoxic T cells, macrophages, brain-reactive antibodies to surface and intracellular receptors, the C5b-9 MAC, MMPs, and reactive oxygen species, ROS.

mediators of neuroinflammation and neuronal apoptosis in these animals (74). Ultrastructural evidence obtained from electron microscopy (76) and a study reporting significant increases in glutamine, glutamate, and lactate concentrations in MRL/lpr brains (84) support the notion of excitotoxic neuronal death. In the case of glutamate toxicity, this hypothesis is supported by evidence of anti-NMDA receptor antibodies resulting in neuronal apoptosis in the mouse brain (111), a similar IgG-mediated mechanism induced by CSF from MRL/lpr mice (99), and the presence of high levels of anti-NMDA receptor antibodies in their CSF (Betty Diamond, personal communication). Considering that anti-CD4 treatment (165) and complement inhibitors (74, 166) ameliorated CNS disease in MRL/lpr mice, one may assume that combination of cellular inflammatory and autoimmune factors (operational at different stages of the disease) underlies brain pathology and aberrant behavior (summarized in Fig. 4).

In comparison to other neurotransmitters, central dopamine system activity (implicated in reward, movement, and cognitive processes) is most profoundly altered in brains of MRL/lpr mice (167). A series of pharmacological studies suggest that damage to central dopaminergic circuits accounts for at least some behavioral deficits in this substrain. In particular, chronic injection with the selective D2/D3 agonist quinpirole induced self-injurious behavior (168), while acute injection with the selective D1/D2 dopamine agonist apomorphine increased rotational behavior (88). In the sucrose preference paradigm, acute injection with the indirect dopamine agonist d-amphetamine failed to alter the response rates of diseased animals to sucrose solutions (102). Taken together, these results link neuropathological findings of dopaminergic cell death in nigrostriatal, mesolimbic, and mesocortical pathways to behavioral deficits in locomotion, motivated behavior, and learning. Although the contribution of peripheral disease manifestations on behavioral performance cannot be excluded, these results support the hypothesis that the dopamine system is affected in MRL/lpr brains and underlies changes in emotional reactivity and motivated behavior.

3. Summary

Compared to other models of systemic autoimmune disease, the MRL model has several key characteristics that render it an indispensable tool in studies of autoimmunity–brain interactions (43). First, compared to "induced" models of CNS SLE, MRL/lpr mice spontaneously develop manifestations that match the human disorder in complexity, chronicity, and severity. This includes a variety of intrathecal BRA and brain atrophy, which are both characteristic of more severe forms of CNS SLE. Second, in behavioral studies, the MRL model is well controlled with $MRL^{+/+}$ (stock 486) and MRL/lpr/JJ groups (stock 6825). The differences in genomes are <0.1 % (when compared to stock 486) and even less in case of stock 6825. Lastly, the MRL model is well defined at genetic, cellular, and behavioral levels. In particular, the *lpr* lesion (encoding for FasR deficiency) on chromosome 19, "double negative" clones of lymphocytes, neurodegeneration, and behavioral deficits are well explored phenomena, replicated by different research groups. This abundance of knowledge allows diverse manipulations at all system levels, thus advancing our understanding of relationships between genes, autoimmunity, and brain dysfunction.

The roles of stress hormones in initial modulation of brain morphology and behavior of MRL/lpr mice appear important (100) and may act similar to iatrogenic effects of sustained corticosteroid therapy on brains of CNS SLE patients (25). Progressive neuronal death and microglial activation are concomitant with the development of more severe systemic autoimmune/inflammatory disease and more diverse AABS. Although other neurotransmitter systems are likely involved, dopaminergic neurons seem to be a specific target of autoimmune reactions, possibly accounting for early deficits in emotional reactivity and motivated behavior. Further interplay among activated microglia, neuroactive cytokines, BRA, and cytotoxic T-cells likely leads to an accumulation of neurotoxic metabolites, edema, and brain atrophy. Although adult neurons and neural progenitors are targeted in diseased MRL/lpr mice (88, 95, 99, 169), the possible effect of autoimmunity on brain cells may be extended into prenatal life and influences from the maternal immune system (170).

While the MRL/lpr substrain displays many characteristics that resemble human CNS SLE, there are limitations which need be considered when studying this model. First, human CNS SLE has relapsing–remitting presentations of symptoms, while MRL/lpr mice show a progressive and unrelenting course of disease. Second, human SLE shows a strong gender preference (i.e., about 9–10 times more female than male patients). Although the disease starts few weeks earlier in female mice, the MRL/lpr substrain does not show such gender bias, possibly due to a different hormonal milieu in human and murine forms of lupus. Lastly, while more sophisticated assessments are administered in diagnosing human CNS SLE, "psychiatric manifestations" in MRL/lpr mice are merely constructs that can be proposed from dissimilar performances in behavioral tests. Despite these limitations, the MRL model remains useful and unique in understanding the complex immuno-neuroendocrine interactions. There is no doubt that deeper understanding of pathogenic pathways and neurotoxic mediators in these animals may help in elucidating CNS SLE etiology and provide a basis for new treatment modalities in brain disorders with autoimmune origin.

Acknowledgments

This work was supported by the grant from the Ontario Mental Health Foundation.

References

1. Ader R, Felten D, Cohen N (2001) Psychoneuroimmunology. Academic Press, New York
2. Goehler LE, Gaykema RP, Hansen MK, Anderson K, Maier SF, Watkins LR (2000) Vagal immune-to-brain communication: a visceral chemosensory pathway. Auton Neurosci 85:49–59
3. Benveniste EN, Huneycutt BS, Shrikant P, Ballestas ME (1995) Second messenger systems in the regulation of cytokines and adhesion molecules in the central nervous system. Brain Behav Immun 9:304–314
4. Dunn AJ (2000) Cytokine activation of the HPA axis. Ann N Y Acad Sci 917:608–617
5. McEwen BS (2000) Allostasis and allostatic load: implications for neuropsychopharmacology. Neuropsychopharmacology 22:108–124
6. Johnson EO, Kamilaris TC, Chrousos GP, Gold PW (1992) Mechanisms of stress: a dynamic overview of hormonal and behavioral homeostasis. Neurosci Biobehav Rev 16:115–130
7. Dantzer R, O'Connor JC, Freund GG, Johnson RW, Kelley KW (2008) From inflammation to sickness and depression: when the immune system subjugates the brain. Nat Rev Neurosci 9:46–56
8. McEwen BS (2003) Mood disorders and allostatic load. Biol Psychiatry 54:200–207
9. McEwen BS, Biron CA, Brunson KW, Bulloch K, Chambers WH, Dhabhar FS, Goldfarb RH, Kitson RP, Miller AH, Spencer RL, Weiss JM (1997) The role of adrenocorticoids as modulators of immune function in health and disease: neural, endocrine and

immune interactions. Brain Res Rev 23: 79–133

10. Cotman CW, Brinton RE, Galaburda A, McEwen B, Schneider DM (1987) The neuro-immune-endocrine connection. Raven, New York
11. Hanly JG (2005) Neuropsychiatric lupus. Rheum Dis Clin North Am 31:273–298, vi
12. Tincani A, Brey R, Balestrieri G, Vitali C, Doria A, Galeazzi M, Meroni PL, Migliorini P, Neri R, Tavoni A, Bombardieri S (1996) International survey on the management of patients with SLE.2. The results of a questionnaire regarding neuropsychiatric manifestations. Clin Exp Rheumatol 14:S23–S29
13. van Dam AP, Wekking EM, Oomen HA (1991) Psychiatric symptoms as features of systemic lupus erythematosus. Psychother Psychosom 55:132–140
14. Colamussi P, Giganti M, Cittanti C, Dovigo L, Trotta F, Tola MR, Tamarozzi R, Lucignani G, Piffanelli A (1995) Brain single-photon emission tomography with Tc-99m-HMPAO in neuropsychiatric systemic lupus erythematosus: relations with EEG and MRI findings and clinical manifestations. Eur J Nucl Med 22: 17–24
15. Handa R, Sahota P, Kumar M, Jagannathan NR, Bal CS, Gulati M, Tripathi BM, Wali JP (2003) In vivo proton magnetic resonance spectroscopy (MRS) and single photon emission computerized tomography (SPECT) in systemic lupus erythematosus (SLE). Magn Reson Imaging 21:1033–1037
16. Huang WS, Chiu PY, Tsai CH, Kao A, Lee CC (2002) Objective evidence of abnormal regional cerebral blood flow in patients with systemic lupus erythematosus on Tc-99m ECD brain SPECT. Rheumatol Int 22:178–181
17. Lopez-Longo FJ, Carol N, Almoguera MI, Olazaran J, Onso-Farto JC, Ortega A, Monteagudo I, Gonzalez CM, Carreno L (2003) Cerebral hypoperfusion detected by SPECT in patients with systemic lupus erythematosus is related to clinical activity and cumulative tissue damage. Lupus 12:813–819
18. Komatsu N, Kodama K, Yamanouchi N, Okada S, Noda S, Nawata Y, Takabayashi K, Iwamoto I, Saito Y, Uchida Y, Ito H, Yoshikawa K, Sato T (1999) Decreased regional cerebral metabolic rate for glucose in systemic lupus erythematosus patients with psychiatric symptoms. Eur Neurol 42:41–48
19. Brooks WM, Sabet A, Sibbitt WL, Barker PB, van Zijl PC, Duyn JH, Moonen CT (1997) Neurochemistry of brain lesions determined by spectroscopic imaging in systemic lupus erythematosus. J Rheumatol 24:2323–2329
20. Volkow ND, Warner N, McIntyre R, Valentine A, Kulkarni M, Mullani N, Gould L (1988) Cerebral involvement in systemic lupus erythematosus. Am J Physiol Imaging 3:91–98
21. Gonzalez-Scarano F, Lisak RP, Bilaniuk LT, Zimmerman RA, Atkins PC, Zweiman B (1979) Cranial computed tomography in the diagnosis of systemic lupus erythematosus. Ann Neurol 5:158–165
22. Kaell AT, Shetty M, Lee BC, Lockshin MD (1986) The diversity of neurologic events in systemic lupus erythematosus. Prospective clinical and computed tomographic classification of 82 events in 71 patients. Arch Neurol 43:273–276
23. Miguel EC, Pereira RM, Pereira CA, Baer L, Gomes RE, de Sa LC, Hirsch R, de Barros NG, de Navarro JM, Gentil V (1994) Psychiatric manifestations of systemic lupus erythematosus: clinical features, symptoms, and signs of central nervous system activity in 43 patients. Medicine 73:224–232
24. Omdal R, Selseth B, Klow NE, Husby G, Mellgren SI (1989) Clinical neurological, electrophysiological, and cerebral CT scan findings in systemic lupus erythematosus. Scand J Rheumatol 18:283–289
25. Ainiala H, Dastidar P, Loukkola J, Lehtimaki T, Korpela M, Peltola J, Hietaharju A (2005) Cerebral MRI abnormalities and their association with neuropsychiatric manifestations in SLE: a population-based study. Scand J Rheumatol 34:376–382
26. Waterloo K, Omdal R, Jacobsen EA, Klow NE, Husby G, Torbergsen T, Mellgren SI (1999) Cerebral computed tomography and electroencephalography compared with neuropsychological findings in systemic lupus erythematosus. J Neurol 246:706–711
27. Sibbitt WL, Sibbitt RR (1993) Magnetic resonance spectroscopy and positron emission tomography scanning in neuropsychiatric systemic lupus erythematosus. Rheum Dis Clin North Am 19:851–868
28. Sibbitt WL, Haseler LJ, Griffey RH, Hart BL, Sibbitt RR, Matwiyoff NA (1994) Analysis of cerebral structural changes in systemic lupus erythematosus by proton MR spectroscopy. AJNR Am J Neuroradiol 15:923–928
29. Jennekens FG, Kater L (2002) The central nervous system in systemic lupus erythematosus. Part 2. Pathogenetic mechanisms of clinical syndromes: a literature investigation. Rheumatology (Oxford) 41:619–630
30. McLean BN, Miller D, Thompson EJ (1995) Oligoclonal banding of IgG in CSF, blood–brain barrier function, and MRI findings in patients with sarcoidosis, systemic lupus

erythematosus, and Behcet's disease involving the nervous system. J Neurol Neurosurg Psychiatry 58:548–554
31. Hirohata S, Hirose S, Miyamoto T (1985) Cerebrospinal fluid IgM, IgA, and IgG indexes in systemic lupus erythematosus. Their use as estimates of central nervous system disease activity. Arch Intern Med 145: 1843–1846
32. Winfield JB, Shaw M, Silverman LM, Eisenberg RA, Wilson HA III, Koffler D (1983) Intrathecal IgG synthesis and blood–brain barrier impairment in patients with systemic lupus erythematosus and central nervous system dysfunction. Am J Med 74: 837–844
33. Yoshio T, Hirata D, Onda K, Nara H, Minota S (2005) Antiribosomal P protein antibodies in cerebrospinal fluid are associated with neuropsychiatric systemic lupus erythematosus. J Rheumatol 32:34–39
34. Greenwood DL, Gitlits VM, Alderuccio F, Sentry JW, Toh BH (2002) Autoantibodies in neuropsychiatric lupus. Autoimmunity 35: 79–86
35. Henn FA, McKinney WT (1987) Animal models in psychiatry. In: Meltzer HY (ed) Psychopharmacology: the third generation of progress. Raven, New York, pp 687–695
36. Dixon FJ, Andrews BS, Eisenberg RA, McConahey PJ, Theofilopoulos AN, Wilson CB (1978) Etiology and pathogenesis of a spontaneous lupus-like syndrome in mice. Arthritis Rheum 21:S64–S67
37. Szechtman H, Sakić B, Denburg JA (1997) Behaviour of MRL mice: an animal model of disturbed behaviour in systemic autoimmune disease. Lupus 6:223–229
38. Sakić B, Szechtman H, Denburg JA (1997) Neurobehavioral alteration in autoimmune mice. Neurosci Biobehav Rev 21:327–340
39. Alexander JJ, Quigg RJ (2007) Systemic lupus erythematosus and the brain: what mice are telling us. Neurochem Int 50:5–11
40. Sherman GF, Galaburda AM, Behan PO, Rosen GD (1987) Neuroanatomical anomalies in autoimmune mice. Acta Neuropathol (Berl) 74:239–242
41. Theofilopoulos AN (1992) Murine models of lupus. In: Lahita RG (ed) Systemic lupus erythematosus, 2nd edn. Churchill Livingstone, New York, pp 121–194
42. Andrews BS, Eisenberg RA, Theofilopoulos AN, Izui S, Wilson CB, McConahey PJ, Murphy ED, Roths JB, Dixon FJ (1978) Spontaneous murine lupus-like syndromes. Clinical and immunopathological manifestations in several strains. J Exp Med 148:1198–1215
43. Gulinello M, Putterman C (2011) The MRL/lpr mouse strain as a model for neuropsychiatric systemic lupus erythematosus. J Biomed Biotechnol 2011:207504
44. Watanabe-Fukunaga R, Brannan CI, Copeland NG, Jenkins NA, Nagata S (1992) Lymphoproliferation disorder in mice explained by defects in Fas antigen that mediates apoptosis. Nature 356:314–317
45. Nagata S (1994) Mutations in the Fas antigen gene in lpr mice. Semin Immunol 6:3–8
46. Singer GG, Carrera AC, Marshakrothstein A, Martineza C, Abbas AK (1994) Apoptosis, fas and systemic autoimmunity: the MRL-Ipr/Ipr model. Curr Opin Immunol 6:913–920
47. Park C, Sakamaki K, Tachibana O, Yamashima T, Yamashita J, Yonehara S (1998) Expression of Fas antigen in the normal mouse brain. Biochem Biophys Res Commun 252:623–628
48. Sakić B, Kolb B, Whishaw IQ, Gorny G, Szechtman H, Denburg JA (2000) Immunosuppression prevents neuronal atrophy in lupus-prone mice: evidence for brain damage induced by autoimmune disease? J Neuroimmunol 111:93–101
49. Sakić B, Denburg JA, Denburg SD, Szechtman H (1996) Blunted sensitivity to sucrose in autoimmune MRL-lpr mice: a curve-shift study. Brain Res Bull 41:305–311
50. Sakić B, Szechtman H, Denburg SD, Denburg JA (1995) Immunosuppressive treatment prevents behavioral deficit in autoimmune MRL-lpr mice. Physiol Behav 58:797–802
51. Ballok DA, Woulfe J, Sur M, Cyr M, Sakić B (2004) Hippocampal damage in mouse and human forms of systemic autoimmune disease. Hippocampus 14:649–661
52. Williams S, Sakić B, Hoffman SA (2010) Circulating brain-reactive autoantibodies and behavioral deficits in the MRL model of CNS lupus. J Neuroimmunol 218:73–82
53. Ballok DA (2007) Neuroimmunopathology in a murine model of neuropsychiatric lupus. Brain Res Rev 54:67–79
54. Sakić B, Szechtman H, Talangbayan H, Denburg SD, Carbotte RM, Denburg JA (1994) Disturbed emotionality in autoimmune MRL-lpr mice. Physiol Behav 56:609–617
55. Sakić B, Szechtman H, Talangbayan H, Denburg S, Carbotte R, Denburg JA (1994) Behavior and immune status of MRL mice in the postweaning period. Brain Behav Immun 8:1–13
56. Sakić B, Szechtman H, Keffer M, Talangbayan H, Stead R, Denburg JA (1992) A behavioral profile of autoimmune lupus-prone MRL mice. Brain Behav Immun 6:265–285

57. Ballok DA, Szechtman H, Sakić B (2003) Taste responsiveness and diet preference in autoimmune MRL mice. Behav Brain Res 140:119–130
58. Sakić B, Gurunlian L, Denburg SD (1998) Reduced aggressiveness and low testosterone levels in autoimmune MRL-lpr males. Physiol Behav 63:305–309
59. Sakić B, Szechtman H, Denburg SD, Carbotte RM, Denburg JA (1993) Spatial learning during the course of autoimmune disease in MRL mice. Behav Brain Res 54:57–66
60. Hess DC, Taormina M, Thompson J, Sethi KD, Diamond B, Rao R, Feldman DS (1993) Cognitive and neurologic deficits in the MRL/lpr mouse: a clinicopathologic study. J Rheumatol 20:610–617
61. Brey RL, Amato AA, Kagan-Hallet K, Rhine CB, Stallworth CL (1997) Anti-intercellular adhesion molecule-1 (ICAM-1) antibody treatment prevents central and peripheral nervous system disease in autoimmune-prone mice. Lupus 6:645–651
62. Sakić B, Szechtman H, Stead R, Denburg JA (1996) Joint pathology and behavioral performance in autoimmune MRL-lpr mice. Physiol Behav 60:901–905
63. Abbott NJ, Mendonca LL, Dolman DE (2003) The blood–brain barrier in systemic lupus erythematosus. Lupus 12:908–915
64. Diamond B (2010) Antibodies and the brain: lessons from lupus. J Immunol 185: 2637–2640
65. Vogelweid CM, Johnson GC, Besch-Williford CL, Basler J, Walker SE (1991) Inflammatory central nervous system disease in lupus-prone MRL/lpr mice: comparative histologic and immunohistochemical findings. J Neuroimmunol 35:89–99
66. Sidor MM, Sakić B, Malinowski PM, Ballok DA, Oleschuk CJ, Macri J (2005) Elevated immunoglobulin levels in the cerebrospinal fluid from lupus-prone mice. J Neuroimmunol 165:104–113
67. Alexander EL, Murphy ED, Roths JB, Alexander GE (1983) Congenic autoimmune murine models of central nervous system disease in connective tissue disorders. Ann Neurol 14:242–248
68. Farrell M, Sakić B, Szechtman H, Denburg JA (1997) Effect of cyclophosphamide on leucocytic infiltration in the brain of MRL/lpr mice. Lupus 6:268–274
69. Ma X, Foster J, Sakić B (2006) Distribution and prevalence of leukocyte phenotypes in brains of lupus-prone mice. J Neuroimmunol 179:26–36
70. McHale JF, Harari OA, Marshall D, Haskard DO (1999) TNF-alpha and IL-1 sequentially induce endothelial ICAM-1 and VCAM-1 expression in MRL/lpr lupus-prone mice. J Immunol 163:3993–4000
71. Zameer A, Hoffman SA (2003) Increased ICAM-1 and VCAM-1 expression in the brains of autoimmune mice. J Neuroimmunol 142:67–74
72. Tomita M, Holman BJ, Williams LS, Pang KC, Santoro TJ (2001) Cerebellar dysfunction is associated with overexpression of proinflammatory cytokine genes in lupus. J Neurosci Res 64:26–33
73. Tomita M, Holman BJ, Santoro TJ (2001) Aberrant cytokine gene expression in the hippocampus in murine systemic lupus erythematosus. Neurosci Lett 302:129–132
74. Alexander JJ, Jacob A, Bao L, Macdonald RL, Quigg RJ (2005) Complement-dependent apoptosis and inflammatory gene changes in murine lupus cerebritis. J Immunol 175: 8312–8319
75. McIntyre KR, Ayer-LeLievre C, Persson H (1990) Class II major histocompatibility complex (MHC) gene expression in the mouse brain is elevated in the autoimmune MRL/Mp-lpr/lpr strain. J Neuroimmunol 28:39–52
76. Ballok DA, Ma X, Denburg JA, Arsenault L, Sakić B (2006) Ibuprofen fails to prevent brain pathology in a model of neuropsychiatric lupus. J Rheumatol 33:2199–2213
77. Ballok DA, Millward JM, Sakić B (2003) Neurodegeneration in autoimmune MRL-lpr mice as revealed by Fluoro Jade B staining. Brain Res 964:200–210
78. Del Bigio MR (1993) Neuropathological changes caused by hydrocephalus. Acta Neuropathol 85:573–585
79. Gerber J, Raivich G, Wellmer A, Noeske C, Kunst T, Werner A, Bruck W, Nau R (2001) A mouse model of Streptococcus pneumoniae meningitis mimicking several features of human disease. Acta Neuropathol 101:499–508
80. Alexander EL, Alexander GE (1983) Aseptic meningoencephalitis in primary Sjogren's syndrome. Neurology 33:593–598
81. Auer RN, Wieloch T, Olsson Y, Siesjo BK (1984) The distribution of hypoglycemic brain damage. Acta Neuropathol 64:177–191
82. Fujioka M, Okuchi K, Hiramatsu KI, Sakaki T, Sakaguchi S, Ishii Y (1997) Specific changes in human brain after hypoglycemic injury. Stroke 28:584–587
83. Denenberg VH, Sherman GF, Rosen GD, Morrison L, Behan PO, Galaburda AM

(1992) A behavior profile of the MRL/Mp lpr/lpr mouse and its association with hydrocephalus. Brain Behav Immun 6:40–49

84. Alexander JJ, Zwingmann C, Quigg R (2005) MRL/lpr mice have alterations in brain metabolism as shown with ((1)H-(13)C) NMR spectroscopy. Neurochem Int 47:143–151

85. Alexander JJ, Bao L, Jacob A, Kraus DM, Holers VM, Quigg RJ (2003) Administration of the soluble complement inhibitor, Crry-Ig, reduces inflammation and aquaporin 4 expression in lupus cerebritis. Biochim Biophys Acta 1639:169–176

86. Hampton DW, Seitz A, Chen P, Heber-Katz E, Fawcett JW (2004) Altered CNS response to injury in the MRL/MpJ mouse. Neuroscience 127:821–832

87. Lawson LJ, Perry VH, Dri P, Gordon S (1990) Heterogeneity in the distribution and morphology of microglia in the normal adult mouse brain. Neuroscience 39:151–170

88. Ballok DA, Earls AM, Krasnik C, Hoffman SA, Sakić B (2004) Autoimmune-induced damage of the midbrain dopaminergic system in lupus-prone mice. J Neuroimmunol 152: 83–97

89. Hess DC (1997) Cerebral lupus vasculopathy. Mechanisms and clinical relevance. Ann N Y Acad Sci 823:154–168

90. Baraczka K, Nekam K, Pozsonyi T, Jakab L, Szongoth M, Sesztak M (2001) Concentration of soluble adhesion molecules (sVCAM-1, sICAM-1 and sL-selectin) in the cerebrospinal fluid and serum of patients with multiple sclerosis and systemic lupus erythematosus with central nervous involvement. Neuroimmunomodulation 9:49–54

91. Chinn RJS, Wilkinson ID, Hallcraggs MA, Paley MNJ, Shorthall E, Carter S, Kendall BE, Isenberg DA, Newman SP, Harrison MJG (1997) Magnetic resonance imaging of the brain and cerebral proton spectroscopy in patients with systemic lupus erythematosus. Arthritis Rheum 40:36–46

92. Rocca MA, Agosta F, Mezzapesa DM, Ciboddo G, Falini A, Comi G, Filippi M (2006) An fMRI study of the motor system in patients with neuropsychiatric systemic lupus erythematosus. Neuroimage 30:478–484

93. Sled JG, Spring S, van Eede M, Lerch JP, Ullal S, Sakić B (2009) Time course and nature of brain atrophy in the MRL mouse model of central nervous system lupus. Arthritis Rheum 60:1764–1774

94. Sakić B, Szechtman H, Denburg JA, Gorny G, Kolb B, Whishaw IQ (1998) Progressive atrophy of pyramidal neuron dendrites in autoimmune MRL-lpr mice. J Neuroimmunol 87:162–170

95. Maric D, Millward JM, Ballok DA, Szechtman H, Barker JL, Denburg JA, Sakić B (2001) Neurotoxic properties of cerebrospinal fluid from behaviorally impaired autoimmune mice. Brain Res 920:183–193

96. Kovac AD, Grammig J, Mahlo J, Steiner B, Roth K, Nitsch R, Bechmann I (2002) Comparison of neuronal density and subfield sizes in the hippocampus of CD95L-deficient (gld), CD95-deficient (lpr) and nondeficient mice. Eur J Neurosci 16:159–163

97. Sakić B, Maric I, Koeberle PD, Millward JM, Szechtman H, Maric D, Denburg JA (2000) Increased TUNEL-staining in brains of autoimmune Fas-deficient mice. J Neuroimmunol 104:147–154

98. Yamashita T, Ninomiya M, Hernandez AP, Garcia-Verdugo JM, Sunabori T, Sakaguchi M, Adachi K, Kojima T, Hirota Y, Kawase T, Araki N, Abe K, Okano H, Sawamoto K (2006) Subventricular zone-derived neuroblasts migrate and differentiate into mature neurons in the post-stroke adult striatum. J Neurosci 26:6627–6636

99. Sakić B, Kirkham DL, Ballok DA, Mwanjewe J, Fearon IM, Macri J, Yu G, Sidor MM, Denburg JA, Szechtman H, Lau J, Ball AK, Doering LC (2005) Proliferating brain cells are a target of neurotoxic CSF in systemic autoimmune disease. J Neuroimmunol 169: 68–85

100. Lechner O, Dietrich H, Oliveira dos SA, Wiegers GJ, Schwarz S, Harbutz M, Herold M, Wick G (2000) Altered circadian rhythms of the stress hormone and melatonin response in lupus-prone MRL/MP-fas(Ipr) mice. J Autoimmun 14:325–333

101. Mirescu C, Gould E (2006) Stress and adult neurogenesis. Hippocampus 16:233–238

102. Anderson KK, Ballok DA, Prasad N, Szechtman H, Sakić B (2006) Impaired response to amphetamine and neuronal degeneration in the nucleus accumbens of autoimmune MRL-lpr mice. Behav Brain Res 166:32–38

103. Brey RL, Cote S, Barohn R, Jackson C, Crawley R, Teale JM (1995) Model for the neuromuscular complications of systemic lupus erythematosus. Lupus 4:209–212

104. Loheswaran G, Stanojcic M, Xu L, Sakić B (2010) Autoimmunity as a principal pathogenic factor in the refined model of neuropsychiatric lupus. Clin Exp Neuroimmunol 1:141–152

105. How A, Dent PB, Liao SK, Denburg JA (1985) Antineuronal antibodies in neuropsy-

chiatric systemic lupus erythematosus. Arthritis Rheum 28:789–795

106. Williams GW, Bluestein HG, Steinberg AD (1981) Brain-reactive lymphocytotoxic antibody in the cerebrospinal fluid of patients with systemic lupus erythematosus: correlation with central nervous system involvement. Clin Immunol Immunopathol 18:126–132
107. Bluestein HG, Zvaifler NJ (1976) Brain-reactive lymphocytotoxic antibodies in the serum of patients with systemic lupus erythematosus. J Clin Invest 57:509–516
108. Bresnihan B, Hohmeister R, Cutting J, Travers RL, Waldburger M, Black C, Jones T, Hughes GR (1979) The neuropsychiatric disorder in systemic lupus erythematosus: evidence for both vascular and immune mechanisms. Ann Rheum Dis 38:301–306
109. Golombek SJ, Graus F, Elkon KB (1986) Autoantibodies in the cerebrospinal fluid of patients with systemic lupus erythematosus. Arthritis Rheum 29:1090–1097
110. Quismorio FP, Friou GJ (1972) Antibodies reactive with neurons in SLE patients with neuropsychiatric manifestations. Int Arch Allergy Appl Immunol 43:740–748
111. DeGiorgio LA, Konstantinov KN, Lee SC, Hardin JA, Volpe BT, Diamond B (2001) A subset of lupus anti-DNA antibodies cross-reacts with the NR2 glutamate receptor in systemic lupus erythematosus. Nat Med 7: 1189–1193
112. Tanaka S, Matsunaga H, Kimura M, Tatsumi K, Hidaka Y, Takano T, Uema T, Takeda M, Amino N (2003) Autoantibodies against four kinds of neurotransmitter receptors in psychiatric disorders. J Neuroimmunol 141:155–164
113. Zandman-Goddard G, Chapman J, Shoenfeld Y (2007) Autoantibodies involved in neuropsychiatric SLE and antiphospholipid syndrome. Semin Arthritis Rheum 36:297–315
114. Isshi K, Hirohata S (1996) Association of anti-ribosomal P protein antibodies with neuropsychiatric systemic lupus erythematosus. Arthritis Rheum 39:1483–1490
115. Denburg SD, Denburg JA (2003) Cognitive dysfunction and antiphospholipid antibodies in systemic lupus erythematosus. Lupus 12: 883–890
116. Hanly JG, Urowitz MB, Siannis F, Farewell V, Gordon C, Bae SC, Isenberg D, Dooley MA, Clarke A, Bernatsky S, Gladman D, Fortin PR, Manzi S, Steinsson K, Bruce IN, Ginzler E, Aranow C, Wallace DJ, Ramsey-Goldman R, van VR, Sturfelt G, Nived O, Sanchez-Guerrero J, Alarcon GS, Petri M, Khamashta M, Zoma A, Font J, Font J, Kalunian K, Douglas J, Qi Q, Thompson K, Merrill JT (2008) Autoantibodies and neuropsychiatric events at the time of systemic lupus erythematosus diagnosis: results from an international inception cohort study. Arthritis Rheum 58:843–853
117. Kowal C, DeGiorgio LA, Nakaoka T, Hetherington H, Huerta PT, Diamond B, Volpe BT (2004) Cognition and immunity; antibody impairs memory. Immunity 21: 179–188
118. Huerta PT, Kowal C, DeGiorgio LA, Volpe BT, Diamond B (2006) Immunity and behavior: antibodies alter emotion. Proc Natl Acad Sci U S A 103:678–683
119. Kowal C, DeGiorgio LA, Lee JY, Edgar MA, Huerta PT, Volpe BT, Diamond B (2006) Human lupus autoantibodies against NMDA receptors mediate cognitive impairment. Proc Natl Acad Sci U S A 103:19854–19859
120. Ndhlovu M, Preuss BE, Dengjel J, Stevanovic S, Weiner SM, Klein R (2011) Identification of alpha-tubulin as an autoantigen recognized by sera from patients with neuropsychiatric systemic lupus erythematosus. Brain Behav Immun 25:279–285
121. Colasanti T, Delunardo F, Margutti P, Vacirca D, Piro E, Siracusano A, Ortona E (2009) Autoantibodies involved in neuropsychiatric manifestations associated with systemic lupus erythematosus. J Neuroimmunol 212:3–9
122. Lefranc D, Launay D, Dubucquoi S, de SJ, Dussart P, Vermersch M, Hachulla E, Hatron PY, Vermersch P, Mouthon L, Prin L (2007) Characterization of discriminant human brain antigenic targets in neuropsychiatric systemic lupus erythematosus using an immunoproteomic approach. Arthritis Rheum 56:3420–3432
123. Williams RC Jr, Sugiura K, Tan EM (2004) Antibodies to microtubule-associated protein 2 in patients with neuropsychiatric systemic lupus erythematosus. Arthritis Rheum 50: 1239–1247
124. Yoshio T, Onda K, Nara H, Minota S (2006) Association of IgG anti-NR2 glutamate receptor antibodies in cerebrospinal fluid with neuropsychiatric systemic lupus erythematosus. Arthritis Rheum 54:675–678
125. Arinuma Y, Yanagida T, Hirohata S (2008) Association of cerebrospinal fluid anti-NR2 glutamate receptor antibodies with diffuse neuropsychiatric systemic lupus erythematosus. Arthritis Rheum 58:1130–1135
126. Stanojcic M, Loheswaran G, Xu L, Hoffman SA, Sakić B (2010) Intrathecal antibodies and brain damage in autoimmune MRL mice. Brain Behav Immun 24:289–297

127. Hoffman SA, Madsen CS (1990) Brain specific autoantibodies in murine models of systemic lupus erythematosus. J Neuroimmunol 30:229–237
128. Hoffman SA, Arbogast DN, Ford PM, Shucard DW, Harbeck RJ (1987) Brain-reactive autoantibody levels in the sera of ageing autoimmune mice. Clin Exp Immunol 70:74–83
129. Crimando J, Hoffman SA (1992) Detection of brain-reactive autoantibodies in the sera of autoimmune mice using ELISA. J Immunol Methods 149:87–95
130. Sakić B, Szechtman H, Denburg SD, Carbotte RM, Denburg JA (1993) Brain-reactive antibodies and behavior of autoimmune MRL-lpr mice. Physiol Behav 54:1025–1029
131. Gao HX, Sanders E, Tieng AT, Putterman C (2010) Sex and autoantibody titers determine the development of neuropsychiatric manifestations in lupus-prone mice. J Neuroimmunol 229:112–122
132. Gao HX, Campbell SR, Cui MH, Zong P, Hee-Hwang J, Gulinello M, Putterman C (2009) Depression is an early disease manifestation in lupus-prone MRL/lpr mice. J Neuroimmunol 207:45–56
133. Hoffman SA, Sakić B (2008) Autoimmunity and brain dysfunction. In: Zalcman S, Siegel A (eds) The neuroimmunological basis of behavior and mental disorders. Springer, New York
134. Meroni PL, Tincani A, Sepp N, Raschi E, Testoni C, Corsini E, Cavazzana I, Pellegrini S, Salmaggi A (2003) Endothelium and the brain in CNS lupus. Lupus 12:919–928
135. Tang B, Matsuda T, Akira S, Nagata N, Ikehara S, Hirano T, Kishimoto T (1991) Age-associated increase in interleukin 6 in MRL/lpr mice. Int Immunol 3:273–278
136. Singh AK, Lebedeva TV (1994) Interleukin-1 contributes to high level IgG production in the murine MRL/lpr lupus model. Immunol Invest 23:281–292
137. Boswell JM, Yui MA, Endres S, Burt DW, Kelley VE (1988) Novel and enhanced IL-1 gene expression in autoimmune mice with lupus. J Immunol 141:118–124
138. Sakić B, Szechtman H, Braciak TA, Richards CD, Gauldie J, Denburg JA (1997) Reduced preference for sucrose in autoimmune mice: a possible role of interleukin-6. Brain Res Bull 44:155–165
139. Kwant A, Sakić B (2004) Behavioral effects of infection with interferon-gamma adenovector. Behav Brain Res 151:73–82
140. Sakić B, Szechtman H, Gauldie J, Denburg JA (2001) Behavioral effects of infection with IL-6 adenovector. Brain Behav Immun 15:25–42
141. Marshall D, Dangerfield JP, Bhatia VK, Larbi KY, Nourshargh S, Haskard DO (2003) MRL/lpr lupus-prone mice show exaggerated ICAM-1-dependent leucocyte adhesion and transendothelial migration in response to TNF-alpha. Rheumatology (Oxford) 42: 929–934
142. Banks WA, Kastin AJ, Gutierrez EG (1994) Penetration of interleukin-6 across the murine blood–brain barrier. Neurosci Lett 179:53–56
143. Banks WA, Kastin AJ, Gutierrez EG (1993) Interleukin-1 alpha in blood has direct access to cortical brain cells. Neurosci Lett 163:41–44
144. Gutierrez EG, Banks WA, Kastin AJ (1993) Murine tumor necrosis factor alpha is transported from blood to brain in the mouse. J Neuroimmunol 47:169–176
145. Tsai CY, Wu TH, Tsai ST, Chen KH, Thajeb P, Lin WM, Yu HS, Yu CL (1994) Cerebrospinal fluid interleukin-6, prostaglandin E2 and autoantibodies in patients with neuropsychiatric systemic lupus erythematosus and central nervous system infections. Scand J Rheumatol 23:57–63
146. Svenungsson E, Andersson M, Brundin L, van Vollenhoven R, Khademi M, Tarkowski A, Greitz D, Dahlstrom M, Lundberg I, Klareskog L, Olsson T (2001) Increased levels of proinflammatory cytokines and nitric oxide metabolites in neuropsychiatric lupus erythematosus. Ann Rheum Dis 60:372–379
147. Hayley S, Merali Z, Anisman H (2003) Stress and cytokine-elicited neuroendocrine and neurotransmitter sensitization: implications for depressive illness. Stress 6:19–32
148. Hu Y, Dietrich H, Herold M, Heinrich PC, Wick G (1993) Disturbed immuno-endocrine communication via the hypothalamo- pituitary-adrenal axis in autoimmune disease. Int Arch Allergy Immunol 102:232–241
149. Rivier C, Rivest S (1993) Mechanisms mediating the effects of cytokines on neuroendocrine functions in the rat. In: Chadwick D, Marsh J, Ackrill K (eds) Corticotropin-releasing factor. Wiley, Chichester, pp 204–225
150. Spangelo BL, Gorospe WC (1995) Role of the cytokines in the neuroendocrine-immune system axis. Front Neuroendocrinol 16:1–22
151. Miller AH, Maletic V, Raison CL (2009) Inflammation and its discontents: the role of cytokines in the pathophysiology of major depression. Biol Psychiatry 65:732–741
152. Del Rey A, Besedovsky HO (2000) The cytokine-HPA axis circuit contributes to prevent or moderate autoimmune processes, Z Rheumatol 59(suppl 2):II/31–II/35
153. Lorton D, Lubahn C, Bellinger DL (2003) Potential use of drugs that target neural-

immune pathways in the treatment of rheumatoid arthritis and other autoimmune diseases. Curr Drug Targets Inflamm Allergy 2:1–30

154. Spangelo BL, Judd AM, Call GB, Zumwalt J, Gorospe WC (1995) Role of the cytokines in the hypothalamic-pituitary-adrenal and gonadal axes. Neuroimmunomodulation 2: 299–312
155. Spangelo BL, Judd AM, Isakson PC, MacLeod RM (1989) Interleukin-6 stimulates anterior pituitary hormone release in vitro. Endocrinology 125:575–577
156. Shanks N, Moore PM, Perks P, Lightman SL (1999) Alterations in hypothalamic-pituitary-adrenal function correlated with the onset of murine SLE in MRL +/+ and lpr/lpr mice. Brain Behav Immun 13:348–360
157. Sakić B, Laflamme N, Crnic LS, Szechtman H, Denburg JA, Rivest S (1999) Reduced corticotropin-releasing factor and enhanced vasopressin gene expression in brains of mice with autoimmunity-induced behavioral dysfunction. J Neuroimmunol 96:80–91
158. McEwen BS (1999) Stress and the aging hippocampus. Front Neuroendocrinol 20:49–70
159. Woolley CS, Gould E, McEwen BS (1990) Exposure to excess glucocorticoids alters dendritic morphology of adult hippocampal pyramidal neurons. Brain Res 531:225–231
160. Ballok DA, Sakić B (2008) Purine receptor antagonist modulates serology and affective behaviors in lupus-prone mice: Evidence of autoimmune-induced pain? Brain Behav Immun 22(8):1208–1216
161. Sapolsky RM (2000) Glucocorticoids and hippocampal atrophy in neuropsychiatric disorders. Arch Gen Psychiatry 57:925–935
162. Peress NS, Roxburgh VA, Gelfand MC (1981) Binding sites for immune components in human choroid plexus. Arthritis Rheum 24: 520–526
163. Schwartz MM, Roberts JL (1983) Membranous and vascular choroidopathy: two patterns of immune deposits in systemic lupus erythematosus. Clin Immunol Immunopathol 29:369–380
164. Reilly CM, Oates JC, Cook JA, Morrow JD, Halushka PV, Gilkeson GS (2000) Inhibition of mesangial cell nitric oxide in MRL/lpr mice by prostaglandin J2 and proliferator activation receptor-gamma agonists. J Immunol 164:1498–1504
165. O'Sullivan FX, Vogelweid CM, Beschwilliford CL, Walker SE (1995) Differential effects of CD4(+) T cell depletion on inflammatory central nervous system disease, arthritis and sialadenitis in MRL/lpr mice. J Autoimmun 8:163–175
166. Jacob A, Hack B, Bai T, Brorson JR, Quigg RJ, Alexander JJ (2010) Inhibition of C5a receptor alleviates experimental CNS lupus. J Neuroimmunol 221:46–52
167. Sakić B, Lacosta S, Denburg J, Szechtman H (2002) Altered neurotransmission in brains of autoimmune mice: pharmacological and neurochemical evidence. J Neuroimmunol 129: 84–96
168. Chun S, McEvilly R, Foster JA, Sakić B (2008) Proclivity to self-injurious behavior in MRL-lpr mice: implications for autoimmunity-induced damage in the dopaminergic system. Mol Psychiatry 13:1043–1053
169. Stanojcic M, Burstyn-Cohen T, Nashi N, Lemke G, Sakić B (2009) Disturbed distribution of proliferative brain cells during lupus-like disease. Brain Behav Immun 23(7): 1003–1013
170. Lee JY, Huerta PT, Zhang J, Kowal C, Bertini E, Volpe BT, Diamond B (2009) Neurotoxic autoantibodies mediate congenital cortical impairment of offspring in maternal lupus. Nat Med 15:91–96

Chapter 15

Interleukin-2 and the Brain: Dissecting Central Versus Peripheral Contributions Using Unique Mouse Models

John M. Petitto, Danielle Meola, and Zhi Huang

Abstract

Although many studies have documented peripheral immune alterations in patients with psychiatric and neurological disorders, almost all these data in humans are correlative. The actions of IL-2 on neurodevelopment, function, and disease are the result of both IL-2's actions in the peripheral immune system and intrinsic actions in the CNS. Determining if, and under what conditions (e.g., development, acute injury) these different actions of IL-2 are operative in the brain is essential to make advances in understanding the multifaceted affects of IL-2 on CNS function and disease. Mouse models have provided ways to obtain new insights into how the complex biology of a cytokine such as IL-2 can have simultaneous, dynamic effects on multiple systems (e.g., regulating homeostasis in the brain and immune system, autoimmunity that can affect both systems). Here we describe some of the relevant literature and our research using different mouse models. This includes models such as congenic IL-2 knockout mice bred on immunodeficient backgrounds coupled with immune reconstitution strategies used to dissect neuroimmunological processes involved in the development of septohippocampal pathology, and test the hypothesis that dysregulation of the brain's endogenous neuroimmunological milieu may occur with the loss of brain IL-2 gene expression and be involved in initiating CNS autoimmunity. Use of animal models like these in the field of psychoneuroimmunology may lead to critical advances into our understanding of the role of brain cytokines and autoimmunity in neurodegenerative diseases (e.g., Alzheimer's disease), neurodevelopmental disorder (e.g., autism, schizophrenia), and autoimmune diseases including multiple sclerosis.

Key words: Cytokines, Chemokines, Neuroimmunology, Congenic mice, Knockout mice, Immunodeficient mice, T cells, Autoimmunity, Neurological diseases, Neuromedicine

1. Introduction: Cytokines and the Brain

Landmark research by Zalcman et al. (1) provided some of the first evidence of the selective actions of brain cytokines, refuting the commonly held view at the time that cytokines acting in the brain had redundant functional properties mirroring their actions in the peripheral immune system. This work and others complemented groundbreaking findings that lymphocytes could secrete

Qing Yan (ed.), *Psychoneuroimmunology: Methods and Protocols*, Methods in Molecular Biology, vol. 934, DOI 10.1007/978-1-62703-071-7_15, © Springer Science+Business Media, LLC 2012

classic neuropeptides and that peripheral immunization signaled hypothalamic neurons (2, 3). These and other studies in psychoneuroimmunology laid the foundation for multidisciplinary research that sought to identify the mechanisms whereby different cytokines may modulate complex neurobiological processes (e.g., complex domains of behaviors such as learning and memory).

In the CNS, many cytokines and cytokine receptors are synthesized by endogenous brain cells, and frequently exhibit neuromodulatory and neurotrophic effects that are limited to specific neural pathways. Cytokines derived from peripheral immune cells (and in some cases perhaps other tissues) do not readily cross the blood–brain barrier. The mechanisms of cytokine transport vary for different cytokines (e.g., active vs. passive transport) as does the degree to which they enter the CNS (4). Goehler et al. (5) have described how the area postrema acts as an anatomical "interface" between the peripheral immune system and the brain. Afferent sensory fibers of the vagus can carry signals initiated by interleukin-1 to brainstem areas (e.g., nucleus tractus solitarius), and vagal sensory activation may occur during infection and provide input to the brain and modify behavior (6, 7). Whether, and how, other cytokines signal the CNS via the vagus or other afferent nerves in the periphery that allow animals to adapt to their environment is unknown and could be an important avenue of research.

Cytokine receptors are typically more readily detectable in the brain than cytokines themselves. It appears that cytokines frequency have more general effects on the brain's endogenous immune-like cells (e.g., microglia). It has proved much more challenging to unequivocally detect cytokines and cytokine receptors using immunohistocytochemistry (or to reliably detect cytokine receptors using radioligand receptor binding or autoradiography) (8). Receptors for IL-1R (9), IL-1R antagonist (10), and IL-6R (11), for example, are also detectable in the rodent dentate gyrus by in situ hybridization. Gene expression for IL-2 receptors has been found throughout CA1–CA4 of the hippocampus and dentate gyrus (8, 12–14). Thus, receptors for these cytokines in the hippocampus place them in a position to influence learning and memory and other related behaviors, and some of these same cytokines that have been found to target receptors in the hippocampus have the capacity to modulate neurobiological processes known to mediate these behaviors. The neuroimmunology of cognition has received considerable attention. Hippocampal long-term potentiation (LTP), an important neurobiological mechanism involved in learning and memory storage, is modulated by several cytokines (15). IL-1 mRNA and protein have been found to be increased in the hippocampus following some forms of peripheral immune system activation such as occurs following LPS administration (16), and learning and memory performance deficits induced by systemic administration of LPS can be antagonized by antibody to

IL-1β (17). This is one mechanism by which pyrogens are known to induce sickness behavior (e.g., fever, decreased activity and exploration, reduced social interaction, depressive signs and symptoms) that impairs cognitive performance (18, 19). IL-1 is the most widely studied cytokine involved in learning and memory, and I.C.V. administration of IL-1β, for example, impaired contextual fear conditioning but did not change auditory-cue fear conditioning—a form of conditioning that is not dependent on the hippocampus (20).

The sections that follow focus on IL-2's actions in the hippocampus and cognition, and particularly on our laboratory's research using an animal model to disentangle the complex actions of peripheral and central IL-2 on brain development and autoimmunity. Some of the pathophysiology and neuropathology observed in this model is reminiscent of abnormalities seen in certain neuropsychiatric disorders.

2. IL-2 and the Brain: The Septohippocampal System and Cognition

There is a large body of research indicating that IL-2 may be involved in CNS development, normal brain physiology, and homeostatic repair mechanisms, as well as brain dysfunction and neurodegenerative processes. The initial clue that IL-2 had CNS actions came from cancer patients where their behavior was found to be altered after prolonged exposure. Treatment with IL-2 induced cognitive dysfunction and other untoward neuropsychiatric side effects at doses significantly above what would be considered physiological (21–23).

Depending on the methodology and conditions, the data suggest that microglia, astrocytes, and neurons can produce this cytokine (24–27). In culture systems, IL-2 provides trophic support to neurons from the hippocampus and medial septum (28, 29), and enhances neurite branching (29, 30). It is noteworthy that IL-2 has been shown to be one of the most potent modulators of acetylcholine (ACh) release from rat hippocampal slices (31). In hippocampal slices, IL-2 modulates acetylcholine in a dose-dependent biphasic manner, potentiating release at very low (fM) concentrations and inhibiting release at higher (nM) concentrations, whereas by contrast, cholinergic interneurons in the striatum do not respond to IL-2 (32). IL-2 gene expression and protein have been identified in the CNS (24, 33). It is localized in discrete areas of perfused normal rat forebrain including the septohippocampal system and related limbic regions (12, 34), and is present in human hippocampal tissue (35).

Preclinical studies in animals have substantiated the effects of IL-2 on septohippocampal circuitry. As the hippocampus is essential for spatial learning and memory consolidation, IL-2 appears to alter memory processing via interactions with septohippocampal cholinergic nerve terminals in the hippocampus (25) where it can modify LTP (36) and various parameters of cognitive performance in animals (26, 37–41). Aged mice were found to be particularly vulnerable to repeated dosing of IL-2, exhibiting both memory deficits and neuronal damage that was selective to the hippocampus (41). There are no studies, to our knowledge, that have systematically examined if elderly humans—such as those receiving IL-2 immunotherapy for cancer treatment—are more vulnerable to the effects of IL-2 than younger adults. Chronic dosing of IL-2, however, has been shown by Anisman's lab to disrupt the working component of spatial memory in nonaged rats in the Morris water-maze (40).

IL-2 has been implicated in the pathogenesis of several major psychiatric and neurological disorders, including those that exhibit neuropathological alterations of the septohippocampal system (26). The predominant effects of IL-2 in the brain occur in the hippocampal formation where receptors for this cytokine are enriched (12–14, 25, 42). In postmortem hippocampi of Alzheimer's disease patients, IL-2 levels were found to be elevated compared to controls (35).

3. Neurotrophic Factors and Septohippocampal Cytoarchitecture Are Altered by IL-2 Deficiency

Most findings are from in vitro studies, and to lesser degree, from studies in animals where IL-2's effects on various target behaviors or functional neurobiological outcomes (e.g., LTP in vivo) are used to make inferences about the action of the endogenous cytokine. Although the literature has documented many actions of IL-2 in the brain ranging from trophic actions on cultured neurons to the modulation of neurotransmitters and behavior, virtually all of these studies have used the strategy of administering exogenous IL-2. Thus, one of the goals of our research has been to study IL-2 knockout mice to better understand the role of endogenous IL-2 on brain function.

Our lab's research has shown that IL-2 gene deletion impaired learning and memory performance, sensorimotor gating, and resulted in reductions in hippocampal infrapyramidal (IP) mossy fiber length in mice (43). Rodent models have shown that mossy fiber length correlates positively with spatial learning ability in a number of studies (44–46). We have found that IL-2 knockout mice also have fewer IP granule cells (47). As IL-2 has been found to have neurotrophic and neuromodulatory actions on hippocampal neurons in vitro, our data suggests that hippocampal IL-2 may provide trophic support for hippocampal neurons. Loss of or dysregulated brain IL-2 function may play a key role in altering the ongoing increase in dentate granule cells during the first year of life (48, 49) and effect the integrity of axons in the dentate gyrus (50).

IL-2 knockout mice had significantly reduced concentrations of brain-derived neurotrophic factor (BDNF) protein and increased concentrations of nerve growth factor (NGF) in the hippocampus compared to wild-type littermates (where possible in our work, we attempt to compare littermates so that intrauterine and postnatal experience is controlled). Although our research had shown that receptors for IL-2 are enriched in the hippocampus, including the granule cell layer (GCL) of the dentate gyrus (DG) (13, 14), it was unclear in the literature if IL-2's trophic effects on neurons in vitro (28–30) operate in vivo, or if IL-2 could modify the expression of brain neurotrophic factors. In fact, we found that the observed differences in the level of BDNF were consistent with our hypothesis that we would find reductions in trophic factors important to hippocampal development and maintenance. BDNF plays a role in the maintenance and repair of septal cholinergic neurons (51–53), and can implement a positive feedback mechanism with these neurons to enhance the release of acetylcholine (54), and can also modulate postnatal neurogenesis (55, 56), thus potentially impacting granule cell number. The mechanism of the interaction between IL-2 gene deletion and the reduction of BDNF levels remains unclear. Though BDNF is expressed in the peripheral immune system by lymphocytes, IL-2 does not stimulate its production or release in these cells. IL-2 can, however, upregulate the expression of TrkB, the receptor for BDNF, in lymphocytes (57). Furthermore, some evidence suggests that BDNF can stimulate a positive feedback mechanism of its own via the TrkB receptor in hippocampal neurons (58, 59). IL-2 deficiency may therefore potentially lead to a downregulation of the TrkB receptor, thereby partially inhibiting the positive feedback production of BDNF. Our data suggest that IL-2 may have direct and/or indirect effects on BDNF.

Moderate lesions of rat septohippocampal projections have been shown to result in increased expression of mRNA for NGF, but not BDNF in hippocampal target cells (60). Opposite to the aforementioned findings with BDNF, NGF protein levels were actually increased in the IL-2 knockout mice. In keeping with our observations of reduced medial septal cholinergic survival in IL-2 knockout mice (47, 61), it is possible that the hippocampal target neurons in these animals may produce higher protein levels of NGF as a compensatory response. Interestingly, the imbalance that we see in IL-2 knockout mice between BDNF and NGF levels (decreased BDNF and increased NGF concentrations) is also found in the postmortem hippocampus of Alzheimer's disease brains (62).

4. IL-2 Deficiency-Induced Autoimmunity and the Brain: Changes in the Brain's Neuroimmunological Milieu Contributes to the Development of CNS Autoimmunity

A number of clinical syndromes and diseases affecting the CNS have a putative link to autoimmunity; however, with the exception of multiple sclerosis and myasthenia gravis, little is known about specific factors and pathways that govern CNS autoimmunity. IL-2 has been implicated in the pathogenesis of CNS autoimmune disease, multiple sclerosis, as well as in schizophrenia and Alzheimer's disease (63–65). Research examining the actions of IL-2 in the brain has focused almost exclusively on the cytokine's neuromodulatory and neurotrophic properties; however until recently, it was unknown if IL-2 deficiency results in the spontaneous development of CNS autoimmunity. In the immune system, IL-2 is indispensable for maintaining immunological homeostasis (e.g., self-tolerance, T regulatory cell development and function). It is now known that IL-2 is essential for normal T regulatory cell function which is critical in self-tolerance (66). IL-2 deficiency in knockout mice produces the spontaneous development of autoimmune disease affecting several organ systems (e.g., intestines, heart) characterized by T cell infiltration, and in some organs autoantibody deposition as well (67–69).

We tested the hypothesis that IL-2 deficient mice develop a unique form of autoimmunity that selectively targets septal cholinergic projection neurons. Autoimmune-mediated loss of brain septal cholinergic neurons has been found in animals immunized with septal cholinergic hybrid cells (70). We had previously found that choline acetyltransferase (ChAT)-positive neurons in the medial septum/vertical diagonal band of Broca (MS/vDB) of IL-2 KO and IL-2 WT littermates on the C57BL/6 background differed as a function of age (47, 61). At 8–12 weeks of age IL-2 KO mice show considerable evidence of peripheral autoimmunity (e.g., marked splenomegaly), whereas 3-week-old IL-2 KO mice do not yet develop autoimmunity. We postulated that the selective loss of septal cholinergic neurons in IL-2 KO mice (i.e., vs. no differences compared to WT mice for ChAT-positive neurons in the striatum or in GABAergic neurons in the MS/vDB) was due to autoimmune-mediated neurodegeneration that occurs postnatally between weaning and early adulthood (development of the medial septum is essentially complete by embryonic day 17 (71)). Thus, we quantified $CD3^{+}$ T cells in the septum, hippocampus, and cerebellum of IL-2 KO and IL-2 WT mice at ages ranging from 2 to 14 weeks. T cells infiltrated the brains of IL-2 deficient mice, but were not selective for the septum. Brain T lymphocyte levels in IL-2 KO mice positively correlated with the degree of peripheral autoimmunity (72). We did not detect $CD19^{+}$ B lymphocytes, IgG-positive lymphocytes, or IgG deposition indicative of autoantibodies in the brains of IL-2 KO mice.

Emerging data from our lab and others suggested that dysregulation of the brain's endogenous neuroimmunological milieu may occur with the loss of brain IL-2 gene expression and be involved in initiating processes that lead to CNS autoimmunity (47, 72, 73). Therefore, in a recent study we sought to test our working hypothesis that IL-2 deficiency induces endogenous changes in the CNS that play a key role in eliciting T cell homing into the brain (74). We used an experimental approach that combined mouse congenic breeding and immune reconstitution to test this hypothesis. In congenic mice without brain IL-2 (two IL-2 KO alleles) that were reconstituted with a normal wild-type immune system, the loss of brain IL-2 doubled the number of T cells that trafficked into the brain in all regions quantified (hippocampus, septum, and cerebellum) compared to mice with two wild-type brain IL-2 alleles and a wild-type peripheral immune system. We found that congenic mice with normal brain IL-2 (two wild-type IL-2 alleles) that were immune reconstituted with autoreactive Treg-deficient T cells from IL-2 KO mice developed the expected peripheral autoimmunity (splenomegaly) and had a comparable doubling of T cell trafficking into the hippocampus and septum, whereas they exhibited an additional twofold proclivity for the cerebellum over the septohippocampal regions. Unlike brain trafficking of wild-type T cells, the increased homing of IL-2 KO T cells to the cerebellum was independent of brain IL-2 gene expression. T cells selective for the cerebellum could shed light on putative autoimmune disease processes associated with cerebellar pathology in certain neurological and neuropsychiatric disease (e.g., autism). Our findings from this study show that brain IL-2 deficiency induces endogenous CNS changes that may lead to the development of brain autoimmunity, and that autoreactive Treg-deficient IL-2 KO T cells trafficking to the brain could have a proclivity to induce cerebellar neuropathology.

5. Concluding Remarks

Psychoneuroimmunology research described in this brief review chapter indicates that IL-2 dysregulation in the brain and immune system may play a role in neuropathology and disease in humans. It is possible, for example, that early neurodevelopmental alterations associated with IL-2 dysregulation may account for pathophysiological abnormalities seen decades later in the mature brain of individuals with neurodevelopmental diseases such as schizophrenia and autism. Considerable interest over several decades has attempted to link prenatal viral infection and/or the maternal immune response to such a putative agent that may serve as an environmental trigger that elicits neuroimmunological and neurobiological changes leading to the expression of schizophrenia in individuals with genetic loading for the disorder. The normal timing during which IL-2 may stimulate neuronal growth and migration during early development may be modified by a developmental event like viral infection or birth trauma in a genetically susceptible individual. In the hippocampus, where IL-2 receptors are enriched, this could contribute to the alterations in this region such as the abnormal orientation of subsets of hippocampal neurons found in the postmortem brains of individuals with schizophrenia.

Immunological disturbances in the peripheral immune system during development could also contribute to abnormalities in neurodevelopment. Using animal models to determine when and under what conditions (e.g., development, injury) these different actions of IL-2 are operative in the brain may help to advance our knowledge of the neuroimmunology of several major mental disorders. The role of autoimmunity in brain disease has been somewhat elusive, with the exception of a few diseases. Despite a plethora of published studies, almost all of this data in humans is correlative and much of the basic research has understandably relied on simpler models (e.g., in vitro models). Thus, informative animal models such those described earlier may provide valuable new insight in understanding how the complex biology of a cytokine like IL-2 can have simultaneous, dynamic effects on multiple systems (e.g., regulating homeostasis in the brain and immune system, autoimmunity that can affect both systems).

Models such as the congenic IL-2 knockout mice bred on immunodeficient backgrounds coupled with immune reconstitution strategies can be valuable to test novel hypotheses such as our postulation that changes in the brain's endogenous neuroimmunological milieu that occur with the loss of brain IL-2 gene expression may be involved in initiating CNS autoimmunity. Thus, further research using this approach may help to delineate further the complexity of IL-2 biology in the brain and immune system. Use of animal models like these in psychoneuroimmunology research may advance our understanding of the role of brain cytokines and autoimmunity in neurodegenerative diseases (e.g., Alzheimer's disease), neurodevelopmental diseases (e.g., autism, schizophrenia), and autoimmune diseases including multiple sclerosis.

Acknowledgements

Funding for this study was provided by NIH RO1 NS055018.

References

1. Zalcman S, Green-Johnson JM, Murray L, Nance DM, Dyck D, Anisman H, Greenberg AH (1994) Cytokine-specific central monoamine alterations induced by interleukin-1, -2, and -6. Brain Res 643:40–49
2. Besedovsky HO, Del Rey A, Klusman I, Furukawa H, Monge Arditi G, Kabiersch A (1991) Cytokines as modulators of the hypothalamus-pituitary-adrenal axis. J Steroid Biochem Mol Biol 40:613–618
3. Blalock JE (1994) The syntax of immune-neuroendocrine communications. Immunol Today 15:504–511
4. Pan W, Kastin AJ (1999) Penetration of neurotrophins and cytokines across the blood–brain/blood–spinal cord barrier. Adv Drug Deliv Rev 36:291–298
5. Goehler LE, Erisir A, Gaykema RP (2006) Neural-immune interface in the rat area postrema. Neuroscience 140:1415–1434
6. Maier SF, Watkins LR (1998) Cytokines for psychologists: implications of bidirectional immune-to-brain communication for understanding behavior, mood and cognition. Psychol Rev 105:83–107
7. Goehler LE, Lyte M, Gaykema RP (2007) Infection-induced viscerosensory signals from the gut enhance anxiety: implications for psychoneuroimmunology. Brain Behav Immun 21:721–726
8. Petitto JM, Huang Z (2001) Cloning the full-length IL-2/15 receptor-β cDNA sequence from mouse brain: evidence of enrichment in hippocampal formation neurons. Regul Pept 98:77–87
9. Cunningham ETJ, Wada E, Carter DB, Tracey DE, Battey JF, De Souza EB (1992) In situ histochemical localization of type I interleukin-1 receptor messenger RNA in the central nervous system, pituitary, and adrenal gland of the mouse. J Neurosci 12:1101–1114
10. Licinio J, Wong ML, Gold PW (1991) Localization of interleukin-1 receptor antagonist mRNA in rat brain. Endocrinology 129:562–564
11. Schobitz B, Voorhuis DA, De Kloet ER (1992) Localization of interleukin-6 mRNA and interleukin-6 receptor mRNA in rat brain. Neurosci Lett 136:189–192
12. Lapchak PA, Araujo DM, Quirion R, Beaudet A (1991) Immunoautoradiographic localization of interleukin 2-like immunoreactivity and interleukin 2 receptors (Tac antigen-like immunoreactivity) in the rat brain. Neuroscience 44: 173–184
13. Petitto JM, Huang Z (1994) Molecular cloning of a partial cDNA of the interleukin-2 receptor-β in normal mouse brain: in situ localization in the hippocampus and expression by neuroblastoma cells. Brain Res 650:140–145
14. Petitto JM, Huang Z, Raizada M, Rinker CM, McCarthy DB (1998) Molecular cloning of the cDNA coding sequence of IL-2 receptor-γ (γ_c) from human and murine forebrain: expression in the hippocampus in situ and by brain cells in vitro. Mol Brain Res 53:152–162
15. Jankowsky J, Patterson P (1999) Cytokine and growth factor involvement in long-term potentiation. Mol Cell Neurosci 14:273–286
16. Laye S, Parnet P, Goujon E, Dantzer R (1994) Peripheral administration of lipopolysaccharide induces the expression of cytokine transcripts in the brain and pituitary of mice. Brain Res Mol Brain Res 27:157–162
17. Gibertini M, Newton C, Klein TW, Friedman H (1995) Legionella pneumophila-induced visual learning impairment reversed by anti-interleukin-1 beta. Proc Soc Exp Biol Med 210:7–11
18. Aubert A, Vega C, Dantzer R, Goodall G (1995) Pyrogens specifically disrupt the acquisition of a task involving cognitive processing in the rat. Brain Behav Immun 9:129–148
19. Dantzer R, Bluthe RM, Gheusi G, Cremona S, Laye S, Parnet P, Kelley KW (1998) Molecular basis of sickness behavior. Ann N Y Acad Sci 856:132–138
20. Pugh CR, Kumagawa K, Fleshner M, Watkins LR, Maier SF, Rudy JW (1998) Selective effects of peripheral lipopolysaccharide administration on contextual and auditory-cue fear conditioning. Brain Behav Immun 3:212–229
21. Denicoff KD, Rubinow DR, Papa MZ, Simpson C, Seipp CA, Lotze MT, Chang AE, Rosenstein D, Rosenberg SA (1987) The neuropsychiatric effects of treatment with interleukin-2 and lymphokine-activated killer cells. Ann Intern Med 107:293–300
22. West WH, Tauer KW, Yannelli JR, Marshall GD, Orr DW, Thurman GB, Oldham RK (1987) Constant-infusion recombinant interleukin-2 in adoptive immunotherapy of advanced cancer. N Engl J Med 316:898–905
23. Capuron L, Ravaud A, Radat F, Dantzer R, Goodall G (1998) Effects of interleukin-2 and alpha interferon cytokine immunotherapy on the mood and cognitive performance of cancer patients. Neuroimmunomodulation 22:9
24. Eizenberg O, Faber-Elman A, Lotan M, Schwartz M (1995) Interleukin-2 transcripts in human and rodent brains: possible expression by astrocytes. J Neurochem 64:1928–1936
25. Hanisch UK, Quirion R (1996) Interleukin-2 as a neuroregulatory cytokine. Brain Res Rev 21:246–284

26. Hanisch U, Neuhaus J, Rowe W, Van-Rossum D, Möller T, Kettenmann H, Quirion R (1997) Neurotoxic consequences of central long-term administration of interleukin-2 in rats. Neuroscience 79:799–818
27. Labuzek K, Kowalski J, Gabryel B, Herman ZS (2005) Chlorpromazine and loxapine reduce interleukin-1beta and interleukin-2 release by rat mixed glial and microglial cell cultures. Eur Neuropsychopharmacol 15:23–30
28. Awatsuji H, Furukawa Y, Nakajima M, Furukawa S, Hayashi K (1993) Interleukin-2 as a neurotrophic factor for supporting the survival of neurons cultured from various regions of fetal rat brain. J Neurosci Res 35:305–311
29. Sarder M, Saito H, Abe K (1993) Interleukin-2 promotes survival and neurite extension of cultured neurons from fetal rat brain. Brain Res 625:347–350
30. Sarder M, Abe K, Saito H, Nishiyama N (1996) Comparative effect of IL-2 and IL-6 on morphology of cultured hippocampal neurons from fetal rat brain. Brain Res 715:9–16
31. Hanisch UK, Seto D, Quirion R (1993) Modulation of hippocampal acetylcholine release: a potent central action of interleukin-2. J Neurosci 13:3368–3374
32. Seto D, Kar S, Quirion R (1997) Evidence for direct and indirect mechanisms in the potent modulatory action of interleukin-2 on the release of acetylcholine in rat hippocampal slices. Br J Pharmacol 120:1151–1157
33. Lapchak PA (1992) A role for interleukin-2 in the regulation of striatal dopaminergic function. Neuroreport 3:165–168
34. Villemain F, Owens T, Renno T, Beaudet A (1991) Localization of mRNA for interleukin-2 (IL-2) in mouse brain by in situ hybridization. Soc Neurosci Abstr 17:1199
35. Araujo DM, Lapchak PA (1994) Induction of immune system mediators in the hippocampal formation in Alzheimer's and Parkinson's diseases: selective effects on specific interleukins and interleukin receptors. Neuroscience 61: 745–754
36. Tancredi V, Zona C, Velotti F, Eusebi F, Santoni A (1990) Interleukin-2 suppresses established long-term potentiation and inhibits its induction in the rat hippocampus. Brain Res 525:149–151
37. Bianchi M, Panerai AE (1993) Interleukin-2 enhances scopolamine-induced amnesia and hyperactivity in the mouse. Neuroreport 4: 1046–1048
38. Bianchi M, Ferrario P, Zonta N, Panerai AE (1995) Effects of interleukin-1 beta and interleukin-2 on amino acids levels in mouse cortex and hippocampus. Neuroreport 6:1689–1692
39. Mennicken F, Quirion R (1997) Interleukin-2 increases choline acetyltransferase activity in septal-cell cultures. Synapse 26:175–183
40. Lacosta S, Merali Z, Anisman H (1999) Influence of acute and repeated interleukin-2 administration on spatial learning, locomotor activity, exploratory behaviors, and anxiety. Behav Neurosci 113:1030–1041
41. Nemni R, Iannaccone S, Quattrini A, Smirne S, Sessa M, Lodi M, Erminio C, Canal N (1992) Effect of chronic treatment with recombinant interleukin-2 on the central nervous system of adult and old mice. Brain Res 591:248–252
42. Araujo DM, Lapchak PA, Collier B, Quirion R (1989) Localization of interleukin-2 immunoreactivity and interleukin-2 receptors in the rat brain: interaction with the cholinergic system. Brain Res 498:257–266
43. Petitto JM, McNamara R, Gendreau PL, Huang Z, Jackson A (1999) Impaired learning and memory and altered hippocampal neurodevelopment resulting from IL-2 gene deletion. J Neurosci Res 56:441–446
44. Schöpke R, Wolfer DP, Lipp HP, Leisinger-Trigona MC (1991) Swimming navigation and structural variations of the infrapyramidal mossy fibers in the hippocampus of the mouse. Hippocampus 3:315–328
45. Schwegler H, Crusio WE, Lipp HP, Heimrich B (1988) Water-maze learning in the mouse correlates with variation in hippocampal morphology. Behav Genet 18:153–165
46. Schwegler H, Crusio WE (1995) Correlations between radial-maze learning and structural variations of septum and hippocampus in rodents. Behav Brain Res 67:29–41
47. Beck RD Jr, King MA, Ha GK, Cushman JD, Huang Z, Petitto JM (2005) IL-2 deficiency results in altered septal and hippocampal cytoarchitecture: relation to development and neurotrophins. J Neuroimmunol 160:146–153
48. Altman J, Bayer SA (1990) Migration and distribution of two populations of hippocampal granule cell precursors during the perinatal and postnatal periods. J Comp Neurol 301: 365–381
49. Cameron HA, McKay RD (2001) Adult neurogenesis produces a large pool of new granule cells in the dentate gyrus. J Comp Neurol 435: 406–417
50. Schwegler H, Crusio WE, Lipp HP, Brust I, Mueller GG (1991) Early postnatal hyperthyroidism alters hippocampal circuitry and improves radial-maze learning in adult mice. J Neurosci 11:2102–2106
51. Alderson RF, Alterman AL, Barde YA, Lindsay RM (1990) Brain-derived neurotrophic factor increases survival and differentiated

functions of rat septal cholinergic neurons in culture. Neuron 5:297–306

52. Morse JK, Wiegand SJ, Anderson K, You Y, Cai N, Carnahan J, Miller J, DiStefano PS, Altar CA, Lindsay RM et al (1993) Brain-derived neurotrophic factor (BDNF) prevents the degeneration of medial septal cholinergic neurons following fimbria transection. J Neurosci 13:4146–4156
53. Ward NL, Hagg T (2000) BDNF is needed for postnatal maturation of basal forebrain and neostriatum cholinergic neurons in vivo. Exp Neurol 162:297–310
54. Knipper M, da Penha Berzaghi M, Blochl A, Breer H, Thoenen H, Lindholm D (1994) Positive feedback between acetylcholine and the neurotrophins nerve growth factor and brain-derived neurotrophic factor in the rat hippocampus. Eur J Neurosci 6:668–671
55. Larsson E, Mandel RJ, Klein RL, Muzyczka N, Lindvall O, Kokaia Z (2002) Suppression of insult-induced neurogenesis in adult rat brain by brain-derived neurotrophic factor. Exp Neurol 177:1–8
56. Lee J, Duan W, Mattson MP (2002) Evidence that brain-derived neurotrophic factor is required for basal neurogenesis and mediates, in part, the enhancement of neurogenesis by dietary restriction in the hippocampus of adult mice. J Neurochem 82:1367–1375
57. Besser M, Wank R (1999) Cutting edge: clonally restricted production of the neurotrophins brain-derived neurotrophic factor and neurotrophin-3 mRNA by human immune cells and Th1/Th2-polarized expression of their receptors. J Immunol 162:6303–6306
58. Canossa M, Griesbeck O, Berninger B, Campana G, Kolbeck R, Thoenen H (1997) Neurotrophin release by neurotrophins: implications for activity-dependent neuronal plasticity. Proc Natl Acad Sci USA 94:13279–13286
59. Saarelainen T, Vaittinen S, Castren E (2001) trkB-receptor activation contributes to the kainate-induced increase in BDNF mRNA synthesis. Cell Mol Neurobiol 21:429–435
60. Hellweg R, Humpel C, Lowe A, Hortnagl H (1997) Moderate lesion of the rat cholinergic septohippocampal pathway increases hippocampal nerve growth factor synthesis: evidence for long-term compensatory changes? Brain Res Mol Brain Res 45:177–181
61. Beck RD Jr, King MA, Huang Z, Petitto JM (2002) Alterations in septohippocampal cholinergic neurons resulting from interleukin-2 gene knockout. Brain Res 955:16–23
62. Hock C, Heese K, Hulette C, Rosenberg C, Otten U (2000) Region-specific neurotrophin imbalances in Alzheimer disease: decreased levels of brain-derived neurotrophic factor and increased levels of nerve growth factor in hippocampus and cortical areas. Arch Neurol 57: 846–851
63. Merrill JE (1990) Interleukin-2 effects in the central nervous system. Ann N Y Acad Sci 594: 188–199
64. Quirion R, Aubert I, Robitaille Y, Gauthier S, Araujo DM, Chabot JG (1990) Neurochemical deficits in pathological brain aging: specificity and possible relevance for treatment strategies. Clin Neuropharmacol 13:73–80
65. Zalcman SS (2002) Interleukin-2-induced increases in climbing behavior: inhibition by dopamine D-1 and D-2 receptor antagonists. Brain Res 944:157–164
66. Turka LA, Walsh PT (2008) IL-2 signaling and CD4+ CD25+ Foxp3+ regulatory T cells. Front Biosci 13:1440–1446
67. Horak I, Lohler J, Ma A, Smith KA (1995) Interleukin-2 deficient mice: a new model to study autoimmunity and self-tolerance. Immunol Rev 148:35–44
68. Kundig TM, Schorle H, Bachmann MF, Hengartner H, Zinkernagel RM, Horak I (1993) Immune responses in interleukin-2-deficient mice. Science 262:1059–1061
69. Schorle H, Holtschke T, Hunig T, Schimpl A, Horak I (1991) Development and function of T cells in mice rendered interleukin-2 deficient by gene targeting. Nature 352:621–624
70. Kalman J, Engelhardt JI, Le WD, Xie W, Kovacs I, Kasa P, Appel SH (1997) Experimental immune-mediated damage of septal cholinergic neurons. J Neuroimmunol 77:63–74
71. Semba K, Fibiger HC (1988) Time of origin of cholinergic neurons in the rat basal forebrain. J Comp Neurol 269:87–95
72. Huang Z, Dauer DJ, Ha GK, Lewis MH, Petitto JM (2009) Interleukin-2 deficiency induced T cell autoimmunity in the mouse brain. Neurosci Lett 463:44–48
73. Cardona AE, Li M, Lui L, Savarin C, Ransohoff RM (2008) Chemokines in and out of the central nervous system: much more than chemotaxis and inflammation. J Leukoc Biol 84: 587–594
74. Huang Z, Danielle M, Petitto JM (2011) Loss of CNS IL-2 gene expression modifies brain T lymphocyte trafficking: Response of normal versus autoreactive Treg-deficient T cells. Neurosci Lett 499:213–218

Chapter 16

Psychoneuroimmunology and Natural Killer Cells: The Chromium Release Whole Blood Assay

Mary Ann Fletcher, Zachary Barnes, Gordon Broderick, and Nancy G. Klimas

Abstract

Natural killer (NK) cells are an essential component of innate immunity. These lymphocytes are also sensitive barometers of the effects of endogenous and exogenous stressors on the immune system. This chapter will describe a chromium (^{51}Cr) release bioassay designed to measure the target cell killing capacity of NK cells (NKCC). Key features of the cytotoxicity assay are that it is done with whole blood and that numbers of effector cells are determined for each sample by flow cytometry and lymphocyte count. Effector cells are defined as CD3−CD56+ lymphocytes. Target cells are the K562 eyrthroleukemia cell line. Killing capacity is defined as number of target cells killed per effector cell, at an effector cell/target cell ratio of 1:1 during a 4 h in vitro assay.

Key words: Natural killer cells, NK cells, Natural killer cell cytotoxicity, NKCC, Lymphocytes, K562 target cells, Chromium release assay, Innate immunity, Flow cytometry

1. Introduction

The natural killer (NK) cell is a large, granular lymphocyte with ability to lyse tumor cells and virus-infected cells without prior exposure and immunization (1). These cells can prolong asymptomatic states in HIV-infected persons with low CD4 counts (2) and protect against malignancy (3). The NK cell is a reliable marker of neuroendocrine–immune interactions. Stressful life events that trigger the fight or flight response, such as a natural disaster, can alter lymphocyte trafficking and function, leading to elevated ($p < 0.001$) natural killer cell cytotoxicity (NKCC) and number of circulating NK cells ($p < 0.000$) as were seen in post Hurricane Andrew samples (4). According to a metaanalysis by Segerstrom and Miller (5), the mobilization of NK cells during acute psychologic stressors is one of the most

Qing Yan (ed.), *Psychoneuroimmunology: Methods and Protocols*, Methods in Molecular Biology, vol. 934, DOI 10.1007/978-1-62703-071-7_16, © Springer Science+Business Media, LLC 2012

Table 1
Friedman test: effect of aerobic exercise on NK cell counts in Gulf War illness cases (T0 = baseline; T1 = VO_2 max; T2 = 4 h)

Column name	Count	Ranked sum	Average rank
T0 CD3-CD56+ cells	37	70.50	1.64
T1 CD3-CD56+ cells	37	119.00	2.77
T2 CD3-CD56+ cells	37	68.50	1.59

Column name	Mean	Std. dev.	Median	25–75	Percentiles
T0 CD3-CD56+ cells	138.13	72.13	127.00	90.00	168.25
T1 CD3-CD56+ cells	461.66	276.09	417.00	252.00	560.00
T2 CD3-CD56+ cells	141.74	73.39	132.00	93.00	173.00

$\chi^2 = 38.03000$
Probability = 0.000000

Table 2
Friedman test: effect of aerobic exercise on NK cell counts in healthy controls (T0 = baseline; T1 = VO_2 max; T2 = 4 h)

Column name	Count	Ranked sum	Average rank
T0 CD3-CD56+ cells	35	59.50	1.42
T1 CD3-CD56+ cells	37	119.00	2.83
T2 CD3-CD56+ cells	37	73.50	1.75

Column name	Mean	Std. dev.	Median	25–75	Percentiles
T0 CD3-CD56+ cells	148.75	80.94	147.00	82.00	204.00
T1 CD3-CD56+ cells	642.74	377.05	602.00	358.00	802.00
T2 CD3-CD56+ cells	176.29	106.73	172.00	109.00	203.25

$\chi^2 = 46.08300$
Probability = 0.000000

replicated and robust findings in human psychoneuroimmunology. For example, 45 first-time tandem parachutists were examined for NK activity 2 h before, immediately after, and 1 h after jumping. Functional capacity of NK cells increased immediately after jumping followed by a decrease significantly below starting values 1 h later (6). In laboratory studies with Gulf War Illness patients and healthy controls, serial measurements showed a significant and rapid positive effect of an aerobic exercise challenge (VO_2 max) on the number of NK cells as shown in Tables 1 and 2. NK cell activity is also affected as shown in Fig. 1 (7, 8).

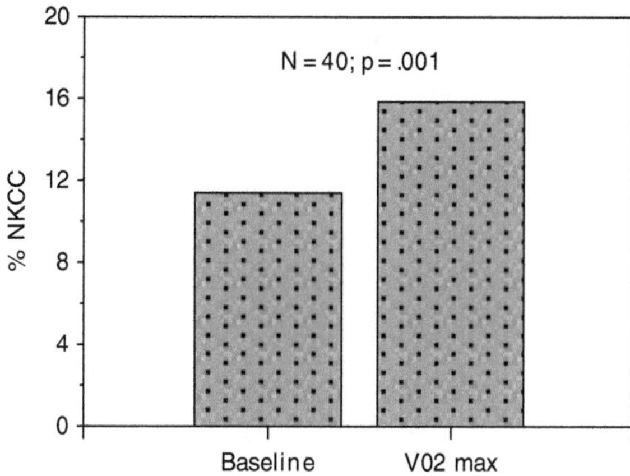

Fig. 1. Effect of exercise challenge to VO_2 max on NKCC (% of target cells killed at a target cell ratio of 1:1) in 40 healthy controls.

Acute psychological stress may result in increased risk of infection, for example development of colds in rhinovirus inoculated volunteers (9). Sustained stress resulted in lower natural killer cell cytotoxicity (NKCC) in Japanese critical care physicians in individuals taking 0–3 days off per month, as compared to those taking 4 or more days off (10). Abnormalities of the stress response are hypothesized as a trigger or mediator of chronic fatigue syndrome (CFS) which is associated with low NKCC (11) (Figs. 2 and 3). The NK cells from patients with CFS have diminished intracellular perforin (12).

The process of cytolysis can be divided into three stages: conjugate formation (binding of the effector cell to the target cell), triggering of the lytic process (signal transduction), and lethal hit (granule exocytosis). Once triggered, the cytolytic process may propagate as effector cells detach from lysed targets and recycle to initiate new lytic interactions. The binding of the NK cell to the target cell involves receptors and ligands, but unlike cytotoxic T cells, does not result from antigen recognition. Following the target-effector cell contact, intracellular granules move to the surface of the NK cell. Perforin from these granules facilitates the release of serine proteases, granzymes, and their passage through the target cell membranes. Granule exocytosis requires binding of the secreted perforin to the target cell membrane and polymerization of this perforin to polyperforin. Intracellular perforin can be quantitatively measured and is a marker for NK cell function (12). Transient expression of CD107a occurs on the NK cell surface following perforin release and can be used as surrogate marker for NK activity (13).

This chapter will describe a chromium (^{51}Cr) release bioassay designed to measure the target cell killing capacity of NK cells. This type of assay was first used over 40 years ago as a quantitative tool to assess lymphocyte-associated cytolysis (14).

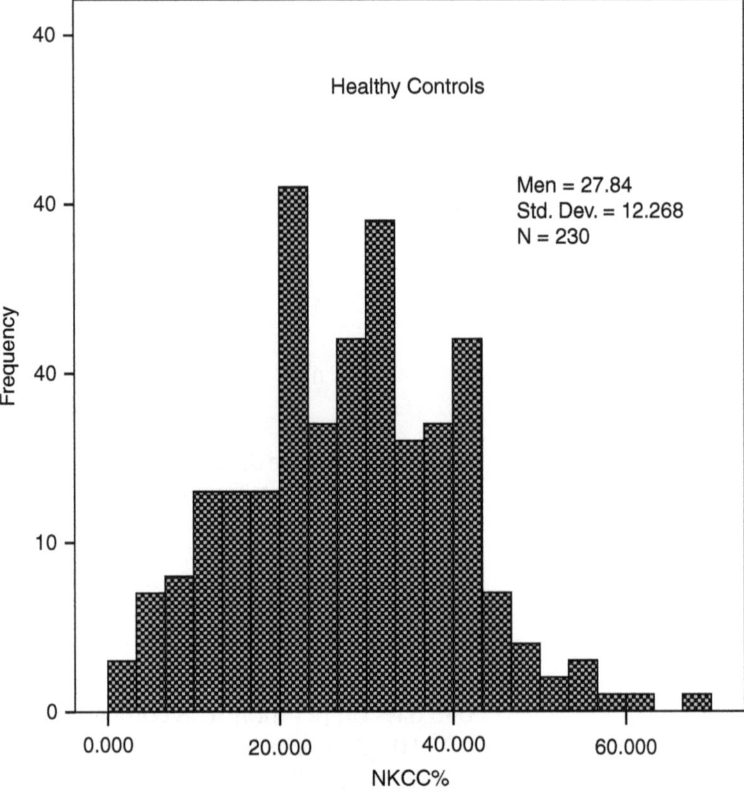

Fig. 2. Histogram of NKCC (% of target cells killed at a target cell ratio of 1:1) for 230 healthy controls.

Radioactive chromium binds to intracellular proteins. Upon lysis of the target cell, the intracellular ^{51}Cr is released in an amount proportional to the amount of cell lysis. Key features of this NKCC assay are that it is done with whole blood and that numbers of effector cells are determined for each sample by flow cytometry and lymphocyte count (15, 16). The use of fresh, whole blood is important for studies in psychoneuroimmunology. The NK cells are not subjected to centrifugation and separation from their soluble and cellular milieu. The whole blood samples are incubated with ^{51}Cr labeled target cells at four target to effector cell ratios, in triplicate for 4 h.

2. Materials and Equipment

2.1. Equipment

1. Multiparameter flow cytometer.
2. Electronic hematology instrument.
3. Automatic gamma counter.
4. Centrifuge with swing-out holders for 96-well culture plates.

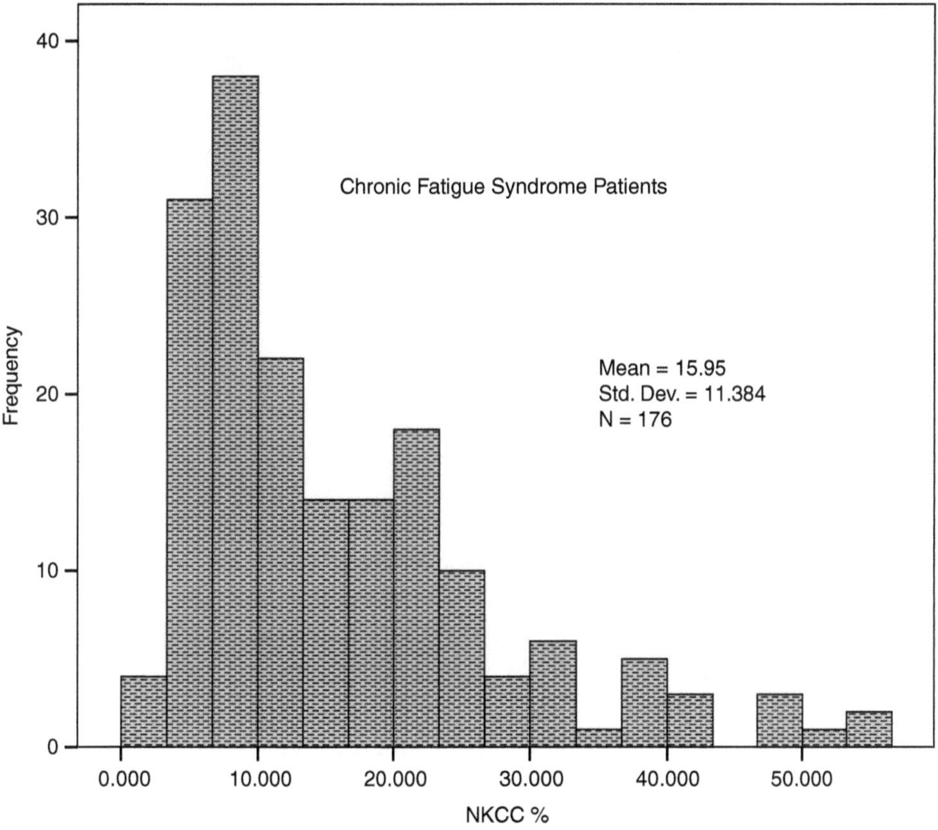

Fig. 3. Histogram of NKCC (% of target cells killed at a target cell ratio of 1:1) for 176 chronic fatigue syndrome cases.

5. Electronic timer.
6. Biological hood.
7. Aerobic filter unit.
8. Water-jacketed incubator (37 °C. 5% CO_2, 95% humidity).
9. Repeat dispenser micropipetter.

2.2. Supplies

1. Sterile polypropylene centrifuge tubes.
2. Sterile micropipettes tip (ranging from 1 μL to 1 mL).
3. Sterile transfer pipettes.
4. Sterile 75 mL tissue culture flasks.
5. Sterile 96-well flat bottom tissue culture plates.

2.3. Reagents

1. Triton X.
2. Fetal bovine serum (FBS).
3. RPMI 1640 medium (1×), without glutamine.
4. Minimum essential medium. Non-essential amino acids (MEM, 10 mM, 100×).

5. Sodium pyruvate (1 mM).
6. L-glutamine 200 mM (100×), aliquoted into 5 mL and stored at −20 °C.
7. Penicillin (5,000 U) and streptomycin (5,000 μg/mL) (100×) aliquoted into 5 mL and stored at −20 °C (Pen-Strep).
8. Trypan blue (0.4%).
9. Triton X-100.
10. ^{51}Cr (5 milliCurrie (mCi)).

3. Methods

3.1. Pre Assay Preparations (in Biohazard Hood with Sterile Technique)

3.1.1. Tissue Culture

1. Stock Media (SM): In a flask mix 500 mL of RPMI, 5 mL of phosphate-buffered saline (PBS), 5 mL MEM, 5 mL sodium pyruvate. Filter through 0.2 μm-pore size filter.
2. Assay Media (AM): Mix and filter (0.2 μm-pore size filter) 90 mL of SM and 10 mL of FBS.
3. Culture Media (CM): Mix and filter (0.2 μm-pore size filter) 85 mL of SM and 15 mL of FBS.
4. Storage Requirements: Chromium in solution, Stock Media, Assay Media, Non-Essential Amino acids, FBS, MEM, Sodium Pyruvate, should all be kept in the refrigerator at 2–8 °C for up to 1 week. L-Glutamine and Pen-Strep should be kept in the freezer at −20 °C.
5. Target cells: The usual target cell is the K562 erythroleukemic cell line available from the ATCC http://www.atcc.org/ . The NK sensitive K562 cell line is maintained in a humidified 5% CO_2 atmosphere at 37 °C in stationary suspension in CM. Cells are subcultured twice weekly to produce log-phase growth (see Note 1, 4×10^6 cells in 20 mL of CM will yield approximately 16×10^6 cells).

3.1.2. Patient Preparation

1. No special preparation is necessary. However, if possible the sample should be collected in the morning so that the assay, which requires several hours to complete, may be done in the same day. Also, NK cell count varies in a circadian rhythm over 24 h (17).

3.1.3. Specimen Collection and Handling Conditions

1. Using standard aseptic technique, collect by venipuncture 3 mL whole blood into a sodium heparin tube and 1 mL of whole blood into an ethylene diamine tetra acetic acid (EDTA) tube. Universal precautions should be observed when handling the blood sample and all biohazardous materials. Chromium used in this procedure is radioactive and should be handled

Table 3
Dilution of target cells

Final concentration (cells/mL)	Amount of initial cell suspension (2×10^6 cells/mL)	Amount of media (mL)
2×10^6	2	0
1×10^6	1	1
0.5×10^6	0.5	1.5
0.25×10^6	0.25	1.75

using appropriate safety standards. Except when stated otherwise, all transfers of cells and biological fluids should be done in the biological hood. However, after the final incubation is complete, samples may be handled outside of the hood, but still with caution as to avoid cross-contamination.

3.2. Assay Procedure

3.2.1. Target Cell Preparation (in Biohazard Hood with Sterile Technique)

1. Pour the entire volume of cultured cells in flask into a 50 mL conical tube. Remove 100 μL of the cell suspension and combine them with100 μL of trypan blue for the initial cell count. Spin 50 mL conical tube at low speed (400 × *g*) for 5 min.
2. Pour off the supernatant into waste, and add 10 mL of room temperature SM to re-suspend the cells. Centrifuge for 5 min at 400 × *g*.
3. Remove the supernatant, add the chromium solution equal to 100 μCi, for each 20×10^6 cells mix. The amount of ^{51}Cr depends on weeks of "age" (time elapsed since the date of calibration of the chromium solution, see Note 2). Incubate for 1 h at 37 °C in a humidified 5% CO_2 atmosphere, with gentle shaking every 15 min.
4. In the same 50 mL tube, add 10 mL of 37 °C AM to the chromium/cell solution, mix gently, and spin at 400 × *g* for 5 min. Pour off the supernatant into the radioactive waste container. Repeat this washing four times.
5. After the fourth wash add 10 mL of 37 °C AM. Remove 50 μL of cell/assay media solution to a test tube; add 50 μL trypan blue for the final cell count in order to determine the volume of assay media needed to produce a cell count of 2×10^6 K562 cells. With remaining solution in the 50 mL tube, centrifuge for 5 min at 400 × *g*.

3.2.2. NKCC Reaction Setup

1. Pour off supernatant from step 5 of 3.2.1 above and add the volume of room temperature AM proscribed by the final cell count, and mix gently. In separate tubes make graded dilutions to produce the four target cell concentration as shown in Table 3.

An assay with four blood samples requires a minimum of 2 mL of each target cell dilution.

2. Add 150 μL well mixed blood from EDTA tube to each well of one row in culture plate.
3. For spontaneous release control (SR), dispense 150 μL AM to one row of 12 wells.
4. For total release control (TR), dispense 150 μL 1% Triton X-100 one row of 12 wells.
5. Add 50 μL cell suspensions to each of three wells for each of the four dilutions (change tips if progressing from stronger to weaker concentration, otherwise tips can be conserved for one row).
6. Cover plate and centrifuge for 10 min at room temperature at 400×*g*.
7. Incubate for plate at 37 °C in a humidified 5% CO_2 atmosphere for 4 h.
8. After 4 h add 100 μL of cold (below 9 C) assay media to all wells to stop the NKCC reaction and centrifuge for 5 min at 400×*g*.

3.2.3. Harvesting and Counting

1. Transfer 100 μL supernatant to counting test tubes without disturbing cell pellet. Start with highest concentration of TR controls, followed by SR controls and finally patient samples. After the last well insert at least three empty test tubes to serve as background.
2. Load the racks into gamma counter and count released ^{51}Cr.

3.2.4. Lymphocyte Count

This information is required for calculation of NKCC using (1). This should be done using an electronic hematology analyser, which will provide the hematocrit that is also needed for (1).

3.2.5. Flow Cytometry

Lymphocytes that are CD45+, CD14−, CD3−, and CD56+ constitute the bulk of the cells capable of NK cell cytotoxic activity. Using four color flow cytometry, determine the percent of cells in the lymphocyte gate that meet this requirement. Multiply this by the lymphocyte count to obtain the number of NK cells for (1).

3.2.6. Calculations

Subtract the background counts (*b*) from all experimental release (ER), SR, and TR and calculate the percent cytotoxicity for each dilution of target cells according to (1).

$$\% \text{ cytotoxicity} = \left[\frac{(\text{ER}-b)\times\{(V_t-(V_b\times\text{HCT}))/V_t\}-(\text{SR}-b)}{(\text{TR}-b)-(\text{SR}-b)}\right]\times 100 \quad (1)$$

V_t is total volume in the well; V_b is the volume of blood in the well; HCT is the hematocrit of blood sample.

When a constant number of NK cells is incubated with various numbers of ^{51}Cr-labled target cells, the numbers of target cells lysed may be expressed as percent cytotoxicity times the number of target cells in the assay. A curve is generated by plotting the number of target cells vs. the number of cells lysed. Because the kinetics of cytotoxicity resemble those of enzyme–substrate interactions, the Michaelis Menten rate equation as developed by Cleland (18) defines the velocity of such reactions (2):

$$v = \frac{V_{max}[T]}{K_m + [T]} \quad (2)$$

where v is the number of target cells lysed; T is the number of target cells in the assay; V_{max} is the number of target cells lysed when the number of target cells is infinite; and K_m is the number of target cells required for ½ $V_{max.}$

Callewaert and Mahle (19) showed that estimates for V_{max} for NKCC are equal to the concentration of NK cells times the mean lytic activity per NK cells. Percent NKCC for the four concentrations of target cells is transformed to the number of target cells killed at each concentration using (3):

$$v = \% \text{ cytotoxicity } [T] \quad (3)$$

The data are then fitted to the Cleland equation. Percent cytotoxicity is determined for effector cell to target cell ratio of 1:1, where the number of effector cells is defined as CD3–CD56+ lymphocytes.

3.2.7. Quality Control for Assay

There is no commercial proficiency test available for this procedure. For quality control, always perform the assay in triplicate and have blinded duplicates submitted to the laboratory. The SR should be <20% of TR and the correlation coefficient (r^2) for the Michaelis Menten equation should be >90%. Each laboratory must determine an expected range for healthy individuals. In our laboratory, the 230 healthy controls shown in Fig. 1 had a mean % cytotoxicity at an effector to target cell ratio of 1:1 of 28%. Table 4 gives the parameters of NKCC for controls and a patient group, CFS

3.2.8. Performance Parameters

Outlying individual scores when found in triplicate data sets (i.e., from three wells from the same tube), should be excluded, and the scores which are closest to one another in the set should be averaged for results.

3.2.9. Limitations of the Procedure

This procedure is done with fresh blood samples. Blood that is <8 h old is preferred. Samples that are <8 but >24 h can be run. However, the results must be compared to the control range determined for samples of that age.

Table 4
Natural killer cell cytotoxicity for chronic fatigue syndrome (CFS) and healthy controls

Subject group and distribution statistics			Statistic	Std. error
CFS	Mean		15.94688	0.858119
	95% Confidence interval for mean	Lower bound	14.25328	
		Upper bound	17.64047	
	Median		12.05000	
	Variance		129.601	
	Std. deviation		11.384233	
	Minimum		1.200	
	Maximum		55.300	
	Range		54.100	
	Interquartile range		13.675	
	Skewness		1.392	0.183
	Kurtosis		1.718	0.364
HC	Mean		27.83922	0.808923
	95% Confidence interval for mean	Lower bound	26.24533	
		Upper bound	29.43310	
	Median		28.00000	
	Variance		150.502	
	Std. deviation		12.267920	
	Minimum		2.000	
	Maximum		69.000	
	Range		67.000	
	Interquartile range		17.025	
	Skewness		0.211	0.160
	Kurtosis		-0.033	0.320

4. Notes

1. Splitting K562 cell cultures. Note: In labs performing the NKCC assay on a daily or weekly basis, the existing cell line of K562 is cultured and continually split using the following procedure which is repeated identically every week, with the exceptions of long weekends or periods when the test is not performed. Tissue culture flasks should always be labeled with the date when they were prepared, written on them.
   (a) *On Monday:* Label four flasks with the date, "K562," and the volumes included; (for example, if 2 mL of cells and 16 of culture media are added, label: "2 +16 media").
   (b) From the Incubator, remove one of the tissue culture flasks from the previous Friday (should be dated), and withdraw 4 mL and put into a flask labeled for Monday's date. Repeat. Then withdraw 2 mL from the same flask from Friday and add this to a third Monday flask. Repeat for a fourth Monday flask.

(c) Complete each of these flasks to 20 mL with Culture Media.

(d) Place the newly composed flasks in the incubator, and discard the Friday one from which transfers were made.

(e) *On Tuesday:* Use the remaining flask from the previous Friday for any NK samples to be done on Tuesday. (No splitting on Tuesday).

(f) *On Wednesday*: Read fully: Repeat the procedure from Monday, except using one of Monday's flasks for transfers, and label the new flasks with Wednesday's date. Note, also, you will this time only compose one flask using 2 mL from the Monday culture, instead of two. The other two new flasks will be 4 mL additions. (Complete to 20 mL with Culture Media).

(g) *On Thursday:* Use the remaining flask from Monday for any NK samples to be done on Tuesday. (No splitting on Thursday).

(h) *On Friday:* Split one of Wednesday's flasks to four new, Friday flasks, with 1.5 mL going to 2 of them, and 0.5 mL going to two other new, Friday flasks. Complete to 20 mL with Culture Media.

(i) Repeat this process weekly. If necessary to do a Saturday NK, make an additional 2 mL flask on Wednesday.

2. Radioactive Chromium-51 usage.
For the addition of Chromium in step 1c, different volumes of the Chromium solution are added depending on the "age," or time elapsed since the date of calibration of the Chromium solution. The Calibration date of the particular solution vial is on the label.

Week 1	90 μL of chromium	Precalibration days
Week 2	100 μL of chromium	Calibration date
Week 3	120 μL of chromium	Post calibration days
Week 4	140 μL of chromium	Post calibration days
Week 5	160 μL of chromium	Post calibration days

Acknowledgements

This work was supported by grants from the NIAAA: R21AA016635 (PI MA Fletcher); NIAID: R01AI065723 (PI MA Fletcher); CFIDS Assoc. of America: (PI N Klimas); NIAID: UO1 AI459940 (PI N Klimas); NIAMSD R01 AR057853-01A1 (PI N Klimas); VA merit awards (PI N Klimas) Dynamic Modeling in GWI, CFS/ME; GW080152 (PI N Klimas).

References

1. Herberman RB, Holden HT (1979) Natural killer cells as antitumor effector cells. J Natl Cancer Inst 62:441–445
2. Solomon GF, Benton D, Harker JO, Bonavida B, Fletcher MA (1994) Prolonged asymptomatic states in HIV-seropositive persons with fewer than 50 CD4+ T cells per MM3. Psychoneuroimmunologic findings. Ann N Y Acad Sci 741:85–90
3. Su DM, Vankayalapati R (2010) A new avenue to cure cancer by turning adaptive immune T cells to innate immune NK cells via reprogramming. J Mol Cell Biol 2:237–239
4. Ironson G, Wyings C, Schneiderman N et al (1997) Post-traumatic stress symptoms, intrusive thoughts, loss and immune function after Hurricane Andrew. Psychosom Med 59:128–141
5. Schedlowski M, Jacobs R, Stratmann G et al (1993) Changes of natural killer cells during acute psychological stress. J Clin Immunol 13:119–126
6. Segerstrom SC, Miller GE (2004) Psychological stress and the human immune system: a meta-analytic study of 30 years of inquiry. Psychol Bull 130:601–630
7. Klimas NG, Rosenthal M, Fletcher MA (2006) Immune effects of an acute exercise challenge in Gulf War Illness. Assoc Military Surgeons US, San Antonio
8. Harvey JM, Barnes Z, Zeng et al (2011) Exercise effects on biomarkers of CFS/ME and GWI. Presented to the International Conference on CFS/ME, Ottawa, Canada
9. Cohen S, Tyrrell DA, Smith AP (1991) Psychological stress and susceptibility to the common cold. N Engl J Med 325:606–612
10. Okamoto H, Tsunoda T, Teruya K et al (2008) An occupational health study of emergency physicians in Japan: health assessment by immune variables (CD4, CD8, CD56, and NK cell activity) at the beginning of work. J Occup Health 50:136–146
11. Fletcher MA, Zeng XR, Maher K et al (2010) Biomarkers in chronic fatigue syndrome: evaluation of natural killer cell function and dipeptidyl peptidase IV/CD26. PLoS One 5(5):e10817
12. Maher K, Klimas NG, Fletcher MA (2005) Chronic fatigue syndrome is associated with diminished intracellular perforin. Clin Exp Immunol 142:505–511
13. Alter G, Malenfant JM, Altfeld M (2004) CD107a as a functional marker for the identification of natural killer cell activity. J Immunol Methods 294:15–22
14. Brunner K, Mauel TJ, Cerottini J-C et al (1968) Quantitative assay of the lytic action of immune lymphoid cells on Cr labeled allogeneic target cells in vitro Inhibition by isoantibody and by drugs. Immunology 14:181
15. Baron GA, Klimas NG, Fischl MA et al (1985) Decreased natural killer cell-mediated cytotoxicity per effector cell. Diagn Immunol 3:197–204
16. Fletcher MA, Baron GA, Ashman MA et al (1987) Use of whole blood methods in assessment of immune parameters in immunodeficiency syndromes. Diagn Clin Immunol 5:69–81
17. Bourin P, Mansour I, Doinel C, Roué R et al (1993) Circadian rhythms of circulating NK cells in healthy and human immunodeficiency virus-infected men. Chronobiol Int 10:298–305
18. Cleland WW (1967) The statistical analysis of enzyme kinetic data. Adv Enzymol Relat Areas Mol Biol 29:1
19. Callewaert DM, Mahle NH (1985) Kinetic models of natural killer cells and their use for studying activated NK cells. In: Herberman RB, Callewaert DM (eds) Mechanisms of cytotoxicity by NK cells. Academic, Orlando, p 381

Chapter 17

The Application of PET Imaging in Psychoneuroimmunology Research

Jonas Hannestad

Abstract

Positron emission tomography (PET) imaging is a research tool that allows in vivo measurements of brain metabolism and specific target molecules. PET imaging can be used to measure these brain variables in a variety of species, including human and non-human primates, and rodents. PET imaging can therefore be combined with various experimental and clinical model systems that are commonly used in psychoneuroimmunology research.

Key words: PET, FDG, PBR, TSPO, Inflammation, Microglia, Endotoxin

1. Introduction

1.1. The Basics of Positron Emission Tomography

Nuclear imaging refers to imaging modalities that measure the amount of radioactivity emitted from a tissue or organ in vivo after the injection of a radiopharmaceutical. The radioactivity measured in the tissue that is being studied, when combined with the measurement of radioactivity in the blood (the so-called input function), is used to quantify a physiologic process or the availability of binding sites of a target molecule. Radiopharmaceuticals are commonly (and interchangeably) called radioligands or *radiotracers*; the latter refers to the fact that the mass dose of the radiopharmaceutical administered is very low. Such "tracer" amounts rarely have any measurable physiologic or biochemical effects, and they do not interfere with the process which they are designed to measure. Radiotracers are designed to measure a specific metabolic process (e.g., glucose metabolism, oxygen uptake, blood flow) or to bind to a specific extra- or intracellular target molecule (e.g., a neurotransmitter receptor or transporter, or a molecule that is found in a specific cell type). Positron emission tomography (PET) is a

Qing Yan (ed.), *Psychoneuroimmunology: Methods and Protocols*, Methods in Molecular Biology, vol. 934, DOI 10.1007/978-1-62703-071-7_17, © Springer Science+Business Media, LLC 2012

type of nuclear imaging in which the radiotracer emits positrons, positively charged particles with characteristics that are very similar to those of the negatively charged electron. This distinguishes PET imaging from another common modality of nuclear imaging—single photon computed tomography (SPECT)—in which the radiotracer emits gamma photons directly. The common terms are summarized in Table 1.

1.2. Radionuclides and Radiotracers

A *nuclide* is an atom that has a specific number of protons and neutrons in its nucleus. While the number of protons determines which element an atom is (e.g., carbon has six protons), an element can have several *isotopes*: nuclides with the same number of protons but different numbers of neutrons (e.g., ^{11}C and ^{12}C have five and six neutrons, respectively). The chemical properties of a nuclide depend on the number of electrons (which equals the number of protons and determines which element it is) but not on the number of neutrons. Therefore, different isotopes of the same element have the same chemical properties, and one can therefore substitute one isotope for another during chemical synthesis. The physical properties (e.g., radioactivity) of a nuclide depend on both the number of protons and neutrons. Some nuclides are unstable and decay by emitting radiation; these are called *radionuclides.* Nuclear imaging is possible because: (1) isotopes are chemically interchangeable and can be substituted in chemical structures, and (2) some nuclides emit radiation. A PET radiotracer is therefore a synthetic or semi-synthetic molecule with certain chemical and biological properties (i.e., affinity for the target molecule, ability to cross the blood–brain barrier (BBB), etc.) in which a positron-emitting isotope has been substituted for an original nuclide in the molecule (e.g., ^{11}C replaces ^{12}C). In PET imaging, the radionuclides used are positron emitters, which are rich in protons relative to neutrons. When the proton in the nucleus decays, it is converted to a neutron, and a positron and a neutrino are emitted. This type of decay is called β^+ decay or positron emission. This differs from β^- decay in which a neutron is converted to a proton, and an electron and an anti-neutrino are emitted. The difference in energy between the pre-decay nuclide and the post-decay nuclide is called transition or decay energy. Positron emitters have a decay energy $\geq$1.022 MeV. When a positron-emitting radionuclide decays, the decay energy is shared between the positron and the neutrino. (Proton-rich nuclides that have a decay energy of less than 1.022 MeV decay by electron capture.)

The radioactivity of a radionuclide is the amount of radiation it emits per unit of time. Radioactivity is measured in disintegrations per second (Becquerels or Bq in the *Système International d'Unités*) and in Curies (Ci) which denotes the radioactivity of 1 g of ^{226}Ra ($3.7\cdot10^{10}$ Bq). For practical purposes, doses of radiotracers administered in PET imaging are often described using the Ci units.

Table 1
Definitions of common terms used in PET imaging

Term	Definition
Activity (radioactivity)	Number of disintegrations per minute of a given radionuclide
Annihilation	The interaction of a positron and electron, which gives rise to two annihilation photons traveling in opposite direction
Attenuation	An annihilation photon interacts with the tissue and does not reach the PET detectors, thus not contributing to the signal
Becquerel (Bq)	Disintegrations per second. A measure of activity. Mostly expressed as megaBq (MBq)
Biological half-life	The time it takes for the body to eliminate half of the radiotracer molecules
Curies (Ci)	The radioactivity of 1 g of radium. Mostly expressed as milliCuries (mCi)
Decay	Emission of radiation due to an unstable configuration of the nucleus
Decay energy	The differential energy of the pre-decay radionuclide and the post-decay nuclide
Dynamic PET imaging	PET imaging that consists of a sequence of contiguous, discrete measurements of emitted radiation
Effective half-life	The combination of the physical and the biological half life
Emission scan	The PET scan that measures radiation emitted from the brain
Input function	The changes in radioactivity in the blood over time as the radiotracer is metabolized, decays and enters tissues
Non-colinearity	The fact that the angle between the two annihilation photons is not exactly 180°
Nondisplaceable binding	Binding of the radiotracer that is not displaceable with an excess of "cold" radiotracer. This is the sum of nonspecific binding and free tissue radiotracer
Nonspecific binding	Binding of the radiotracer to molecules other than the target molecule
Normalization	The use of a positron-emitting phantom to calibrate each PET detector pair
Physical half-life	The time it takes for the radioactivity to be halved. Constant for each radionuclide
Positron range	The distance a positron travels before annihilation
Radiotracer	A pharmaceutical or other molecule in which a radionuclide has been substituted for the original nuclide
Radionuclide	A nuclide that decays and therefore emits radiation. Radionuclides used in PET imaging are positron emitters
Scatter	The process in which a photon interacts with tissue and changes direction
Specific binding	Binding or the radiotracer to the target molecule
Static PET imaging	The measurement of total emission radiation from a tissue over a period of time
Transmission scan	A scan that uses an external source of radiation to measure the attenuation of the organ or tissue to be imaged. This information is then used for attenuation-correction during image reconstruction

For example, doses of radiotracer that are injected into human subjects during PET imaging are mostly in the 5–20 mCi range. Most journals require the use of Bq. Atoms decay randomly; however, the *physical half-life*, i.e., the time it takes for a given radioactivity to be reduced by 50%, is constant for each radionuclide. The *effective half-life* of a radiotracer takes into account the physical half-life of the radionuclide and also the *biological half-life*, which depends on metabolism and elimination. Therefore, the effective half-life is the time it takes to eliminate from an organism half of the radioactivity administered. This halving of radioactivity is a combination of decay (physical half-life) and metabolism/excretion (biological half-life). For radionuclides with a very long physical half-life (e.g., ^{124}I or ^{76}Br), the effective half-life is for practical purposes identical to the biological half-life. In other words, the radiotracer is metabolized and excreted before the radionuclide loses any significant amount of radioactivity. Conversely, for radionuclides with a very short physical half-life (e.g., ^{15}O or ^{82}Rb), the effective half-life is practically identical to the physical half-life. That is, the radionuclide decays so fast that the radioactivity is close to zero before any significant amount of radiotracer has been metabolized and eliminated from the body. Radionuclides with long half-lives (e.g., ^{124}I) can be purchased from a vendor, and the nuclide can be incorporated in the radiotracer molecule during on-site synthesis (if the facility has a radiochemistry lab). Radionuclides with intermediate half-lives (e.g., ^{18}F) can be incorporated into a radiotracer by a vendor, and the radiotracer can be shipped that same day for use at a PET facility that does not have the ability to synthesize radiotracers (this is commonly done in clinical medicine). For radionuclides with short half-lives (e.g., ^{11}C), the nuclide must be produced on-site using a cyclotron and incorporated into the radiotracer molecule in the radiochemistry lab. One important advantage of radiotracers with short half-lives is that multiple PET scans can be performed in 1 day.

1.3. Annihilation and Photon Interactions

When a positron-emitter decays in a tissue, the positron travels a short distance (usually <1 mm) before losing energy and interacting with an electron. This interaction leads to the annihilation of both the positron and the electron. Because the momentum at the time of interaction is almost zero and momentum has to be conserved, the annihilation cannot give rise to a single photon. Rather, two photons traveling in approximately opposite direction from the site of annihilation arise (Fig. 1). These photons, called annihilation photons, are in the gamma spectrum of energy and therefore have the same properties as “real” gamma photons, i.e., photons that arise directly from decay of the nucleus. Because of their high energy, many of these photons will escape the body, and the PET camera can detect them as described in detail below; however, some of these photons will interact with atoms in the tissue through

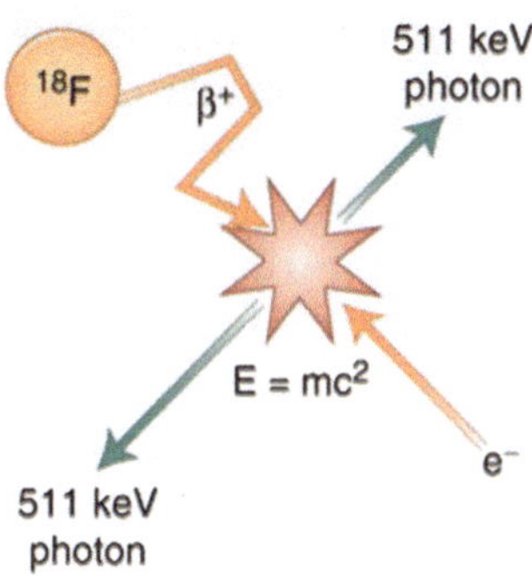

Fig. 1. Positron annihilation. The positron emitted during decay of a positron-emitting nuclide (^{18}F in this case) travels a short distance before interacting with an electron. Both are annihilated and two annihilation photons emerge. These travel in opposite directions and will either be detected by the PET system's detector crystals, or interact with the tissue. Adapted from: Dilsizian V, Di Carli F, Narula J (2009) Essential atlas of cardiovascular disease, vol 1, Chap 14. Copyright 2009 by Current Medicine, Inc. Reproduced with kind permission from Springer Science+Business Media B.V.

which they travel. Interactions with atoms in the tissue contribute to two important phenomena: Attenuation and scatter. *Attenuation* refers to the fact that deeper parts of an organ appear to emit less radioactivity than superficial parts because the photons from, e.g., the thalamus must traverse more tissue before reaching the PET camera detectors than photons from the cortex. Therefore, fewer photons (per volume of tissue) from the thalamus will reach the detectors. *Scatter* refers to the fact that some photons will collide with other particles, changing their direction. During the reconstruction of the final PET image, both attenuation and scatter are accounted for (see below). There are three ways the annihilation photons interact with the tissue: the photoelectric process, Compton scattering, and pair production. The *photoelectric process* occurs when a lower energy photon ejects an electron from an atom, and all the energy of the photon is transferred to the electron. The resulting X-ray photon does not escape the tissue and therefore the annihilation photon is completely "absorbed," i.e., there is no detectable trace of this when measuring radiation from the tissue with a PET camera. Therefore, the photoelectric process contributes to attenuation. In *Compton scattering*, which is the prevalent form of interaction between annihilation photons and a tissue, a higher energy photon interacts with an outer shell electron. This electron is ejected together with a scattered photon with less energy than the incident photon. Compton scatter contributes to attenuation if the scattered photon never reaches the PET camera, or to background noise, if the photon is detected by the PET camera. If the PET camera detects and "counts" a scattered photon, it will misread the localization of the annihilation event because the photon changed direction. To reduce the likelihood of detecting scattered photons as "true" counts, the PET camera has a specific energy window; Compton scattering leads to a loss of energy so that scattered photons are more likely to have energy below the lower limit of this window. In addition, correction for scatter is done during image reconstruction in an attempt to reduce the background signal from scatter. The last type of interaction an annihilation photon can have with the tissue is *pair production*, which occurs when the photon has an energy ≥1.022 MeV and it interacts with the nucleus of an atom, producing a positron and an electron. This new positron will undergo annihilation as described above and gives rise to a new pair of annihilation photons which can be detected by the PET camera, but which do not represent the localization of a radiotracer molecule. These three types of interactions reduce the signal-to-noise ratio. Therefore, an annihilation photon which interacts with the tissue can contribute to attenuation (i.e., it does not continue on the path it started and is therefore not able to "inform" the PET camera of the amount of radioactivity where it originated) and to scatter (if Compton scattering or pair-production gives rise to gamma-energy photons that provide "wrong" information to the PET camera). The aim of the PET detection system and subsequent corrections is therefore to avoid (as much as possible) counting photons that are produced by these three types of interactions, and to count as many of the photons that are produced during annihilation of the positron that emits from the radiotracer and that reach the detection material without interacting with the tissue ("true counts" or "trues").

1.4. PET Detection Systems

PET systems detect annihilation photons using a solid scintillation detector, a crystal material with which the photon interacts to produce visible-light photons (scintillations). The most commonly used solid scintillation crystals in PET imaging are bismuth germanate (BGO), lutetium oxyorthosilicate with cerium (LSO), and yttrium oxyorthosilicate with cerium (YSO). These crystals vary in some important properties including: (1) stopping power (the distance the annihilation photon travels in the crystal before it interacts with an atom and deposits its energy), (2) scintillation decay time (the time, in nanoseconds, it takes from when the annihilation photon excites an atom in the detector crystal until this atom emits a visible-light photon), (3) the light output (how much light is emitted when an annihilation photon excites a crystal atom), and (4) the energy resolution (the fraction of the 511 keV energy that is "converted" to visible light). In addition, these crystals should have a high ratio of photoelectric to Compton interactions (the opposite of what tissue has). This is because photoelectric interactions will deposit the energy in the crystal (desired), whereas Compton scattering may result in photons entering adjacent detectors, contributing to misreads.

The visible-light photons that are produced in the detector crystals are in turn detected by a photomultiplier tube, which converts the energy of these photons into an electrical pulse. This pulse is amplified and sorted by a pulse-height analyzer. The photomultiplier tube only accepts photons within a certain energy window (usually 350–650 keV) to avoid scattered photons (which lose energy during Compton interactions as described above). The narrower this window, the more precise the energy discrimination is, but the lower the detection efficiency (the ability of the detector material to detect as many of the annihilation photons as possible). High detection efficiency allows scan times to be shorter and radiotracer doses to be lower. The detector elements are connected by a coincidence circuit with a window of 6–20 ns to ensure that a photon pair originates from the same positron annihilation. The pair of photons must be detected along a line, i.e., by two detectors that are facing each other. This line does not pass exactly through the site where the decay occurred because the positron travels ~1 mm before annihilation. For radionuclides with high energy (e.g., ^{15}O) the positron range is higher, and this can cause a blurring effect of several millimeters. For more commonly used radionuclides (e.g., ^{11}C and ^{18}F), the positron range is lower and the blurring effect is less than 0.2 mm. In this case, the photon range is therefore not a limiting factor in the resolution of PET systems used for humans.

An annihilation can arise anywhere along the line connecting a pair of detectors, i.e., the PET camera is not able to determine the exact location where the event occurred, only that it occurred somewhere along a certain line connecting two detectors. Although the annihilating photons will be at close to a 180° angle, this is approximate because any residual momentum that the positron–electron pair has before annihilation will cause the angle to be slightly less than or more than 180°, a phenomenon called noncolinearity. The blurring effect of noncolinearity is amplified in large diameter PET cameras, and for human cameras the blurring effects due to noncolinearity can be up to 2 mm.

All the counts from all the detector pairs over the course of a PET scan are combined through a process called computed tomography, an algorithm that computes cross-sectional images that approach the actual concentration of radioactivity in the tissue. This allows the event count for each pixel to be determined, which in turn is used to construct a three-dimensional image of radioactivity in the organ or tissue. The PET image can be co-registered to a magnetic resonance (MR) image of the same brain, and, because MR has higher resolution, facilitate region-of-interest analysis.

PET measurements of radiation emitted from a radiotracer in the brain can be static (a continuous measure of radioactivity during a certain amount of time) or dynamic, i.e., a sequence of contiguous acquisitions which can each last anywhere from 10 s to over 20 min.

Longer acquisition times have better counting statistics but poor temporal resolution, while shorter acquisitions have better temporal resolution, but are noisier. In dynamic PET imaging, data from each "frame" is independently reconstructed to form a set of images. This allows for a measurement of the change in radioactivity in the brain over time. List-mode data acquisitions directly use the arrival time to estimate a dynamic range, and this approach provides extremely high temporal resolution with full spatial resolution.

1.5. Data Correction

As mentioned above, several corrections must be applied to ensure that each voxel value represents (as close as possible) the real tissue radioactivity concentration. Because detector pairs may have different detection efficiencies, a calibration process called *normalization* is used. A "phantom" (a cylinder that emits positrons in a homogeneous manner) is placed in the PET camera and any differences in measured radioactivity will be used to calibrate (normalize) the detector pairs before the PET camera is used for brain scans. As described above, annihilation photons undergo attenuation when traversing a tissue. A *transmission scan*, in which an external radioactive beam goes through the organ to be imaged (e.g., the head), is acquired to measure how much different parts of the organ attenuate radioactivity. This is often done before the emission scan (the scan which measures radioactivity emitted from the radiotracer). If no direct measurement of attenuation is performed (i.e., no transmission scan), attenuation correction can be done using a mathematical model. Several methods are used to correct for scatter, and a description of these is beyond the scope of this chapter. Additional corrections are performed for *random coincidences* (two photons that reach a detector pair within the time window, but which do not originate from the same annihilation event) and for *dead time* (the time it takes for the PET camera to process an event, a time during which another event cannot be detected).

In Subheading 2 of this chapter we provide two protocols, one for a radiotracer used in functional brain imaging (i.e., imaging of a metabolic or biochemical process) and one for a radiotracer used in molecular imaging (i.e., imaging of a target molecule). The following sections apply mostly to radiotracers used in molecular imaging.

1.6. Radiotracer Kinetics

After intravenous administration, a radiotracer will distribute throughout the body according to its biophysical and biochemical properties (e.g., lipophilicity, protein binding, etc.), and it will undergo metabolism depending on its chemical structure. Metabolism of most radiotracers, as is the case with most pharmaceuticals, occurs in the liver; rarely a radiotracer can undergo metabolism in the brain. When a radiotracer is metabolized, sometimes a lipophilic radioactive metabolite can cross the BBB and contribute to non-specific binding. If the radiometabolite does not cross the BBB, the measurements of radioactivity in blood and plasma will determine how much is due to the "parent" radiotracer and how much is due to the metabolite. Parent radiotracer in the blood that is "free" (i.e., non-protein-bound) is available to diffuse across the BBB into the brain parenchyma. Similarly, free (non-target-bound) radiotracer in the brain parenchyma can diffuse back across the BBB and enter the bloodstream again. At equilibrium, those two will be equal (i.e., free plasma radiotracer concentration = free tissue radiotracer concentration). Since the plasma concentration can be measured, we can calculate how much of radioactivity in the brain is due to free tissue radiotracer concentration and how much is due to bound radiotracer. The *input function* is a measure of the time-course of radioactivity in the blood or plasma (usually obtained through arterial and/or venous blood sampling). The input function is used to calculate how much radiotracer is available for uptake into the brain, so that the measurements of radioactivity in the brain can be used to estimate the total binding, which, when taking into account the amount of non-specific binding, can be used to estimate the availability of the target molecule.

If a radiotracer does not undergo metabolism in the brain and radioactive metabolites do not cross the BBB, the concentration of the radiotracer in the brain (and hence the amount of radiation emitting from the brain that will be measured by the PET camera) will depend on: (1) how much radiotracer is available to enter the brain from the blood, and (2) the affinity of the radiotracer for the target molecule. However, not all the radioactivity in the brain represents specific binding because in addition to binding to the target molecule, the radiotracer also binds to other molecules; the latter is called non-specific binding (see below). The ratio of specific and non-specific binding will influence the signal-to-noise ratio of a radiotracer. That is, an ideal radiotracer should bind specifically to the target molecule with high affinity and have very low affinity for all other molecules. With such a radiotracer, the level of radioactivity in the brain relative to that in blood would correlate very closely with the density of the target molecule in the brain.

1.7. Specific, Non-specific, and Non-displaceable Binding

Non-specific binding refers to the fact that radiotracers bind to molecules other than the target. This binding will contribute to the overall radioactive signal from the brain and therefore must be taken into account to allow a more precise estimate of specific binding and target molecule availability. One way of determining the fraction of total binding that is attributable to non-specific binding is to administer "cold" (i.e., non-radioactive) radiotracer that will displace the "hot" radiotracer from the target molecule by competitive binding. That is, such displacement only reduces specific binding, while it has minimal effect on non-specific binding and on free tissue radiotracer concentration. The difference in total binding between when only "hot" radiotracer is administered and when a high dose of "cold" radiotracer is co-administered indicates the specific (or displaceable) binding. The binding that remains, also known as non *non-displaceable binding* because high doses of cold radiotracer is not able to further decrease total binding by displacing the hot radiotracer, is the sum of non-specific binding and free tissue concentration. During the characterization of a new radiotracer, studies are conducted mostly in non-human primates to determine the level of non-displaceable binding. This information is later included in mathematical models of tracer kinetics (tracer kinetic modeling) that are used to quantify the level of specific binding in a PET study.

For certain target molecules, endogenous molecules compete with the radiotracer. For instance, if a neurotransmitter binds to a receptor, it will compete with and displace the radiotracer (and vice versa) depending on each molecule's affinity for the receptor. This phenomenon can be used to estimate changes in levels of endogenous ligands, e.g., dopamine. If an experimental intervention increases endogenous levels of dopamine, this will cause a reduction in the binding of a dopamine receptor radiotracer (because more dopamine displaces more radiotracer), and this can be measured using PET imaging (see for example ref. (1)).

Several measures of radiotracer binding are used in the literature; however, increasingly the field is moving towards a consensus nomenclature (2). A detailed description of measures of binding is beyond the scope of this chapter; however, one frequently used measure is *volume of distribution* (V_T), which refers to the ratio of how many milliliters of blood contain the same amount of radiotracer as 1 cm^3 of brain tissue. For instance, a $V_T = 20$ mL/cm^3 means that 20 mL of plasma has the same amount of radiotracer as 1 cm^3 of brain, i.e., the concentration in the brain is 20 times higher than in plasma. (Even though mL and cm^3 are both measures of volume and V_T is therefore technically unitless, the units of V_T are maintained.) As described above, the reason the concentration is higher in the brain is because the radiotracer binds to molecules in the brain and less free radiotracer is available to diffuse back into the bloodstream. However, V_T does not indicate whether the radiotracer in the brain is specifically bound. Within the brain, binding may occur to the target molecule, to other molecules, or not at all (free tissue radiotracer); therefore, V_T indicates the total amount of radiotracer in the tissue (specifically bound, non-specifically bound, and free). For a radiotracer that diffuses freely across the BBB, at equilibrium the concentration of free tissue radiotracer equals the concentration of free (non-protein-bound) plasma radiotracer. Therefore, at equilibrium, V_T = specific + non-specific binding. For a detailed discussion of the relationship between V_T and binding potential, please see ref. (2).

1.8. Basics of Psychoneuro-immunology

This brief overview of brain-immune interactions is provided so that this chapter can be a stand-alone resource. Readers familiar with this area may skip this part and continue with the Subheading 2.

It is well known that systemic inflammation can have profound effects on the brain. The impact on the brain, and the pathways through which this occurs, depends in part on the severity of systemic inflammation. For instance, in severe systemic inflammation, e.g., sepsis, the BBB can be disrupted, and leukocytes, inflammatory cytokines, and bacterial toxins can enter the brain parenchyma from the blood. This may lead to significant disruption of brain function, including neuronal death (3), which may explain why sepsis in humans is associated with long-term cognitive decline (4). In mild systemic inflammation, even though the BBB remains intact, there are measurable effects on the brain. This happens because the brain receives information from the rest of the body, including the immune system, so that it can coordinate the activities of various systems and organs. The immune system, when faced with "danger signals" (e.g., pathogen-associated molecules or molecules indicative of tissue damage) releases inflammatory cytokines which have both local and systemic effects. The systemic effects include fever, activation of the hypothalamic-pituitary-adrenal (HPA) axis and the autonomic nervous system, and changes in behavior, emotions, and cognition, all effects that are mediated by the brain (5). The evolutionary purpose of these responses is believed to be the optimization of the ability of the immune system to fight off the pathogen, while minimizing collateral damage to tissues and organs, optimizing the chances of survival (6). The notion that the brain receives and interprets information from the immune system is supported by several lines of evidence. For instance, inflammatory cytokines released during viral infections are associated with changes in mood (7). After experimental exposure of human subjects to rhinovirus or influenza virus, blood levels of inflammatory cytokines predicted a reduction in positive affect the following day (8). Other mild immune stimuli are associated with an increase in depressive symptoms in humans (9–13). In the rodent literature, support for this is substantial and it shows us how the immune system communicates with the brain (14–17). One commonly used experimental paradigm in rodents is systemic administration of *endotoxin*, a component of the wall of gram-negative bacteria. Endotoxin binds to the Toll-like 4 receptor on innate immune cells, initiating an intracellular cascade that eventually leads to the release of inflammatory cytokines, e.g., tumor necrosis factor (TNF) and interleukin-6 (IL-6). These cytokines then signal to the brain, leading to a constellation of behaviors similar to depression in humans: anhedonia, decreases in novelty-induced and social behaviors, reduced food intake, and sleep disturbance (18). Depending on the dose of endotoxin used, depressive-like behaviors in rodents may continue after the acute sickness behavior ends (19). Such delayed effects from immune stimuli may occur because increased brain and peripheral levels of cytokines can last for several weeks (20, 21). Endotoxin administration in humans also produces depressive-like symptoms, e.g., fatigue and anhedonia (22). The endothelium of the BBB plays an essential role in mediating inflammatory signals from the bloodstream to the brain parenchyma (23, 24). The luminal surface of BBB endothelial cells has receptors for inflammatory cytokines and for endotoxin; binding of any of these triggers a nuclear factor κB-dependent pathway (25, 26), which allows transduction of the signal across the BBB. In addition to the endothelium, the brain can also detect peripheral inflammatory signals through afferent vagal fibers (27–29). Ultimately, systemic inflammation in rodents induces expression of inflammatory mediators in brain parenchyma (16). This has also been demonstrated in human and non-human primates (30, 31). It is therefore reasonable to assume that immune-to-brain pathways are similar in rodents and humans. In addition to the effects of the immune system on the brain, the brain can modulate immune responses. One important anti-inflammatory pathway is the HPA axis, activation of which leads to release of cortisol, which has potent anti-inflammatory effects (32). The efferent vagus also exerts anti-inflammatory effects through the release of acetylcholine, which may act directly on nicotinic receptors on immune cells (33) or through the activation of the splenic nerve with release of anti-inflammatory norepinephrine in the spleen (34). Therefore, the communication between the brain and the immune system can be viewed as a loop, in which the immune system provides information to the brain about immune events in the body, and the brain uses this information to modulate the immune system. Whether dysregulation in these pathways plays a role in the pathogenesis of psychiatric disorders, in particular depression, is a topic of great interest and controversy (5).

2. Materials

2.1. Materials Required for the Molecular Imaging Protocol

1. Nitrogen gas containing 1% oxygen (for generation of (^{11}C)CO_2 in the cyclotron).
2. Helium (carrier gas for the cyclotron).
3. Hydrogen (reagent for the reduction of (^{11}C)CO_2 to (^{11}C)CH_4).
4. Shimalite-Ni (catalyst for the above reduction).
5. Gas-phase iodine (reagent for the MicroLab for the generation of (^{11}C)CH_3I).
6. *N*,*N*-Dimethylformamide (anhydrous).
7. Tetrabutylammonium hydroxide (1.0 M solution in methanol).
8. Aqueous HCl (0.3 N and 1 mN).

9. HPLC mobile phase (32% acetonitrile/68% buffer solution of 10 mM ammonium formate with 10 mM formic acid, v/v).
10. Semi-preparative HPLC columns (Onyx Monolithic C18, 100 mm × 10.0 mm, Phenomenex).
11. Waters Classic C18 SepPak cartridges.
12. USP absolute ethanol.
13. USP 0.9% NaCl solution.
14. USP 4.2% sodium bicarbonate solution.
15. Deionized water.
16. Liquid nitrogen (for cooling of reactor during trapping of $(^{11}C)CH_3I$ in the precursor solution).
17. Sterile membrane filters (33 mm diameter, 0.22 μm pore size, Millex® GV, Millipore).
18. Sterile empty collection vial, 10 mL.
19. Analytical HPLC mobile phase (44% acetonitrile/56% 0.1 M ammonium formate (v/v)).
20. HPLC column for quality control analysis (Gemini C18(2), 4.6 mm × 250 mm, 5 μm, Phenomenex).

3. Methods

3.1. Functional Imaging with FDG-PET

Functional imaging refers to a brain imaging modality that is used to obtain an estimate of cellular (neuronal) activity. If a disease state or an experimental intervention is associated with changes in neuronal activity, one can use functional imaging to measure this and identify the brain regions involved. An important caveat is that functional imaging cannot distinguish between neuronal activity and that of other cells in the brain (e.g., astrocytes). One commonly used form of functional imaging is functional MR imaging (fMRI), in which MR is used to measure changes in oxygenated blood in the brain. The assumption is that an increase in regional blood flow (which is under tight physiologic control) is indicative of increased metabolic demand and therefore increased cellular activity in a brain region. Functional imaging can also be performed with PET. In this case, a molecule that is used metabolically by cells, e.g., oxygen or glucose, is labeled with a radionuclide, and PET imaging is used to measure changes in the utilization of this molecule. For instance, fluorine-18-labeled 2-deoxy-d-glucose (FDG) is commonly used, both clinically (oncology) and in research (neuroscience). Deoxyglucose, like glucose, is transported across the BBB and taken up by cells in the brain. Inside cells both the molecules are phosphorylated by the enzyme hexokinase and converted to FDG-6-PO_4 and glucose-6-PO_4, respectively. Unlike glucose-6-PO_4 which enters the process of glycolysis, FDG-6-PO_4 is not a substrate of the enzyme phosphoglucose isomerase or any other enzyme inside the cell; it therefore gets "stuck" inside the cell. The biological half-life of FDG is therefore very long, which means that the effective half-life is equivalent to the physical half-life of ^{18}F (110 min). In other words, FDG will emit positrons for several hours after it was administered to the subject, and this radioactivity will occur in the cells which took up FDG shortly after it was administered. This is an advantage in study design (see below). The amount of FDG taken up by a given cell depends approximately on how much glucose that cell needs in that moment, a process that is believed to be tightly regulated. That is, the degree of FDG uptake is proportional to the metabolic activity of the cell at the time of FDG administration. Therefore, the radioactive signal detected from a certain brain region is an indication of the metabolic activity in that region at the time of FDG administration. The underlying assumption is that a significant proportion of this emission is due to neuronal activity. Although astrocytes are less metabolically active than neurons, because astrocytes are up to ten times more numerous than neurons, they account for a large proportion of the FDG signal. A detailed discussion of the theoretical underpinnings of FDG imaging is beyond the scope of this chapter, but there are several excellent review papers available, e.g., ref. (35).

The fact that the signal from FDG can be detected with a PET camera several hours after injection, while the amount of radiation (e.g., the FDG uptake) depends on the metabolic activity at the moment of injection, is an advantage of FDG-PET over fMRI. This allows us to use FDG-PET imaging to measure neuronal activity while the subject is not in the scanner. One can take advantage of this property of FDG and design research studies in which a subject undergoes an experimental intervention that cannot be performed in the scanner but during which the injection of FDG can allow us to "capture" metabolic activity at that time. Another factor in the decision to use FDG-PET over fMRI for functional imaging is whether the measurement of absolute metabolism, rather than relative changes in blood flow, is important for the study question. With FDG-PET, provided that one has an appropriate input function (either through an arterial line or cardiac imaging; see below) one can obtain precise estimates of absolute glucose utilization in brain regions of interest. (fMRI compares blood flow between two different states, but does not give an absolute value of metabolism.) One important advantage of fMRI over FDG-PET is cost; the latter is several times more expensive.

FDG was approved by FDA in 1994; therefore, unlike most other PET radiotracers, its use in human subjects does not require an FDA investigational new drug application (IND). There are a few examples in the literature of the use of FDG-PET imaging in psychoneuroimmunology research. For instance, Semmler et al.

used FDG-PET in rats that received high doses of endotoxin and found that systemic inflammation was associated with a global reduction in metabolism, especially in the cortex, and that this correlated with necrosis in post-mortem samples (3). Capuron et al. used FDG-PET to measure changes in glucose metabolism in patients who received treatment with interferon-alpha, a mild, iatrogenic, inflammatory stimulus that is associated with emergence of depressive symptoms, and found that changes in glucose metabolism in the nucleus accumbens and putamen correlated with interferon-induced fatigue (36). Our group used FDG-PET to measure changes in glucose metabolism in human subjects who received endotoxin, which induces a state of transient systemic inflammation as described above. We found increased metabolism in the insula and reduced metabolism in the cingulate.

3.1.1. Protocol for FDG-PET

In addition to common exclusion criteria used in human subjects research, some additional screening procedures that are specific to PET and MRI include:

1. Ensure that the subjects are medically healthy and that the PET imaging procedures will not put them at undue risk.
2. Exclude subjects with any medical or psychiatric condition that may affect brain glucose metabolism.
3. Use a pregnancy test for women at screening and before each radiotracer injection, and advise women subjects to avoid getting pregnant while participating in the study.
4. Screen for MR contraindications, e.g., metal implants, a history of metalwork, etc., since an MR is required to properly analyze the PET scan.

3.1.2. Endotoxin Administration in Human Subjects

Endotoxin administration in humans requires a physician-sponsored IND application with FDA. For alternatives to endotoxin in human subjects research, see Note 1. Endotoxin for human use is provided by the NIH Clinical Center upon request (contact Dr. Anthony Suffredini). For the background on Clinical Center Reference Endotoxin (CCRE), see Note 2. Endotoxin vials should be stored in the refrigerator (2–8°C). The preparation of endotoxin for human use should be performed by a pharmacist.

1. Reconstitute vials with 5 mL of Sterile Water for Injection, USP. (When reconstituted as recommended, each milliliter contains 200 ng of Reference Endotoxin, 2 mg of lactose, and 200 μg of polyethylene glycol 6000. The vials do not contain a preservative; the reconstituted solution should be used within 24 h. Unused portions should be stored at –70°C).
2. Because endotoxin does not go into solution readily, intermittently shake the vial for 30 min by hand, or use a vortex shaker or equivalent.

3. Dilute the dose further with 0.9% sodium chloride for injection to a final volume of 3 mL so that the volume in the syringe is the same for each subject and with placebo.
4. Draw the reconstituted solution up in a syringe for administration.
5. Label syringe with subject name, date of birth, date of administration, and study ID number.
6. Use immediately or store in the refrigerator (2–8°C) for up to 24 h.
7. Administer the desired endotoxin dose as a 1-min IV bolus after subject preparation is complete and monitoring equipment is in place.

3.1.3. Subject Preparation and Monitoring

In advance of the PET sessions, each subject needs an MRI scan to allow for co-registration and PET image analysis.

1. Ask the subject fast overnight, but to drink plenty of water.
2. Ask the subject not to ingest any alcohol or take any over-the-counter medications for 48 h prior to the scan.
3. Record blood pressure, heart rate, and temperature upon arrival to the PET center.
4. Obtain urine for a pregnancy test for women subjects.
5. Obtain urine for drug and alcohol testing.
6. Insert one IV catheter in each forearm (see Notes 3 and 4).
7. Administer 500 mL of normal saline over 20 min to ensure hydration (this is required for endotoxin administration but not for FDG-PET).
8. Place cardiac leads and continuously monitor heart rate (this is required for endotoxin administration but not for FDG-PET).
9. Obtain any baseline blood samples or behavioral ratings.
10. Administer endotoxin or placebo as an IV bolus and flush with saline.
11. Record blood pressure and heart rate every 15 min for the first 2 h after endotoxin administration, then every 30 min thereafter, and record body temperature hourly (this is required for endotoxin administration but not for FDG-PET).
12. Perform behavioral ratings and obtain blood draws at desired intervals.

3.1.4. FDG-PET Image Acquisition

The following FDG-PET protocol is adapted from the one used at the Yale PET Center. The input function is derived from cardiac imaging rather than from an arterial line. If (^{18}F)FDG needs to be purchased, please see Note 5 for vendors.

1. Place subject in the PET camera feet first, supine, with arms outside the scanner so that the heart is in the field-of-view (FOV).
2. Select correct orientation for cardiac images ("supine" and "feet first").
3. Acquire 2-min positioning scan to ensure that the FOV contains the left ventricle (LV).
4. Display image in a "volume tool" window.
5. Adjust bed if necessary.
6. Immobilize chest with a belt to minimize movement so that the region-of-interest (ROI) can be accurately placed in the LV during image analysis.
7. Acquire a 5-min transmission scan (for attenuation correction).
8. Inject 5.0 mCi ^{18}F-FDG via a pump over 1 min.
9. Acquire a 35-min dynamic 2D emission scan of the heart as ten 30-s frames followed by ten 180-s frames.
10. Starting at 15 min after FDG injection, obtain venous blood samples in heparinized (purple top) tubes every 5 min for a total of TEN samples (see details in Subheading 3.1.5 below).
11. Immediately after the end of the cardiac scan, move the subject out of the camera, turn the subject around so that the head is in the field of view and the arms along the side.
12. Immobilize patient's head using a chinstrap.
13. Acquire a 1-min positioning scan of the brain.
14. Display the image in a "volume tool" window to ensure the brain is in the FOV.
15. Adjust bed if necessary.
16. Acquire a 10-min 3D emission scan of the brain.
17. Acquire a 5-min transmission scan of the brain.
18. Remove the subject from the scanner. (At that time, depending on whether the subject requires further monitoring or the experiment involves further assessments, the IV lines may be removed and the subject can leave.)

3.1.5. Blood Processing

1. Prepare and weigh 20 Wizard gamma counter tubes (10 for whole blood and 10 for plasma).
2. At 15 min post-FDG injection, initiate venous blood sampling (~3 mL each) every 5 min (15, 20, 25, 30, 35, 40, 45, 50, 55, 60 min).

3. Obtain three samples for glucose determination during the FDG portion of the study. Standard glucose sample times are 15, 35, and 50 min post injection.
4. Put 2–3 drops of whole blood in pre-weighed Wizard tubes.
5. Weigh tubes with whole blood.
6. Centrifuge the rest of the whole blood samples for 10 min to separate plasma.
7. Pipette ~1 mL of plasma into pre-weighed Wizard tubes.
8. Weigh tubes with plasma.
9. Run whole blood samples on the gamma counter.
10. Run plasma samples in gamma counter.

3.1.6. FDG-PET Image Analysis

Reconstruction of the brain scan can be built into the protocol and is done after the brain transmission scan. The images are corrected for decay, attenuation, and scatter. Reconstruction parameters for the 3D brain scan are: method = iterative; image size = 128; iterations = 6; subsets = 16; zoom = 2; brain mode = off; offset (cm): *X* = 0.0, *Y* = 0.0; filter = butterworth; kernel FWHM(cm) = 6.0; butterworth filter order = 5; axial filtering = On; scatter correction = On.

Reconstruction of the dynamic heart emission scan is done after the acquisition of the brain scan. This reconstruction may take 2 h and needs to be done offline. Reconstruction parameters for the 2D heart scan are: method = iterative; image size = 256; iterations = 6, subsets = 16; zoom = 1; brain mode = off; offset (cm): *X* = 0.0, *Y* = 0.0; filter = butterworth; kernel FWHM(cm) = 6.0; butterworth filter order = 5; axial filtering = On; scatter correction = On.

1. Identify four non-adjacent (every other) left ventricular slices for region of interest (ROI) placement.
2. Draw an ROI in each of the four LV slices. The circular ROI should have a diameter of approximately 6 pixels (<2 cm).
3. Calculate the average LV time–activity curve from the time–activity curves derived from the ROI in each of the four slices.
4. Average the activity of plasma samples taken at 20, 25, 30, and 35 min.
5. Average the 25–35 min PET frames and allow identification of myocardial FDG uptake.
6. Divide 6 by 7.
7. Use this ratio to scale the 40–60-min blood sample concentrations.
8. Append the scaled 40–60-min samples to the LV curve to complete the input function.
9. Smooth the tail of the input function by fitting sum of exponentials starting at the 5-min post FDG injection time-point.

10. Reslice individual MPRAGE MR data to match the spatial orientation of brain PET image data and extract non-brain tissue.
11. Co-register the individual PET image to the subject's MR using a six-parameter linear registration.
12. Define ROIs manually in each individual, or use an automated anatomical labeling (AAL) template, e.g., (37).
13. Generate parametric images of rCMRGlu using the input function and the reconstructed brain tomographic data.
14. Calculate whole-brain FDG uptake using the MR-based template.
15. Generate regional CMRGlu (rCMRGlu; mg·100/g min) values for ROIs (for absolute vs. relative glucose metabolism, see Note 6).

3.2. Molecular PET Imaging

Molecular or receptor imaging refers to the use of PET (or SPECT) imaging to measure the availability of specific receptors or other molecules of interest (e.g., neurotransmitter transporters, cell-specific markers). These radiotracers are designed to bind to a specific molecule so that its distribution and density can be measured in vivo. Although some radiotracers are commercially available, the majority of radiotracers that have been developed at PET facilities around the world require on-site synthesis. The molecular imaging protocol described here involves (^{11}C)PBR28, a radiotracer that binds to a molecule found mostly in microglia; a brief description of these cells and the molecular target is therefore provided next as background.

3.2.1. Microglia

Microglia (resident macrophages of the brain) are involved in a variety of physiologic and pathologic processes; most importantly, in the initiation and maintenance of neuroinflammation. When provided with molecular signals from neurons, astrocytes, pathogens, or tissue damage, resting microglia become activated and release substances that can cause neuronal dysfunction and damage, e.g., inflammatory cytokines and reactive oxygen species (38), by interfering with neurotransmission, inhibiting neuroplasticity, and causing neuronal death (39). Microglia can also be activated by systemic inflammation. For instance, peripheral administration of endotoxin in rodents is associated with activation of microglia (3, 20). Once stimulated, microglia can stay activated for several months and continue to express inflammatory mediators (20, 39, 40). Activation of microglia by endotoxin or inflammatory cytokines leads to further release of inflammatory cytokines and other potentially neurotoxic substances (39), while exposure to anti-inflammatory cytokines induces a neuroprotective microglial phenotype (41–43). Because of the pivotal role that microglia play in a variety of neurodegenerative,

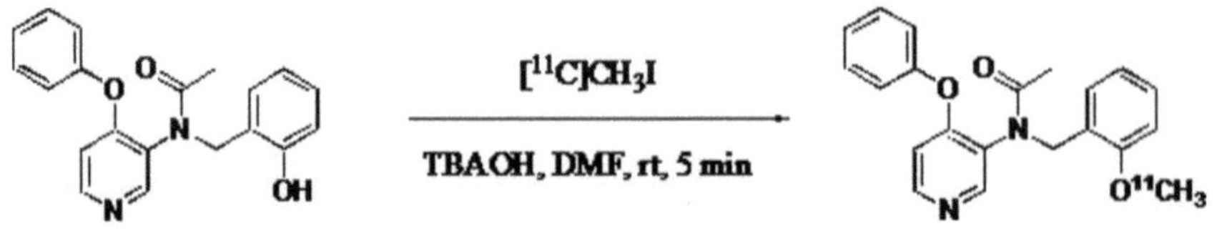

Fig. 2. Synthesis of (^{11}C)PBR28. The radiotracer (^{11}C)PBR28 is synthesized by ^{11}C-methylation of its precursor, *N*-(2-hydroxybenzyl)-*N*-(4-phenoxypyridin-3-yl)acetamide, or desmethyl PBR28, with (^{11}C)CH_3I generated from cyclotron-produced (^{11}C)CO_2. *DMF* dimethylformamide; *TBAOH* tetrabutylammonium hydroxide.

neuroinflammatory, and ischemic disorders of the brain, the ability to measure the activation of microglia in vivo with PET imaging is an area of great interest.

3.2.2. Translocator Protein

The Translocator Protein (TSPO) is an 18-kDa mitochondrial protein that is expressed in steroid-synthesizing cells, in which its role is to allow transport of cholesterol across the mitochondrial membranes. The expression of TSPO is very low in healthy brain tissue, but it increases in pathologies associated with microglial activation including stroke, trauma, infection, and autoimmune and neurodegenerative disorders (44, 45); therefore PET imaging of TSPO can be used to measure microglial activation in various disease states (46). Several PET radiotracers that bind to TSPO are available (47). One such radiotracer recently developed at NIH is (^{11}C)PBR28 (48, 49). The 20-min half-life of ^{11}C permits multiple measurements of microglial activation within a short time period, which allows for a variety of research design options. Our group used this radiotracer to measure binding to TSPO at various times after endotoxin administration in baboons, an example of which is illustrated in Fig. 2. The protocol for this is described below.

3.2.3. (^{11}C)PBR28 Synthesis

(^{11}C)PBR28 is a 348.40-kDa TSPO-specific radiotracer developed by Robert Innis' group at NIMH (48). The precursor can be obtained by request. Due to the short half-life of ^{11}C, (^{11}C)PBR28 must be synthesized on-site (for an ^{18}F alternative, see Note 7). The synthesis described (Fig. 3) is an adaptation used at the Yale PET Center radiochemistry lab, under the direction of Yu-Shin Ding, PhD.

1. In a cyclotron, produce no-carrier-added (^{11}C)CO_2 using the $^{14}N(p,\alpha)^{11}C$ reaction (bombardment of a target of nitrogen gas containing 1% oxygen).
2. Produce (^{11}C)CH_3I from (^{11}C)CO_2 via catalytic hydrogenation to (^{11}C)CH_4 followed by reaction with gas phase iodine in a MicroLab (^{11}C)CH_3I generation apparatus.
3. Synthesize (^{11}C)PBR28 by ^{11}C-methylation of the desmethyl precursor, *N*-(2-hydroxybenzyl)-*N*-(4-phenoxypyridin-3-yl) acetamide, with (^{11}C)CH_3I in a TRACERLab™ FxC automated

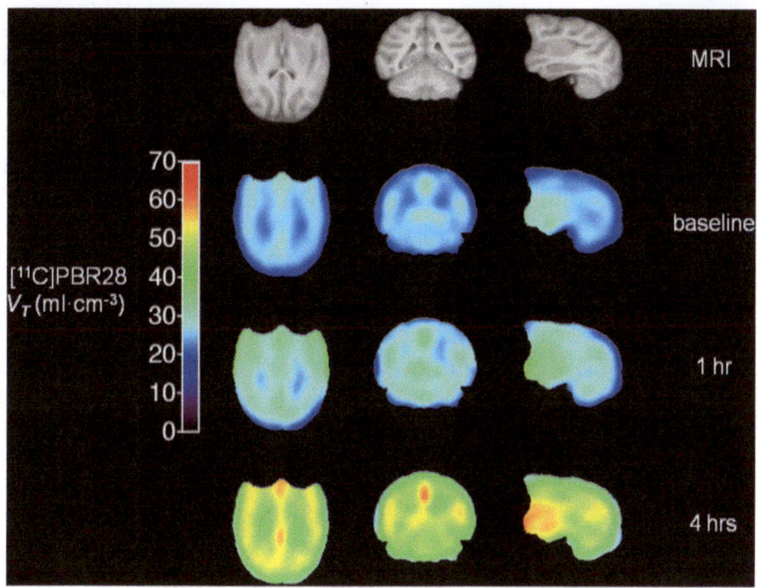

Fig. 3. Changes in (^{11}C)PBR28 binding after endotoxin administration. A baboon was scanned with (^{11}C)PBR28 at baseline, and again 1 and 4 h after receiving intravenous endotoxin administration (0.1 mg/kg). The total volume of distribution increased approximately twofold 4 h after endotoxin administration, indicating an increase in microglial activation.

synthesis module (GE Medical Systems) or equivalent system (see Note 8 for synthesis in an AutoLoop module).

4. Deliver (^{11}C)CH_3I into a solution consisting of the desmethyl PBR28 precursor (0.5 ± 0.1 mg) in dimethylformamide (0.15 mL) and tetrabutylammonium hydroxide (1.0 M solution in methanol).
5. When radioactivity peaks in the reactor vial, allow the reaction to proceed for 5 min at room temperature.
6. Dilute the reaction mixture with a mixture of 0.5 mL of 0.3 N aqueous HCl and 0.5 mL of semi-preparative HPLC mobile phase (32% acetonitrile/68% buffer solution of 10 mM ammonium formate with 10 mM formic acid, v/v).
7. Load the diluted mixture onto a semi-preparative HPLC column (Onyx Monolithic C18, 100 mm × 10.0 mm, Phenomenex) and elute with the mobile phase at a flow rate of 3 mL/min.
8. Monitor the HPLC eluent by tandem radioactivity and UV ($\lambda = 254$ nm) detectors.
9. Collect the radioactivity fraction eluted between 15 and 17 min.
10. Dilute this fraction with 50 mL of water and load onto a Waters Classic C18 SepPak cartridge.
11. Rinse the SepPak cartridge with 10 mL of 1 mM aqueous HCl and dry with inert gas flow.

12. Elute the product off the SepPak cartridge with 1 mL of USP absolute ethanol, followed by 3 mL of USP saline, into a product vial containing 7 mL of USP saline and 40 μL of 4.2% sodium bicarbonate, USP.
13. Filter the content in the product vial through a sterile membrane filter (33 mm diameter, 0.22 μm pore size, Millex® GV, Millipore) into a sterile assembly comprised of a 1 mL sterile quality control vial connected to a vented 10 mL sterile dose vial.

3.2.4. PBR28 Quality Control

Determine specific activity, chemical purity, and radiochemical purity of the radiotracer by HPLC analysis. A Shimadzu LC-20AT Prominence system equipped with a SPD-M20A Diode Array detector or SPD-20A UV/Vis detector (230 nm) connected in series with a Bioscan Flow-Count gamma-detector can be used for quality control analysis.

1. Elute the Gemini C18 analytical column (5 μm, 4.6 mm × 250 mm) with 44% acetonitrile/56% 0.1 M ammonium formate (v/v) at a flow rate of 2 mL/min.
2. Monitor the product for radioactivity and UV absorbance at 230 nm ($t_R = 6.7$ min).
3. Determine the specific activity of (^{11}C)PBR28 at 230 nm by counting an aliquot in a dose calibrator for radioactivity and determine the mass by HPLC against a calibration curve of authentic reference standard.
4. Confirm the identity of the product by co-injecting the product with the reference standard and co-eluting the UV and radioactivity peaks on the HPLC chromatogram.

3.2.5. Protocol for Animal Preparation

The protocol described is for use in baboons because the dose of endotoxin is high; however, (^{11}C)PBR28 can also be used for lower dose endotoxin experiments in humans if an IND is obtained (both for the use of endotoxin and for the use of the radiotracer). The use of baboons (as opposed to rodents) in PET imaging is advantageous because of the similarity with human brain size and receptor systems, and because the body size, peripheral metabolism, and clearance allow for quantification through kinetic modeling; however, PET imaging of microglial activation can also be performed in rodents.

1. Equipment needed: physiological monitor, anesthesia machine/vaporizer, heating pad, emergency drug kit, stereotactic head holder, lines for vacuum pumps, oxygen tanks.
2. Fast the animal overnight prior to each study day.
3. Anesthetize with ketamine (10 mg/kg i.m.).
4. In the same syringe, administer glycopyrrolate (5–10 μg/kg), a peripheral antimuscarinic agent that reduces secretions.

5. Connect monitoring equipment (heart rhythm, respiratory rate, blood pressure, rectal temperature).
6. Perform endotracheal intubation and maintain on ~2% isoflurane.
7. Monitor end-tidal pCO_2 continuously.
8. Insert an arterial line in the femoral artery for measurement of the input function.
9. Insert an i.v. catheter in the posterior tibial vein for administration of fluids, radiotracer, and endotoxin.
10. Monitor heart rate, oxygen saturation, and end-tidal pCO_2 continuously.
11. Record blood pressure at least every 15 min.
12. Record body temperature every 30 min.

3.2.6. Protocol for Endotoxin Administration

The baboon endotoxin model was chosen because it is physiologically and immunologically very similar to human sepsis (50). Female baboons (*Papio anubis*) were ovariohysterectomized at least 3 months prior to the study because estrogen can affect TSPO expression (45). Endotoxin preparation is similar to that for humans described above; however, the source of endotoxin is different.

1. Prepare a solution of endotoxin sufficient to administer a dose of 0.1 mg/kg body weight.
2. Dissolve endotoxin (lipopolysaccharides from *E. coli* serotype O111:B4, Sigma, St. Louis, MO) in saline.
3. A vortex will facilitate dissolution (this may take up to 30 min).
4. Administer as an i.v. bolus in a leg vein and flush with saline to ensure complete delivery.

3.2.7. Protocol for PET Imaging in Baboons

1. Position the anesthetized baboon's head using a modified Rhesus stereotaxic head holder with a #3 mouth bite.
2. Acquire a 6-min transmission scan (for attenuation correction).
3. Immediately before radiotracer injection, obtain 5 mL venous blood to estimate plasma protein binding. Keep sample at room temperature.
4. Administer 5 mCi of (^{11}C)PBR28 with an infusion pump (max mass per injection: 0.25 μg/kg).
5. Acquire dynamic PET images (33 frames over 2 h).
6. Acquire a second 6-min transmission scan after the emission scan.
7. Draw blood samples at 0.75, 1.5, 2.25, 3, 3.75, 4.5, 5.25, 6, 8, 19, 15, 20, 25, 30, 40, 50, 60, 75, 90, 105, and 120 min after (^{11}C)PBR28 injection to measure the time course of

radiotracer and its radioactive metabolites in blood. Maximum total volume of blood = 1% of body weight.

8. Label and pre-weigh 64 Wizard tubes and divide into five groups: whole blood ($n=21$), plasma ($n=21$), acetonitrile extraction ($n=7$), saline standard ($n=6$), and blood standard ($n=9$). The two standards will be created and processed as if they were blood samples.
9. For the saline standard, there will be a total of six samples: three samples of "plasma" and three ultrafiltrate samples (see below). For the blood standard, there will be nine samples: three whole blood, three plasma, and three ultrafiltrate.
10. Count ~5 drops (or 100 μL) of whole blood on the Wizard gamma counter in a pre-weighed tube. Be sure to get blood in the bottom. Counting time is 120 s with a 10,000 counts per second (cps) threshold.
11. Centrifuge whole blood samples collected in potassium EDTA tubes at 3,900 × g for 5 min to separate plasma.
12. After centrifugation, take 0.1 mL of plasma to count directly on the Wizard Counter in a pre-weighed tube. Counting time is 120 s with a 10,000 cps threshold.

3.2.8. Metabolite HPLC Analysis

1. Mix the plasma sample with urea.
2. Load the clear sample onto filter.
3. Take 0.1 mL of filtrated sample and count on the Wizard Counter.
4. After filtration, the filter should also be counted.
5. Inject 5 mL into the HPLC loop.
6. The mobile phase consists of: 1:99% 10 mM ammonium bicarbonate:1% acetonitrile; 2:65% 0.1% ammonium hydroxide: 35% acetonitrile.

For each run, count all fractions on the same counter. Count time: 60 s for 5, 15, and 30 min samples, and 90 s for 60 and 90 min samples.

3.2.9. Protein Binding

This will be performed in triplicate on the saline standard and the blood standard, after centrifugation. Pipette ~0.1 mL of whole blood into the three tubes for the blood standard and spin. For both standards:

1. Pipette 0.1 mL of spiked plasma into each tube.
2. Pipette 0.3 mL of spiked plasma into the top of three ultrafiltrate tubes (Centrifree Micropartion Devices No. 4104, Amicon).
3. Centrifuge at 1,100 × g for 20 min.

4. Pipette ≥0.2 mL of filtrate (from the bottom of the ultrafiltrate unit, the top part pops off and can be discarded) from each unit and place into tubes.
5. Weigh and count these tubes.

3.2.10. PET Image Analysis

1. Prior to PET scans, acquire a T1-weighted coronal MR sequence for each baboon with a 3 T scanner. The MR will be used to assist with anatomical localization of ROIs.
2. Create a template MR image by averaging several individual baboon MR images after spatial normalization, using a normalized-mutual-information (NMI) linear plus nonlinear registration.
3. Warp the individual MRI to a baboon MRI template using a linear plus nonlinear NMI registration.
4. Reconstruct dynamic images from sinograms and correct for measured attenuation, normalization, random events, scatter, and deadtime with the attenuation-weighted ordered-subset-expectation-maximization (OSEM) algorithm (51).
5. Use blood samples to measure the time-course of total radioactivity and the parent fraction in plasma, i.e., the fraction of plasma radioactivity attributable to (^{11}C)PBR28.
6. Register the PET image to the MR image using the automated image registration algorithm as an initialization step.
7. Follow by two iterative registrations based on NMI.
8. Combine transformation parameters from the individual registrations (template-to-MRI and MRI-to-PET) and apply to the PET dynamic data.
9. Calculate mean radioactivity in each ROI for each frame as a function of time.
10. Generate each regional time–activity curve (TAC; results expressed as KBq/mL).
11. Fit TACs to the two-tissue compartmental model using the metabolite-corrected arterial plasma curve as input function.
12. Calculate volume of distribution (V_T) from the estimated model parameters for each ROI.

4. Notes

1. (From Subheading 3.1.2) Endotoxin administration is one of several methods that can be used to induce mild systemic inflammation in human subjects for research purposes (see for

review ref. (5)). Other immune stimuli that are frequently used include *typhoid vaccination* and *interferon-alpha* (which can be used as treatment or it can be administered to healthy subjects). The latter two are approved by FDA for human administration and do not therefore require approval beyond that of the local institutional review board.

2. (From Subheading 3.1.2) CCRE injectable dosage forms are manufactured by the Bureau of Biologics. CCRE is a purified lipopolysaccharide prepared from *Escherichia coli* O:113 (US Standard Reference Endotoxin) and vialed under good manufacturing practice guidelines. CCRE comes in 5-mL clear-glass vials, each containing a white, lyophilized powder which consists of 10,000 endotoxin units (approximately 1 μg of reference endotoxin), 10 mg of lactose, and 1 mg of polyethylene glycol 6000. The dose of endotoxin used in humans ranges from 0.2 to 4 ng/kg body weight. If the main purpose is to induce a state of mild systemic inflammation with subtle symptoms of depression, a dose of less than 1 ng/kg is recommended (5).
3. (From Subheading 3.1.3) When using two IV lines, use the one with the best flow for blood sampling and the other one for administration of the radiotracer and other drugs (e.g., endotoxin).
4. (From Subheading 3.1.3) If an arterial line is used for blood sampling for the input function in lieu of a cardiac scan, only one IV is required (for administration of radiotracer and drugs).
5. (From Subheading 3.1.4) If (^{18}F)FDG cannot be synthesized on site, it can be purchased from:
   (a) PETNET Solutions (http://www.petnetsolutions.com/index.html) with many locations throughout the US and in Great Britain.
   (b) IBA (http://www.iba-molecular.com/delivery-network) with locations in the US, Western Europe, Turkey, India, and South Korea.
6. (From Subheading 3.1.6) If there is no significant difference in whole-brain glucose metabolism between experimental or disease conditions, one can normalize regional absolute glucose metabolism to global absolute glucose metabolism to obtain relative values. In follow-up studies, relative glucose metabolism can be used, which obviates the need for an input function (i.e., the brain scan can be performed without a cardiac scan or arterial line).
7. (From Subheading 3.2.3) Due to the short half-life of ^{11}C, (^{11}C)PBR28 must be synthesized on-site. PBR06 (52) is a new, TSPO-specific radiotracer which, because the radionuclide is ^{18}F, could be synthesized at another facility and shipped to the

PET center (as is often done with FDG). Although PBR06 is not commercially available, this may be possible to arrange by collaboration with a different site that has the ability to synthesize (^{18}F)PBR06. Using (^{18}F)PBR06 does not allow multiple scans in 1 day, due to the long half-life of ^{18}F.

8. (From Subheading 3.2.3) (^{11}C)PBR28 can be synthesized using an AutoLoop™ module, which in our experience increases radioactivity yield by 2.5-fold compared to the FxC module. Dissolve the desmethyl PBR28 precursor (0.2–0.4 mg) in dimethylformamide (80–90 μL) and treat with tetrabutylammonium hydroxide (1.0 M solution in methanol). Vortex the mixture and mix well. At 3–5 min before the delivery of (^{11}C)CH_3I, load the solution into the stainless steel loop of an AutoLoop module housed within a hot cell. (^{11}C)CH_3I, prepared from a Microlab or an alternative generation device, is swept into the loop in a stream of argon gas (flow rate of 30 mL/min) until the radioactivity in the loop reaches a maximum. Allow the reaction to proceed in the loop for 5 min at room temperature. Flush the crude reaction mixture from the loop with the semi-preparative HPLC mobile phase (32% acetonitrile/68% buffer solution of 10 mM ammonium formate with 10 mM formic acid, v/v, at a flow rate of 3 mL/min) onto a HPLC column (Onyx Monolithic C18, 100 mm × 10.0 mm, Phenomenex). The subsequent steps are identical to the FxC synthesis described in Subheading 3.2.3.

Acknowledgments

The author thanks the following colleagues at the Yale PET Center for valuable inputs during the preparation of this chapter: Henry Huang, PhD; Keunpoong Lim, PhD; Jean-Dominique Gallezot, PhD; Beata Planeta-Wilson, MS; and Maria Corsi CNMT.

References

1. Morris ED, Constantinescu CC, Sullivan JM et al (2010) Noninvasive visualization of human dopamine dynamics from PET images. Neuroimage 51:135–144
2. Innis RB, Cunningham VJ, Delforge J et al (2007) Consensus nomenclature for in vivo imaging of reversibly binding radioligands. J Cereb Blood Flow Metab 27:1533–1539
3. Semmler A, Hermann S, Mormann F et al (2008) Sepsis causes neuroinflammation and concomitant decrease of cerebral metabolism. J Neuroinflammation 5:38
4. Iwashyna TJ, Ely EW, Smith DM et al (2010) Long-term cognitive impairment and functional disability among survivors of severe sepsis. JAMA 304:1787–1794
5. DellaGioia N, Hannestad J (2010) A critical review of human endotoxin administration as an experimental paradigm of depression. Neurosci Biobehav Rev 34:130–143

6. Raison CL, Capuron L, Miller AH (2006) Cytokines sing the blues: inflammation and the pathogenesis of depression. Trends Immunol 27:24–31
7. Bucks RS, Gidron Y, Harris P et al (2008) Selective effects of upper respiratory tract infection on cognition, mood and emotion processing: a prospective study. Brain Behav Immun 22:399–407
8. Janicki-Deverts D, Cohen S, Doyle WJ et al (2007) Infection-induced proinflammatory cytokines are associated with decreases in positive affect, but not increases in negative affect. Brain Behav Immun 21:301–307
9. Hermann DM, Mullington J, Hinze-Selch D et al (1998) Endotoxin-induced changes in sleep and sleepiness during the day. Psychoneuroendocrinology 23:427–437
10. Reichenberg A, Yirmiya R, Schuld A et al (2001) Cytokine-associated emotional and cognitive disturbances in humans. Arch Gen Psychiatry 58:445–452
11. Wright CE, Strike PC, Brydon L et al (2005) Acute inflammation and negative mood: mediation by cytokine activation. Brain Behav Immun 19:345–350
12. Eisenberger NI, Inagaki TK, Rameson LT et al (2009) An fMRI study of cytokine-induced depressed mood and social pain: the role of sex differences. Neuroimage 47:881–890
13. Capuron L, Fornwalt FB, Knight BT et al (2009) Does cytokine-induced depression differ from idiopathic major depression in medically healthy individuals? J Affect Disord 119:181–185
14. De La Garza R II (2005) Endotoxin- or pro-inflammatory cytokine-induced sickness behavior as an animal model of depression: focus on anhedonia. Neurosci Biobehav Rev 29:761–770
15. Dunn AJ, Swiergiel AH, de Beaurepaire R (2005) Cytokines as mediators of depression: what can we learn from animal studies? Neurosci Biobehav Rev 29:891–909
16. Pecchi E, Dallaporta M, Jean A et al (2009) Prostaglandins and sickness behavior: old story, new insights. Physiol Behav 97:279–292
17. Anisman H (2009) Cascading effects of stressors and inflammatory immune system activation: implications for major depressive disorder. J Psychiatry Neurosci 34:4–20
18. Larson SJ, Dunn AJ (2001) Behavioral effects of cytokines. Brain Behav Immun 15:371–387
19. Frenois F, Moreau M, O'Connor J et al (2007) Lipopolysaccharide induces delayed FosB/DeltaFosB immunostaining within the mouse extended amygdala, hippocampus and hypothalamus, that parallel the expression of depressive-like behavior. Psychoneuroendocrinology 32:516–531
20. Qin L, Wu X, Block ML et al (2007) Systemic LPS causes chronic neuroinflammation and progressive neurodegeneration. Glia 55:453–462
21. Moreau M, Andre C, O'Connor JC et al (2008) Inoculation of Bacillus Calmette-Guerin to mice induces an acute episode of sickness behavior followed by chronic depressive-like behavior. Brain Behav Immun 22:1087–1095
22. Hannestad J, DellaGioia N, Ortiz N et al (2011) Citalopram reduces endotoxin-induced fatigue. Brain Behav Immun 25:256–259
23. Gosselin D, Rivest S (2008) MyD88 signaling in brain endothelial cells is essential for the neuronal activity and glucocorticoid release during systemic inflammation. Mol Psychiatry 13:480–497
24. Ching S, Zhang H, Belevych N et al (2007) Endothelial-specific knockdown of interleukin-1 (IL-1) type 1 receptor differentially alters CNS responses to IL-1 depending on its route of administration. J Neurosci 27:10476–10486
25. Dauphinee SM, Karsan A (2006) Lipopolysaccharide signaling in endothelial cells. Lab Invest 86:9–22
26. Magder S, Neculcea J, Neculcea V et al (2006) Lipopolysaccharide and TNF-alpha produce very similar changes in gene expression in human endothelial cells. J Vasc Res 43:447–461
27. Kapas L, Hansen MK, Chang HY et al (1998) Vagotomy attenuates but does not prevent the somnogenic and febrile effects of lipopolysaccharide in rats. Am J Physiol 274:R406–R411
28. Opp MR, Toth LA (1998) Somnogenic and pyrogenic effects of interleukin-1beta and lipopolysaccharide in intact and vagotomized rats. Life Sci 62:923–936
29. Konsman JP, Luheshi GN, Bluthe RM et al (2000) The vagus nerve mediates behavioural depression, but not fever, in response to peripheral immune signals; a functional anatomical analysis. Eur J Neurosci 12:4434–4446
30. Reyes TM, Coe CL (1996) Interleukin-1 beta differentially affects interleukin-6 and soluble interleukin-6 receptor in the blood and central nervous system of the monkey. J Neuroimmunol 66:135–141
31. Raison CL, Borisov AS, Majer M et al (2009) Activation of central nervous system inflammatory pathways by interferon-alpha: relationship to monoamines and depression. Biol Psychiatry 65:296–303
32. Bierhaus A, Wolf J, Andrassy M et al (2003) A mechanism converting psychosocial stress into mononuclear cell activation. Proc Natl Acad Sci U S A 100:1920–1925
33. Pavlov VA, Tracey KJ (2005) The cholinergic anti-inflammatory pathway. Brain Behav Immun 19:493–499

34. Vida G, Pena G, Deitch EA et al (2011) Alpha7-cholinergic receptor mediates vagal induction of splenic norepinephrine. J Immunol 186: 4340–4346
35. Wienhard K (2002) Measurement of glucose consumption using ((18)F)fluorodeoxyglucose. Methods 27:218–225
36. Capuron L, Pagnoni G, Demetrashvili MF et al (2007) Basal ganglia hypermetabolism and symptoms of fatigue during interferon-alpha therapy. Neuropsychopharmacology 32:2384–2392
37. Tzourio-Mazoyer N, Landeau B, Papathanassiou D et al (2002) Automated anatomical labeling of activations in SPM using a macroscopic anatomical parcellation of the MNI MRI single-subject brain. Neuroimage 15:273–289
38. Tambuyzer BR, Ponsaerts P, Nouwen EJ (2009) Microglia: gatekeepers of central nervous system immunology. J Leukoc Biol 85:352–370
39. Block ML, Zecca L, Hong JS (2007) Microglia-mediated neurotoxicity: uncovering the molecular mechanisms. Nat Rev Neurosci 8:57–69
40. Maeda J, Higuchi M, Inaji M et al (2007) Phase-dependent roles of reactive microglia and astrocytes in nervous system injury as delineated by imaging of peripheral benzodiazepine receptor. Brain Res 1157: 100–111
41. Li L, Lu J, Tay SS et al (2007) The function of microglia, either neuroprotection or neurotoxicity, is determined by the equilibrium among factors released from activated microglia in vitro. Brain Res 1159:8–17
42. Hanisch UK, Kettenmann H (2007) Microglia: active sensor and versatile effector cells in the normal and pathologic brain. Nat Neurosci 10:1387–1394
43. Pinteaux E, Rothwell NJ, Boutin H (2006) Neuroprotective actions of endogenous interleukin-1 receptor antagonist (IL-1ra) are mediated by glia. Glia 53:551–556
44. Cosenza-Nashat M, Zhao ML, Suh HS et al (2009) Expression of the translocator protein of 18 kDa by microglia, macrophages and astrocytes based on immunohistochemical localization in abnormal human brain. Neuropathol Appl Neurobiol 35:306–328
45. Batarseh A, Papadopoulos V (2010) Regulation of translocator protein 18 kDa (TSPO) expression in health and disease states. Mol Cell Endocrinol 327:1–12
46. Venneti S, Lopresti BJ, Wiley CA (2006) The peripheral benzodiazepine receptor (translocator protein 18 kDa) in microglia: from pathology to imaging. Prog Neurobiol 80:308–322
47. Rupprecht R, Papadopoulos V, Rammes G et al (2010) Translocator protein (18 kDa) (TSPO) as a therapeutic target for neurological and psychiatric disorders. Nat Rev Drug Discov 9: 971–988
48. Brown AK, Fujita M, Fujimura Y et al (2007) Radiation dosimetry and biodistribution in monkey and man of 11 C-PBR28: a PET radioligand to image inflammation. J Nucl Med 48:2072–2079
49. Imaizumi M, Briard E, Zoghbi SS et al (2008) Brain and whole-body imaging in nonhuman primates of ((11)C)PBR28, a promising PET radioligand for peripheral benzodiazepine receptors. Neuroimage 39:1289–1298
50. Redl H, Bahrami S (2005) Large animal models: baboons for trauma, shock, and sepsis studies. Shock 24(suppl 1):88–93
51. Reader AJ, Visvikis D, Erlandsson K et al (1998) Intercomparison of four reconstruction techniques for positron volume imaging with rotating planar detectors. Phys Med Biol 43:823–834
52. Fujimura Y, Kimura Y, Simeon FG et al (2010) Biodistribution and radiation dosimetry in humans of a new PET ligand, (18)F-PBR06, to image translocator protein (18 kDa). J Nucl Med 51:145–149

Chapter 18

The Vaccination Model in Psychoneuroimmunology Research: A Review

Anna C. Phillips

Abstract

This chapter explores the reasoning behind using the vaccination model to examine the influence of psychosocial factors on immunity. It then briefly discusses the mechanics of the vaccination response and the protocols used in Psychoneuroimmunology vaccine research, before giving examples from the research literature of the studies examining relationships such as the association between stress and the vaccination response. It also explores the ways the vaccination model can be used to answer key questions in Psychoneuroimmunology, such as: "does it matter when stressful life events occur relative to when the vaccine is received?" "what are the effects of prior exposure to the antigen?" and "do other psychosocial factors influence vaccine response besides stress?" Finally, it briefly considers the mechanisms underlying psychosocial factors and vaccination response associations and the future research needed to understand these better, and indeed to use current and future knowledge to improve and enhance vaccine responses in key at risk populations.

Key words: Caregiving, Influenza, Interventions, Social support, Stress, Vaccine, Psychoneuroimmunology

1. Introduction: Why Study Vaccination in the Context of PNI Research?

1.1. Alternative Approaches: Enumerative Measures

There are many methods for examining the effects of psychological factors on immunity. Early work concentrated on the influence of psychosocial stress on enumerative measures of immunity. For example, individuals exposed to chronic stress showed reduced numbers of certain immune cells including reduced numbers of B-lymphocytes (1, 2), helper T-lymphocytes (1, 3, 4), cytotoxic T-lymphocytes (1, 5), natural killer (NK) cells (1, 5), and lowered concentrations of secretory immunoglobulin A in saliva (6–9), compared to matched controls. However, it is difficult to determine the clinical significance of such enumerative changes, given

Qing Yan (ed.), *Psychoneuroimmunology: Methods and Protocols*, Methods in Molecular Biology, vol. 934, DOI 10.1007/978-1-62703-071-7_18, that they lie within the normal range for healthy participants (10) and may simply reflect cell migration and recirculation rather than increased production or better function (10). Additionally, cell number changes could be a consequence of shifts in plasma volume and hemoconcentration; in such circumstances, changes in cell number would reflect increased density of a lymphocyte population rather than signal a true increase in absolute cell numbers. Further, even absolute changes in cell number might not necessarily reflect alteration in the capacity of the immune system to mount an effective response to antigenic challenge (10). Consequently, measuring changes in cell number is perhaps not the optimal means of determining variations in the functional capacity of the immune system, and hence the likely clinical implications of psychosocial variables for disease resistance and susceptibility.

1.2. In Vitro Measures

In vitro measures of immune function, such as cell proliferation to stimulation with an antigen (foreign material e.g., bacteria), or cell cytotoxicity (killing ability), have been argued to provide a better indication of the functional capacity of the immune system (10). These measures have been demonstrated to be susceptible to impairment by chronic stress in many studies, e.g., (11–15). Nevertheless, the isolated testing of any particular network of immune cells provides only limited information about the overall status of what is a highly integrated and complex system (10), and an imperfect understanding of the relationship between psychosocial factors and vulnerability to disease (16).

2. The Vaccination Model

2.1. Benefits of the Vaccination Model

A clinically relevant model which examines the impact of psychosocial factors on the integrated response of the immune system to a challenge would avoid these disadvantages. The antibody response to vaccination provides us with such a model. Vaccines act as real immune system challenges, although they are altered in such a way so not to induce disease either by being inactivated or killed, or only a component of the actual pathogen, so are really "imitation infections." Therefore, by measuring the antibody levels in response to vaccination we can assess directly how well the immune system responds to infectious challenge. It is also clinically relevant in that antibody levels or titers are directly related to susceptibility and resistance to infectious disease.

2.2. The Vaccination Response

The vaccination response involves the coordination of a wide variety of immune cells. Antigen is initially recognized and presented by professional antigen presenting cells, such as dendritic cells. Thus presented, the antigen is then recognized by specific helper T cells which process and present the antigen to B-cells, the antibody factories of the immune system; this is termed a thymus-dependent response. There are other types of vaccination which are also recognized by B-cells without the necessity for T-cell help, thus termed a thymus-independent response, which do not elicit as strong or maintained a response as thymus-dependent vaccines. A final type of vaccination, called a conjugate vaccination, is used to improve the response to thymus-independent antigens by attaching a protein to the antigen, which then stimulates an immune response involving helper T-cell recognition.

When stimulated by an antigen, B-lymphocytes replicate and mature into short lived plasma cells which produce the earliest antibody or immunoglobulin, IgM. In a primary response to an antigen not previously encountered, the peak IgM response occurs around 5 days after vaccination. Interaction between activated T- and B-cells leads to the production of high affinity or very specific antibodies in bodily fluids: IgG (found mainly in the blood) and IgA (found mainly at mucosal surfaces, e.g., in saliva). This more specific response peaks around 28 days after vaccination. Other types of antibody include IgE (part of the allergic response) and IgD. IgG is particularly important, as being the most prolific antigen in the blood and a more specific match to the particular antigen makes it more effective at antigen elimination. Secondary antibody responses, in which the immune system has been previously exposed to the antigen, are more rapid and of greater magnitude; this is because some activated T- and B-cells become long lived resting memory cells, remaining in the immune system ready to respond quickly to challenge with previously encountered antigens.

Not all individuals react with a strong antibody response to vaccination, particularly older adults who are only protected against influenza disease in 30–50% of cases following vaccination (17–20). Further, the increase in vaccination availability has not been paralleled by decreased influenza-related mortality (21). This variation in the vaccination response allows for the investigation of other factors which might influence this aspect of immunity between individuals. The relevance of the response to infectious disease risk provides the clinically relevant imperative to do so beyond the interest in increasing knowledge on how various factors affect immune function. As well as age, psychosocial factors, such as stress, may alter both the quantity and quality of antibody present at different times after immunization, meaning that individuals suffering higher levels of stress are more at risk of infectious disease.

3. Stress and the Vaccination Response

3.1. Stress Questionnaires

The most common psychosocial factor examined in the context of the vaccination response is stress. This is usually assessed via life events checklists or perceived stress measures. Life events checklists consist of a list of major and minor life events, e.g., bereavement, moving house, and usually require participants to indicate which have occurred during the past month or year (22). Some also ask participants to indicate how stressful each event was on a rating scale. Life events have been shown to predict a variety of important physical health outcomes, including infectious disease (23), and mortality, particularly in the context of little emotional support (24). In contrast, perceived stress scales measure individuals' feelings about how stressful their lives are rather than the direct occurrence of events (25). Thus these measures are more susceptible to subjective bias, and are better predictors of subjective health outcomes, such as angina, rather than objective outcomes, such as myocardial infarction (26).

3.2. Caregiver Control Models

Another common way of assessing stress in the context of vaccination is to examine antibody responses among those with a key chronic stressor vs. a socio-demographically matched control group, for example, older adults caregiving for a spouse with dementia. The stress of caregiving has been shown to relate to poor health and mortality (27), and can thus be considered an important source of ongoing psychological stress.

3.3. Protocol for Stress and Vaccination Studies

In order to fully test the impact of psychosocial factors on the response to vaccination, both pre-vaccination and post-vaccination blood samples are required for assessment of antibody levels. This is due to the impact that prior vaccination or environmental exposure to the infectious agent can have on pre-vaccination antibody levels, and consequently post-vaccination levels. Without taking a pre-vaccination baseline, it is difficult to state whether stress is affecting the antibody response to a vaccination administered during a research study or simply on the maintenance of previous antibody levels. For example, in 37 nursing home residents, those who reported higher levels of perceived stress had lower pre-vaccine antibody titers to two influenza vaccine components (28). However, it is not clear what this means, given that pre-vaccine titers could reflect differences in prior vaccine history or exposure. In this same study, social support was also negatively correlated with pre- and post-vaccination titers against the A/Panama influenza strain yet positively with pre-vaccination antibody titers against the A/New Caledonia strain (28), making interpretation of the findings very difficult. However, some of the early studies of stress and vaccination in students were opportunistic, in other words they collected stress data from students who opportunistically had already received a prior vaccination. Although more complex to interpret, given lack of baseline or prior exposure information, these studies are able to show that psychological stress does seem to affect the maintenance of antibody titers over time. For example, one study examined the association between life events stress and hepatitis B antibody titer in medical students, vaccinated either in the past 12 months or at least 13 months previously (29). Whereas life events exposure was not related to antibody response in the recently vaccinated cohort, participants in the earlier vaccinated cohort who reported higher life events over the past year were over twice as likely to show an inadequate antibody titer as those with lower life events exposure, providing some evidence that psychosocial stress can have effects on the rate of deterioration of antibody protection (16).

3.4. Key Stress and Vaccination Findings

One of the most common vaccinations studied in the context of stress and antibody response is the influenza vaccination, particularly in undergraduate student and older caregiver samples. The influenza vaccination is a commonly utilized vaccine and consists of three components or strains, usually two A strains and one B strain, which change each year depending on the key circulating varieties. A recent meta-analysis of 13 studies of psychological stress and influenza vaccination concluded that there is a significant negative relationship between psychological stress and antibody titer following influenza vaccination (30). These studies included five in caregivers and eight assessing the impact of stressful life events or perceived stress. The meta-analysis concluded that psychological stress, however measured, had a similar negative impact on influenza vaccine response, but that antibody responses to A/H1N1 and B-influenza types were more sensitive to the influence of stress (30). However, it is difficult at this stage to explain why antibodies against influenza strains are differentially associated with stress. One possibility is that strain novelty influences the associations observed (10, 31), with more novel strains being more susceptible to stress effects.

The impact on certain A-strains and on B-strains is clearly shown in several studies of students. For example, those reporting higher stressful life event exposures and/or higher perceived stress prior to vaccination showed poorer responses to the A-strains of the vaccine at 5 weeks (around the time of the peak response) and 5 months post-vaccination (indicating the decay in antibody response over time) (32). This was replicated for the numbers and severity of stressful life events prior to vaccination with the response to the B/Shangdong influenza strain at both 5 weeks and 5 months post-vaccination (33). Similarly, in a study of the effects of daily stress and feelings of being overwhelmed during the 10 days following vaccination, higher stress ratings were associated with lower antibody titers to the A/New Caledonia strain at both 1 and 4 months following vaccination (34). In older adults too, we observed that the stress of bereavement in the year prior to influenza vaccination was associated with a poorer antibody response to two of the influenza strains in a community sample of 184 adults aged 65 and over (35). Although overall negative life events exposure was not associated with vaccine response in this study, the effect found for bereavement suggests that stress is related to pervasive immune effects throughout the life course, although what constitutes life events stress will vary depending on the age of the sample studied. Taken together, these studies provide evidence that stressful life events both preceding and in the period immediately following vaccination can influence the antibody response. They also show that both the peak antibody response at around 4 weeks and the decay in antibody protection over time are susceptible to influence by stressful life events.

On the whole, the vaccination response in older adults has mainly been considered in the context of the chronic stress of caregiving for a spouse with dementia. Studies have shown that caregivers have poorer antibody responses to vaccination in comparison to matched control participants (36–38). Similarly, caregivers who exhibited repetitive negative thoughts about their situation had lower antibody titers following influenza vaccination (39). However, in younger populations, such as Multiple Sclerosis spousal caregivers, there was no difference in antibody response to influenza vaccination between caregivers and controls (40). This raises the issue of whether the poor antibody response observed in older caregivers is, to an extent, a function of an interaction between chronic stress exposure and immunosenescence (41).

There is an alternative explanation for the discrepancy in outcomes among the caregiver vaccination studies. Rather than immune aging, perhaps it is the intensity of the stress experienced that determines whether caregiving becomes an issue for immunity (40). Dementia is a disease characterized by much more severe cognitive and behavioral disturbances than multiple sclerosis (42–45), and older spousal caregivers of dementia patients have been found to report greater distress than younger multiple sclerosis caregivers (40). Further, the results of two recent meta-analyses indicate that caregivers of dementia patients generally experience greater burden and report more symptoms of depression than those caring for non-dementia, e.g., cancer, patients (46, 47). Thus, it might be hypothesized that, irrespective of the caregiver's age, caring for someone with severe cognitive and behavioral problems will compromise immunity.

We have been able to test this hypothesis recently using a caregiving model in younger adults; young parents caring for children with developmental disabilities. Dealing with severe cognitive difficulties and behaviors that are problematic and distressing are the main challenges of such caring (48–51). In our own studies of 30 caregivers for a child with a developmental disability (mainly Autism) vs. matched controls, we have demonstrated that caregivers report high levels of stress, anxiety, depression, child problem behaviors, and low levels of social support. These caregivers also exhibited a poorer antibody response to a pneumonia vaccination than parents caring for typically developing children at both 1 and

6 months post-vaccination (52). Of the psychological variables considered, child problem behaviors mediated this effect. In addition, within the caregivers, parents reporting more child conduct problems, a component of the child problem behavior measure, mounted a poorer antibody response at 1-month than parents reporting less conduct problems (52). Similarly, these parents mounted a poorer antibody response to the B/Malaysia strain of an influenza vaccine at 1 and 6 months post-vaccination, which again appeared to be mediated by differences in child problem behaviors (53).

These recent findings in younger caregivers reinforce the hypothesis that an aging immune system is not a pre-requisite for a poor response to medical vaccination in caregivers. Nevertheless, among our parental caregivers, older caregivers tended to have a poorer antibody response to B/Malaysia at 1-month, suggesting that we cannot dismiss the hypothesis that chronic stress and immunosenescence may have synergistic effects (41).

4. Different Vaccine Factors

Vaccination studies also have the advantage of being able to incorporate research questions such as "does it matter when stressful life events occur relative to when the vaccine is received?" and "what are the effects of prior exposure to the antigen?" The next section of this chapter will address some of these issues of timing.

4.1. Timing of Stress Measurement

This issue of the timing of stress assessment has been developed in studies of various vaccinations including hepatitis B, which is useful in this context, as the vaccination schedule consists of three inoculations over a 6 month period. The largest of these studies examined the association between life events stress and the final antibody titer in students, vaccinated either in the past 12 months or at least 13 months previously (29). Whereas life events exposure was not related to antibody response in the recently vaccinated cohort, participants in the earlier vaccinated cohort who reported higher life events over the past year were over twice as likely to show an inadequate antibody titer as those with lower life events exposure. This finding suggests that the immunogenicity, the ability to induce a strong vaccination response, of hepatitis B vaccination may initially override the influence of life events stress, although there was also more power to detect effects in the earlier vaccinated cohort as more participants exhibited inadequate antibody titers (29). Nevertheless, this study provides some evidence that psychosocial stress in the period following vaccination can have effects on the rate of deterioration of antibody protection (16).

In a study where a low dose of hepatitis B vaccine was administered, a higher stress index, comprising life events exposure and psychological symptoms, measured at 2 months post-vaccination (thus considering the period post-vaccination) was associated with a poorer final 6 month antibody response, and the stress index at 6 months also tended to relate negatively to antibody response (54). However, as only the final antibody titer was measured, it is difficult to determine whether, in this instance, stress predominantly influenced initial formation or maintenance of antibody levels. Also, the inclusion of psychological symptoms in the composite stress index makes it difficult to ascribe this finding to any specific aspect of stress (16). A similar study using the full dosage hepatitis B vaccination did not yield any significant stress effects (55), although it is possible that this was due to the absence of a 2-month assessment of stress, which was the main predictor of antibody response in the previous study by this group. In a study measuring perceived stress and anxiety during the vaccination period, i.e. post-vaccination, these were not associated with the final antibody response to hepatitis B (36). Further, life events stress prior to vaccination and perceived stress at the time of the initial vaccination were not related to antibody status 5 months following the initial inoculation in a more recent study (56). On the whole, this would suggest either that stress prior to vaccination is less detrimental to the antibody response than stress post-vaccination, or that it is difficult to observe stress effects early on with the full dose hepatitis B vaccination, due to its immunogenicity. Given the findings with the influenza vaccination and stress, this latter seems the more likely explanation.

In contrast to the studies of hepatitis B discussed thus far, one study reported a positive association between perceived life event stress, depression and anxiety during the vaccination period, and hepatitis B antibody status 9 months following the initial vaccination (57). This anomalous result has been attributed to the relatively low levels of stress experienced by the participants in this study, suggesting that moderate levels of life change stress experienced *during* the initial stages of antibody formation may be beneficial to the antibody response, although high levels may be detrimental (57). Such an interpretation receives support from animal research where moderate stress at the time of vaccination has been associated with an enhanced antibody response (*see* e.g., (58)). This will be discussed further in the section on acute stress below.

4.2. Primary and Secondary Exposure to Vaccine Antigens

Vaccination with an antigen to which the participant has not been previously exposed induces a primary antibody response whereas vaccination against more common pathogens such as influenza induces a secondary immune response. By examining the effect of stress on both primary and secondary immune responses, we can begin to determine which aspects of the immune response are most susceptible to stress-induced modulation.

Hepatitis B vaccination has been used in this context due to the vaccination schedule and the low likelihood of prior naturalistic exposure to this pathogen. In an earlier study, individuals reporting higher mean perceived stress and anxiety over the vaccination period were less likely to have sero-converted (produced a protective antibody level) by the time of the second inoculation (36). Whereas, an emotional disclosure intervention group did not differ from controls in antibody levels at the time of the second inoculation (59). However, psychological stress levels were not measured, making it difficult to interpret these data. More recently, we have used hepatitis A as a primary antigen. Students who reported a higher number and severity of life events had a poorer antibody response to hepatitis A at the 18-week, but not 4-week, follow-up, suggesting stress can impact upon the maintenance of antibody levels (60). Early studies using the vaccination model used novel non-pathogenic antigens to examine the antigen-specific antibody response. Keyhole limpet hemocyanin (KLH), a protein, has been used in this context; the KLH-specific IgG antibody response was lower at 8 weeks, but not 3 weeks, post-vaccination in participants reporting fewer positive life events prior to vaccination (61).

The consensus of this evidence suggests that stress can influence the primary antibody response, particularly the maintenance of responses to novel antigens. It also supports the idea that life events stress effects are more likely to be evident with novel vaccine types (33). As discussed above, the secondary antibody response to hepatitis B vaccination has produced mixed results, but there appears to be stronger evidence for a negative effect of psychological stress on the secondary response to this antigen (16, 62), in line with the findings for the influenza vaccine.

4.3. Thymus-Dependent Versus -Independent Vaccines

A further advantage to the vaccination model is that there are different types of vaccination, which can be used to help elucidate which cells involved in the vaccination response are influenced by psychological factors. Most vaccinations, which consist of inactivated or dead viruses like influenza, induce a thymus-dependent antibody response, as described above. A few vaccinations, however, protect against bacterial infections or toxins, like meningococcal A or tetanus, respectively, which do not require T-cell help. There are also conjugate vaccines, in which substances that elicit a T-cell response are conjugated to a thymus-independent pathogen, such as a protein, in order to boost the efficiency of the antibody response against the thymus-independent pathogen. If psychological factors are consistently associated with the response to thymus-dependent and conjugate vaccinations but not with thymus-independent response, this would imply that it is T-cells that are particularly liable to psychological influence.

Indeed, there is evidence to suggest that stress may exert its effects mainly on T-cells; we showed that higher frequency and intensity of stressful life events were associated with a poorer response to influenza and meningococcal C (following previous conjugate meningococcal C vaccination), but not to thymus-independent meningococcal A (33). Similarly, no association was found between stress and antibody response to a thymus-independent pneumonia vaccination in pre-school children (63). However, as older caregivers have been reported to show poorer maintenance of antibody levels over time following pneumonia vaccination than controls (37), it is possible that other factors such as age and severity of stress may interact to impair antibody-mediated immunity more generally than just the T-cell response.

It should be noted that in the study of caregivers and the pneumonia vaccination, perceived stress did not differ between the caregiver and controls, but there was a significant difference in social support. This might suggest that thymus-dependent vaccinations are susceptible to the effects of stressful life events, but that thymus-independent vaccinations are more vulnerable to other psychosocial factors such as lower social support. There is some evidence for this suggestion. In our own laboratory, we found that social support, but not life events stress, was positively associated with the response to a thymus-independent pneumococcal vaccine in young healthy students (60, 64).

The comparison between thymus-dependent and -independent vaccination responses suggest that both types of response are susceptible to psychosocial influence, but that there are key variables which influence whether an effect on vaccination response is observed. These include: the type of psychosocial factor studied (i.e. stress vs. social support), and the age of the population sampled.

4.4. Acute Versus Chronic Stress

Following on from the discussion above in Subheading 4.1 regarding when stress is measured, such that moderate or less severe stress at the time of vaccination might actually have a beneficial effect, it has been suggested in recent years that acute (minutes or hours) stress may be immune enhancing when experienced close to the immune challenge. Such immune enhancement by acute stress would be an adaptive mechanism, and might be regarded as an integral component of the fight or flight response, and circumstances that elicit such a response are likely to also involve exposure to antigens and, therefore, a robust immune response would be adaptive for survival (58). Recently, our laboratory examined the effect of acute psychological stress on antibody response to vaccination in humans. Participants completed a 45 min time pressured, socially evaluated mental arithmetic task, or a resting control period, immediately prior to influenza vaccination. An enhancement of the antibody response to one of the influenza viral strains was found in women in the psychological stress group compared to control (65).

4.5. Timing of Vaccination

As well as the timing and duration of stress measurements associated with the vaccine response, other behavioral factors have recently been found to impact upon the antibody response. One such factor is that of the time of day of vaccination. In our study of the effects of psychological stress on vaccination responses in the 184 older adults (35), we observed that the time of day of vaccine administration significantly influenced antibody titer (66). Men responded better in the morning than the afternoon; 41% of men showed a twofold response when vaccinated in the morning vs. 24% of men vaccinated in the afternoon. This effect was independent of current illnesses, medication, vaccination history, and our reported findings of the effects of bereavement and marital quality. Women tended to show the reverse pattern. We have also recently observed the same pattern in a study of younger adults' antibody response to the hepatitis A vaccination (66). However, these studies were not fully randomized, and there was little opportunity to examine the biological mechanisms, such as cytokine and stress hormone levels. Consequently, there is a clear and pressing need for a properly randomized controlled trial of the impact of time of influenza vaccination on antibody response and vaccine efficacy in older adults in a National Health Service (NHS) setting. We are currently conducting a cluster-randomized trial of this sort within the NHS in Birmingham, UK, and hope to confirm that a simple manipulation of the time of vaccination will improve the immune response against influenza in older adults. This would yield an intervention, easy to adopt and implement within the health services, at little or no added cost. The benefits will be a decreased incidence of influenza infection and influenza-related mortality in older adults.

5. Other Psychosocial Factors and the Vaccination Model

5.1. Social Support

The support of friends and loved ones is an important determinant of immune health, and is relatively easily measured in vaccination studies via validated questionnaires. Studies have assessed both functional social support, a measure of the quality and availability of social resources a person has, and structural social support, the number of friends a person can call on, in the context of vaccination. First, students reporting greater social support demonstrated a stronger combined immune response to the third inoculation of the three-dose hepatitis B vaccination (36). Second, loneliness and smaller social network size were associated with a poorer antibody response to the A/New Caledonian strain of the influenza vaccination in college students (67). Third, students with greater functional social support showed higher titers to the A/Panama influenza strain at both 5 weeks and 5 months following vaccination (33). In older nursing home residents, social support was also negatively correlated with pre- and post-vaccination titers against the A/Panama influenza strain yet positively with pre-vaccination antibody titers against the A/New Caledonia strain (28), a finding which even the authors were unable to explain. Along with the caregiver study discussed above, these studies generally show that a lack of social support has a strong negative impact on antibody levels following vaccination.

Marriage is also a source of social support. In our own work, older adults who were married, and particularly those who were happily married, showed a better antibody response to the influenza vaccination than those who were unmarried or less happily married (35). However, more general functional social support and social network size were not associated with antibody response in this older population (35). These findings perhaps lend weight to the suggestion that the population studied influences which psychosocial factors are important for the vaccination response.

5.2. Personality

Personality factors, although often examined in the context of health outcomes, again using validated questionnaires (see e.g., (68)), have scarcely been investigated relative to the vaccination response. First, among a group of 12-year old girls, those characterized by higher internalizing scores and lower self-esteem at baseline exhibited lower antibody titers following rubella vaccination (69). A similar concept, neuroticism, was negatively associated with both the peak antibody response to the A/Panama strain of an influenza vaccination, and the maintenance of antibody titers to this strain in students (70). Among female graduate students, trait negative affect/mood was negatively associated with the antibody response to the second hepatitis B injection (56). Further, independently of negative affect, trait positive affect was associated with a better antibody response following a second hepatitis B vaccination in graduate students (71). Thus, both negative and positive traits appear to be able to influence this aspect of immune function and disease protection. However, in exercising and sedentary elderly individuals, dispositional optimism was not found to be associated with antibody titers following influenza vaccination (72). Inconsistencies in these results could be attributable to the different measures of personality studied, or the different ages of the populations used, which will now be discussed in more detail.

6. Future Directions: Mechanisms and Interventions

The studies reviewed above outline the different methods of examining associations between psychological factors and the antibody response to vaccination. These studies show the strong associations between psychological stress, other psychosocial factors and the immune response to vaccination, such that stressful psychological circumstances are associated with poorer antibody responses, while positive factors such as social support relate to a better immune response to vaccination. Taken together, these findings suggest two main directions for future research. First, despite the range of vaccinations used in such studies, as yet little is known about the exact mechanisms by which stress and other factors can influence antibody responses to vaccination. Research incorporating a range of measurements, such as stress hormones, immune system messengers (cytokines), and the function of key cells in the vaccination response, such as antigen presenting cells, would be necessary to further our understanding regarding exactly how stress gets inside the body to affect this clinically relevant immune outcome. Second, the clinical implications, in terms of susceptibility to disease, arising from a better understanding of the relationships between psychological factors and the vaccination response are important, particularly in the context of older adults who already display poor vaccination responses. Psychological interventions to improve vaccination response in these populations could include techniques such as stress management, relaxation, cognitive behavioral therapy, and emotional disclosure.

Regarding such interventions, one study showed an improvement in the ability of older caregivers for a spouse with dementia to mount a fourfold increase in antibody titer following influenza vaccination relative to matched controls, although the mechanisms of effect were unclear and the intervention group was not randomly sampled (73). Similarly, participants taking part in a written emotional disclosure intervention, where they wrote about their emotions about a previously undisclosed stressful event, showed significantly higher antibody titers at 4 and 6 months following vaccination with hepatitis B compared to a control non-intervention group (59). A different clinical application of the vaccination model has arisen from the positive immune effects demonstrated in response to acute stress (65). These preliminary findings suggest that the development of such a behavioral challenge that could be applied in General Practitioner settings could be a way forward for improving the vaccination response. This would be particularly important for groups at risk of infectious disease such as older adults, the bereaved, and caregivers. At this stage, more work is required to establish exactly what types of intervention in which age groups and are likely to be the most beneficial for psychological, and hence immunological, health. Behavioral interventions, such as the time of day of vaccination may also be important in this context.

7. Conclusion

In conclusion, vaccination has had a substantial impact on public health, although not everyone mounts a satisfactory and protective antibody response to vaccination. This increasingly appears to be the case with progressing age. Studying antibody responses to vaccination is now contributing to the understanding of how psychosocial exposures can influence immunity and, consequently, resistance to disease. The current challenges are to build upon the methodology that has been developed through these studies to unravel the underlying mechanisms and to develop and apply feasible behavioral interventions to boost the response to vaccination and, thus, optimize our resistance against infectious disease.

References

1. McKinnon W, Weisse CS, Reynolds CP, Bowles CA, Baum A (1989) Chronic stress, leukocyte subpopulations, and humoral response to latent viruses. Health Psychol 8:389–402
2. Schaeffer MA, Baum A, Reynolds CF, Rikli P, Davidson LM, Fleming I (1985) Immune status as a function of chronic stress at Three Mile Island. Psychosom Med 47:85
3. Futterman AD, Wellisch DK, Zighelboim J, Luna-Raines M, Weiner H (1996) Psychological and immunological reactions of family members to patients undergoing bone marrow transplantation. Psychosom Med 58:472–480
4. Kiecolt-Glaser JK, Glaser R, Shuttleworth EC, Dyer CS, Ogrocki P, Speicher CE (1987) Chronic stress and immunity in family caregivers of Alzheimer's disease victims. Psychosom Med 49:523–535
5. De Gucht V, Fischler B, Demanet C (1999) Immune dysfunction associated with chronic professional stress in nurses. Psychiatry Res 85:105–111
6. Deinzer R, Kleineidam C, Stiller-Winkler R, Idel H, Bachg D (2000) Prolonged reduction of salivary immunoglobulin A (sIgA) after a major academic exam. Int J Psychophysiol 37:219–232
7. Jemmott JB III, Borysenko JZ, Borysenko M, McClelland DC, Chapman R, Meyer D, Benson H (1983) Academic stress, power motivation, and decrease in secretion rate of salivary secretory immunoglobulin A. Lancet 1:1400–1402
8. Jemmott JB III, Magloire K (1988) Academic stress, social support, and secretory immunoglobulin A. J Pers Soc Psychol 55:803–810
9. McClelland DC, Alexander C, Marks E (1982) The need for power, stress, immune function, and illness among male prisoners. J Abnorm Psychol 91:61–70
10. Vedhara K, Fox JD, Wang ECY (1999) The measurement of stress-related immune dysfunction in psychoneuroimmunology. Neurosci Biobehav Rev 23:699–715
11. Arnetz BB, Wasserman J, Petrini B, Brenner SO, Levi L, Eneroth P, Salovaara H, Hjelm R, Salovaara L, Theorell T et al (1987) Immune function in unemployed women. Psychosom Med 49:3–12
12. Bartrop RW, Luckhurst E, Lazarus L, Kiloh LG, Penny R (1977) Depressed lymphocyte function after bereavement. Lancet 1:834–836
13. Esterling BA, Kiecolt-Glaser JK, Glaser R (1996) Psychosocial modulation of cytokine-induced natural killer cell activity in older adults. Psychosom Med 58:264–272
14. Irwin M, Patterson T, Smith TL, Caldwell C, Brown SA, Gillin JC, Grant I (1990) Reduction of immune function in life stress and depression. Biol Psychiatry 27:22–30
15. Schleifer SJ, Keller SE, Camerino M, Thornton JC, Stein M (1983) Suppression of lymphocyte stimulation following bereavement. JAMA 250:374–377
16. Burns VE, Carroll D, Ring C, Drayson M (2003) Antibody response to vaccination and psychosocial stress in humans: relationship and mechanisms. Vaccine 21:2523–2534
17. Allsup S, Haycox A, Regan M, Gosney M (2004) Is influenza vaccination cost effective for healthy people between ages 65 and 74 years? A randomised controlled trial. Vaccine 23:639–645
18. Patriarca PA (1994) Editorial: a randomized controlled trial of influenza vaccine in the elderly: scientific scrutiny and ethical responsibility. JAMA 272:1700–1701
19. Goodwin K, Viboud C, Simonsen L (2006) Antibody response to influenza vaccination in the elderly: a quantitative review. Vaccine 24:1159–1169
20. Nichol KL, Margolis KL, Wuorenma J, Von Sternberg T (1994) The efficacy and cost effectiveness of vaccination against influenza among elderly persons living in the community. N Engl J Med 331:778–784
21. Simonsen L, Reichert TA, Viboud C, Blackwelder WC, Taylor RJ, Miller MA (2005) Impact of influenza vaccination on seasonal mortality in the US elderly population. Arch Intern Med 165:265–272
22. Brown GW, Harris TO (1989) Social origins of depression: a study of psychiatric disorder in women. Routledge, London

23. Cohen S, Tyrell DAJ, Smith AP (1991) Psychological stress and susceptibility to the common cold. N Engl J Med 325:606–612
24. Rosengren A, Orth-Gomer K, Wedel H, Wilhelmsen L (1993) Stressful life events, social support, and mortality in men born in 1933. BMJ 307:1102–1105
25. Cohen S, Kamarck T, Mermelstein R (1983) A global measure of perceived stress. J Health Soc Behav 24:385–396
26. Macleod J, Davey Smith G, Heslop P, Metcalfe C, Carroll D, Hart C (2002) Psychological stress and cardiovascular disease: empirical demonstration of bias in a prospective observational study of Scottish men. BMJ 324:1247–1251
27. Schulz R, Beach SR (1999) Caregiving as a risk factor for mortality: the Caregiver Health Effects Study. JAMA 282:2215–2219
28. Moynihan JA, Larson MR, Treanor J, Duberstein PR, Power A, Shore B, Ader R (2004) Psychosocial factors and the response to influenza vaccination in older adults. Psychosom Med 66:950–953
29. Burns VE, Carroll D, Ring C, Harrison LK, Drayson M (2002) Stress, coping and hepatitis B antibody status. Psychosom Med 64:287–293
30. Pedersen AF, Zachariae R, Bovbjerg DH (2009) Psychological stress and antibody response to influenza vaccination: a meta-analysis. Brain Behav Immun 23:427–433
31. Gulati U, Keitel WA, Air GM (2007) Increased antibodies against unfolded viral antigens in the elderly after influenza vaccination. Influenza Other Respi Viruses 1:147–156
32. Burns VE, Carroll D, Drayson M, Whitham M, Ring C (2003) Life events, perceived stress and antibody response to influenza vaccination in young healthy adults. J Psychosom Res 55:569–572
33. Phillips AC, Burns VE, Carroll D, Ring C, Drayson M (2005) The association between life events, social support and antibody status following thymus-dependent and thymus-independent vaccinations in healthy young adults. Brain Behav Immun 19:325–333
34. Miller GE, Cohen S, Pressman S, Barkin A, Rabin BS, Treanor JJ (2004) Psychological stress and antibody response to influenza vaccination: when is the critical period for stress, and how does it get inside the body? Psychosom Med 66:215–223
35. Phillips AC, Carroll D, Burns VE, Ring C, Macleod J, Drayson M (2006) Bereavement and marriage are associated with antibody response to influenza vaccination in the elderly. Brain Behav Immun 20:279–289
36. Glaser R, Kiecolt-Glaser JK, Bonneau RH, Malarkey W, Kennedy S, Hughes J (1992) Stress-induced modulation of the immune response to recombinant hepatitis B vaccine. Psychosom Med 54:22–29
37. Glaser R, Sheridan JF, Malarkey W, MacCallum RC, Kiecolt-Glaser JK (2000) Chronic stress modulates the immune response to a pneumococcal pneumonia vaccine. Psychosom Med 62:804–807
38. Vedhara K, Cox NK, Wilcock GK, Perks P, Hunt M, Anderson S, Lightman SL, Shanks NM (1999) Chronic stress in elderly carers of dementia patients and antibody response to influenza vaccination. Lancet 353:627–631
39. Segerstrom SC, Schipper LJ, Greenberg RN (2008) Caregiving, repetitive thought, and immune response to vaccination in older adults. Brain Behav Immun 22:744–752
40. Vedhara K, McDermott MP, Evans TG, Treanor JJ, Plummer S, Tallon D, Cruttenden KA, Schifitto G (2002) Chronic stress in non-elderly caregivers: psychological, endocrine and immune implications. J Psychosom Res 53:1153–1161
41. Graham JE, Christian LM, Kiecolt-Glaser JK (2006) Stress, age, and immune function: toward a lifespan approach. J Behav Med 29:389–400
42. Keegan BM, Noseworthy JH (2002) Multiple sclerosis. Annu Rev Med 53:285–302
43. Poser CM, Paty DW, Scheinberg L, McDonald WI, Davis FA, Ebers GC, Johnson KP, Sibley WA, Silberberg DH, Tourtellotte WW (1983) New diagnostic criteria for multiple sclerosis: guidelines for research protocols. Ann Neurol 13:227–231
44. Gregory CA, Hodges JR (1996) Clinical features of frontal lobe dementia in comparison to Alzheimer's disease. J Neural Transm Suppl 47:103–123
45. Neary D, Snowden JS, Gustafson L, Passant U, Stuss D, Black S, Freedman M, Kertesz A, Robert PH, Albert M, Boone K, Miller BL, Cummings J, Benson DF (1998) Frontotemporal lobar degeneration: a consensus on clinical diagnostic criteria. Neurology 51:1546–1554
46. Pinquart M, Sorensen S (2003) Associations of stressors and uplifts of caregiving with caregiver burden and depressive mood: a meta-analysis. J Gerontol B Psychol Sci Soc Sci 58: P112–P128
47. Pinquart M, Sorensen S (2003) Differences between caregivers and noncaregivers in psychological health and physical health: a meta-analysis. Psychol Aging 18:250–267
48. Floyd FJ, Gallagher EM (1997) Parental stress, care demands, and use of support services for school-age children with disabilities and behavior problems. Family Relations 46:359–371
49. Hastings RP, Daley D, Burns C, Beck A (2006) Maternal distress and expressed emotion: cross-sectional and longitudinal relationships with

behavior problems of children with intellectual disabilities. Am J Ment Retard 111:48–61

50. Higgins DJ, Bailey SR, Pearce JC (2005) Factors associated with functioning style and coping strategies of families with a child with an autism spectrum disorder. Autism 9:125–137
51. Maes B, Broekman TG, Dosen A, Nauts J (2003) Caregiving burden of families looking after persons with intellectual disability and behavioural or psychiatric problems. J Intellect Disabil Res 47:447–455
52. Gallagher S, Phillips AC, Drayson MT, Carroll D (2009) Parental caregivers of children with developmental disabilities mount a poor antibody response to pneumococcal vaccination. Brain Behav Immun 23:338–346
53. Gallagher S, Phillips AC, Drayson MT, Carroll D (2009) Care-giving for a child with intellectual disabilities is associated with a poor antibody response to influenza vaccination. Psychosom Med 71:341–344
54. Jabaaij L, Grosheide PM, Heijtink RA, Duivenvoorden HJ, Ballieux RE, Vingerhoets AJJM (1993) Influence of perceived psychological stress and distress on antibody response to low dose rDNA hepatitis B vaccine. J Psychosom Res 37:361–369
55. Jabaaij L, Van Hattum J, Vingerhoets AJJM, Oostveen FG, Duivenvoorden HJ, Ballieux RE (1996) Modulation of immune response to rDNA hepatitis B vaccination by psychological stress. J Psychosom Res 41:129–137
56. Marsland AL, Cohen S, Rabin BS, Manuck SB (2001) Associations between stress, trait negative affect, acute immune reactivity, and antibody response to hepatitis B injection in healthy young adults. Health Psychol 20:4–11
57. Petry J, Weems LB, Livingstone JNI (1991) Relationship of stress, distress, and the immunologic response to a recombinant hepatitis B vaccine. J Fam Pract 32:481–486
58. Dhabhar FS, McEwen BS (1996) Stress-induced enhancement of antigen-specific cell-mediated immunity. J Immunol 156:2608–2615
59. Petrie KJ, Booth RJ, Pennebaker JW, Davison KP, Thomas MG (1995) Disclosure of trauma and immune response to a hepatitis B vaccination program. J Consult Clin Psychol 63: 787–792
60. Gallagher S, Phillips AC, Ferraro AJ, Drayson MT, Carroll D (2008) Psychosocial factors are associated with the antibody response to both thymus-dependent and thymus-independent vaccines. Brain Behav Immun 22:456–460
61. Snyder BK, Roghmann KJ, Sigal LH (1990) Effect of stress and other biopsychosocial factors on primary antibody response. J Adolesc Health Care 11:472–479
62. Cohen S, Miller GE, Rabin BS (2001) Psychological stress and antibody response to immunization: a critical review of the human literature. Psychosom Med 63:7–18
63. Boyce WT, Adams S, Tschann JM, Cohen F, Wara D, Gunnar MR (1995) Adrenocortical and behavioral predictors of immune response to starting school. Pediatr Res 38:1009–1017
64. Gallagher S, Phillips AC, Ferraro AJ, Drayson MT, Carroll D (2008) Social support is positively associated with the immunoglobulin M response to vaccination with pneumococcal polysaccharides. Biol Psychol 78:211–215
65. Edwards KM, Burns VE, Reynolds T, Carroll D, Drayson M, Ring C (2006) Acute stress exposure prior to influenza vaccination enhances antibody response in women. Brain Behav Immun 20:159–168
66. Phillips AC, Gallagher S, Carroll D, Drayson M (2008) Morning vaccine administration is associated with an enhanced response to vaccination in men. Psychophysiology 45:663–666
67. Pressman SD, Cohen S, Miller GE, Barkin A, Rabin BS, Treanor JJ (2005) Loneliness, social network size, and immune response to influenza vaccination in college freshmen. Health Psychol 24:297–306
68. Smith TW, Glaser K, Ruiz JM, Gallo LC (2004) Hostility, anger, aggressiveness, and coronary heart disease: an interpersonal perspective on personality, emotion, and health. J Pers 72:1217–1270
69. Morag M, Morag A, Reichenberg MA, Lerer B, Yirmiya R (1999) Psychological variables as predictors of rubella antibody titers and fatigue—a prospective double blind study. J Psychiatr Res 33:389–395
70. Phillips AC, Carroll D, Burns VE, Drayson M (2005) Neuroticism, cortisol reactivity, and antibody response to vaccination. Psychophysiology 42:232–238
71. Marsland AL, Cohen S, Rabin BS, Manuck SB (2006) Trait positive affect and antibody response to hepatitis B vaccination. Brain Behav Immun 20:261–269
72. Kohut ML, Cooper MM, Nickolaus MS, Russell DR, Cunnick JE (2002) Exercise and psychosocial factors modulate immunity to influenza vaccine in elderly individuals. J Gerontol 57:557–562
73. Vedhara K, Bennett PD, Clark S, Lightman SL, Shaw S, Perks P, Hunt MA, Philip JM, Tallon D, Murphy PJ, Jones RW, Wilcock GK, Shanks NM (2003) Enhancement of antibody responses to influenza vaccination in the elderly following a cognitive-behavioural stress management intervention. Psychother Psychosom 72:245–252

Chapter 19

Using Vaccinations to Assess In Vivo Immune Function in Psychoneuroimmunology

Victoria E. Burns

Abstract

Finding clinically relevant measures of immune function is an important challenge in psychoneuroimmunological research. Here, we discuss the advantages of the vaccination model, and provide guidance on the methodological decisions that are important to consider in the use of this technique. These include the choice of vaccination, timing of assessments, and the available outcome measures.

Key words: Antibody response, In vivo, Methods, Psychological Stress, Vaccination, Psychoneuroimmunology

1. Introduction

Antibody response to vaccination has received increasing attention in the field of psychoneuroimmunology as a useful measure of in vivo immune function (1–3). The immune system is a multifaceted network of organs, cells, and molecules, which continually interact to recognize and eradicate foreign and/or dangerous entities. To add another layer of complexity, there are also clear structural and chemical pathways through which these immune cells and molecules interact with the neuroendocrine system (4, 5). Although no single measure of "immune function" can profess to capture the state of this system in its entirety, antibody response to vaccination provides a useful model for studying integrated immune responses.

Strong evidence now exists that the magnitude of these responses is associated with a wide range of psychosocial factors. Both young and older adults who have been exposed to chronic stress have poorer antibody responses to a variety of vaccinations (2, 6). Further, reduced antibody responses have been found in participants with higher rates of neuroticism (7) and loneliness (8), whereas both

Qing Yan (ed.), *Psychoneuroimmunology: Methods and Protocols*, Methods in Molecular Biology, vol. 934,
DOI 10.1007/978-1-62703-071-7_19,

social support (9–11) and positive affect (12) predict better antibody responses. There are also preliminary findings suggesting that both chronic and acute psychological interventions can alter the efficacy of vaccinations (13–15), indicating that antibody response to vaccination is a useful marker of immune function that is sensitive to psychosocial influence. The success of its use as a research tool, however, relies on careful decision making about the type of vaccination administered, the sampling protocol, and the laboratory analysis. This chapter will highlight some key methodological considerations for researchers considering adopting this approach.

2. Advantages of Vaccination Response as an In Vivo Method of Measuring Immune Function

2.1. Integrated Measure of Immune Function

In order to appreciate the benefits of a vaccination approach, it is important to understand the immunological process involved in producing an antibody response. The infectious agent, or antigen, contained in the vaccine is recognized and internalized by professional antigen presenting cells, and then displayed on their cell surface. Chemokines direct these APCs to the lymphoid tissues, where the antigen is presented to T cells. If a specific T cell recognizes this antigen, and the necessary co-stimulatory signals are present, it becomes activated and proliferates. These T cells are now able to activate B cells that have recognized and presented the same antigen. With this T cell help, the B cells can then proliferate and become plasma cells which produce antigen-specific antibodies. These antibodies can be measured in serum, providing a quantifiable measure of the final product of this cascade of reactions (16). A successful antibody response, therefore, reflects optimal functioning of a wide variety of immunological components, rather than a single cell type or molecule. Further, the lymphoid organs are innervated and immune cells are found by the nerve terminals (17), the immune cells display receptors for many neuroendocrine products (18), and there is considerable evidence that immune processes are dramatically altered by this close interaction (19). Many immune assays are conducted in vitro, isolated from these influences, and therefore may not reflect how the cells function in vivo (3). In contrast, as an in vivo process, antibody response to vaccination occurs within this dynamic neuroendocrine environment and, therefore, provides a much better estimation of naturalistic immune functioning (2).

2.2. Control of the Timing of Administration

Vaccination allows the safe administration of antigen at a selected time point, and the assessment of immune status both pre- and post-exposure. This has clear advantages for study design and is a further strength of the vaccine model. For example, by administering a vaccine during or after participation in a psychological or control intervention, it is possible to examine the immune effects of enhanced psychological functioning. Recent studies using this approach have demonstrated that antibody response to vaccination can be improved by mindfulness meditation (14) and cognitive-behavioral stress management (15). This careful control over exposure can also be used to begin to understand mechanisms underpinning the influence of stress on immune function. Miller and colleagues conducted a study in which participants completed daily stress questionnaires for 13 days before, during, and after administration of the influenza vaccination (20). The strongest associations between daily stress and antibody response occurred 8–10 days after vaccine administration, which suggested for the first time that there may be a critical period during which stress influences the antibody response.

2.3. Clinical Relevance

Antibody response to vaccination has clear clinical implications for both vaccination efficacy and as a marker of susceptibility to infection. Specific antibody level is the most commonly used measure of vaccine efficacy in clinical practice and most vaccines are designed to maximize this response (21). This is based on evidence that the greater the antibody response, the better the protection against infection; for example, the level of serum antibody against both influenza and hepatitis B vaccinations has been associated with the extent of resistance to illness (22–24). As there is still considerable variation in vaccine efficacy, particularly in vulnerable populations such as older adults (25), interventions designed specifically to enhance antibody response to vaccination may be particularly beneficial. One such study was based on the proposition that, in the short term, immunological changes associated with the fight or flight response may be beneficial, rather than detrimental, for survival (26, 27). Participants completed a 45-min socially evaluated mental arithmetic task immediately prior to vaccination and showed augmented antibody responses to the influenza (13) and meningitis A+C (28) vaccines. These effects were apparent for sub-groups and strains where the corresponding control group had relatively poor responses, suggesting that populations with the greatest immune impairment may benefit the most from these interventions.

Antibody response to vaccination can also be used as an indicator of the immune system's general ability to respond to an antigen. In this case, the aim is not so much to understand how psychological processes impact on vaccine efficacy per se, but rather to use the antibody response to this one particular antigen as indicative of the general way that it would respond to any infectious agent to which it is naturalistically exposed. Early research, which focuses on the effect of stress on self-reported incidence of upper respiratory tract infections (29, 30), was hampered by the subjective nature of the outcome measure and the uncontrollable variations in antigen exposure that influence infection rates. One way to address these issues is the experimental administration of live viruses, as with the groundbreaking series of studies by Sheldon Cohen and colleagues (31, 32). However, this is only possible in certain specialist facilities, and cannot be conducted with vulnerable populations such as pregnant women (33). In contrast, there are a wide variety of approved vaccines that can be used to model individual susceptibility to many types of infection.

As such, measuring the antibody response to vaccination yields results that are scientifically robust and have easily interpretable clinical implications for both vaccination efficacy and susceptibility to infection. One caveat to add to this discussion, however, is that studies examining the associations between both chronic and acute psychosocial factors and antibody response to vaccination have typically only reported small to medium effect sizes. It remains unclear whether changes of this magnitude equate to substantial alterations in disease susceptibility; elucidating this issue should be a priority for future research.

3. Methodological Considerations in Using the Vaccination Model

3.1. Choice of Vaccination

Vaccines differ in terms of the type of antibody response they elicit, the relative novelty of the antigen (i.e., whether the participants are likely to have been exposed to the antigen before), and the typical efficacy of the vaccination in the general population. Further, depending on your study population, some vaccines may provide more clinically relevant outcome measures. All these factors influence your choice of vaccination, and each will be addressed here in turn.

3.1.1. Type of Vaccination for Your Immunological Question

The earlier section on the general processes involved in an antibody response to vaccination actually describes a thymus-dependent response to a protein antigen, such as influenza or hepatitis B. This is the most common type of vaccine, and it was illustrated that T helper lymphocytes are an essential stimulus for successful B lymphocyte proliferation and maturation to antibody-secreting plasma cells. Other vaccines, such as those containing fragments of the polysaccharide capsule that coats bacteria such as pneumococci and meningococci, are able to evoke antibody responses without T lymphocyte help, and are known as thymus-independent antibody responses. There is also a third type of vaccination in which a polysaccharide antigen, that alone would produce a thymus-independent response, is conjugated to a protein molecule in order to invoke a thymus-dependent, and therefore more robust, antibody response. By comparing the relative susceptibility of thymus-dependent and independent responses, it is possible to begin to determine which aspects of the immune system are most affected by psychosocial factors. For example, if an intervention changes the response to a thymus-dependent, but not -independent, vaccines, this would suggest that the effect is likely to be due to changes in T cell function. Alternatively, if all types of vaccinations are equally susceptible, then it could be surmised that stress affects more general processes such as antigen presentation or B-lymphocyte clonal expansion and production of immunoglobulins.

The relative susceptibility to stress of these different types of vaccines has only been systematically examined in a limited number of studies. Although there was initially some evidence that stress was detrimental to thymus-dependent, but not thymus-independent, antibody responses (11), more recent research suggests that both types of vaccines are associated with psychosocial factors (10). For example, caregivers of children with developmental disabilities, who are characterized by high levels of chronic stress, showed a diminished antibody response to both influenza (34) and the polysaccharide pneumococcal (35) vaccinations, compared to parents of normally developing children. Whether the somewhat less consistent findings in thymus-independent vaccines reflect a relative robustness to psychosocial influence warrants further attention.

3.1.2. Clinical Relevance in Your Population

The clinical relevance of the vaccination for the prospective study population should also be a consideration. While any vaccination will act as a theoretical model of in vivo immunity, the clinical implications are enhanced where the vaccine is carefully chosen in order to reflect pressing concerns in the selected group of participants. For example, the influenza virus causes high levels of morbidity and mortality in older adults (36) and, therefore, studies finding an influence of psychosocial stress in this context have a particular resonance. Similarly, examples of stress-induced decrements in hepatitis B vaccine efficacy in medical students may have ramifications for clinical practice (37). There are also ethical benefits to carefully selecting your vaccine on the basis of clinical relevance; it is easier to persuade ethics committees, and indeed potential study participants, of the benefits of your research if you will be administering vaccines that will be of direct benefit to your cohort.

3.1.3. Antigen Novelty in Your Population

It is also important to consider the novelty of the vaccine antigen in your population. The first time the immune system encounters an antigen, it produces a slower, “primary” immune response. In contrast, if it is a familiar antigen, a more rapid and effective “secondary” immune response is generated. The three-dose hepatitis B vaccination course administered over a period of 6 months, would therefore allow the assessment of the initial primary response to the first vaccination, and then secondary responses to the subsequent doses. This could help elucidate which aspects of the immune response are more susceptible to psychosocial influence. This model assumes, however, that the participants are naïve to the hepatitis B antigen at study entry. In the UK, this would be likely in most young, healthy adults, as it is rare for them to have been exposed to the blood-borne hepatitis B virus naturalistically and there is no routine vaccination programme for those outside high risk groups such as medical practitioners or drug users. However, in many countries, hepatitis B vaccine is given routinely in childhood, and therefore such a model would not be possible. This illustrates how important it is to be aware of the vaccination and exposure history of your potential cohort.

Some researchers circumvent the issues of naturalistic exposure or previous vaccination entirely, by using a non-clinical vaccination such as keyhole limpet hemocyanin (KLH) (38, 39). KLH is a novel copper-containing protein, derived from the giant keyhole limpet mollusc. It is non-pathogenic and is not encountered naturally, but when given as a vaccine it induces a pronounced primary immune response in humans. This gives many advantages for study design, as it is possible to give repeated doses and therefore control whether you are examining a primary or secondary response; this allows much more mechanistic studies. In addition, as a non-clinical vaccine, KLH is not affected by changes in vaccine composition that hamper, for example, research using the influenza vaccination. At least some of the three strains contained in this trivalent vaccine change each year to reflect the current naturalistic prevalence of different strains of influenza. This makes it difficult to conduct a study over more than one season and combine the data, particularly if the analysis uses the absolute antibody levels, the magnitude of which will vary dependent on strain. Although this can be dealt with statistically to some extent, the use of KLH abrogates this issue entirely. However, antibody responses to non-pathogenic novel antigens are less easy to interpret in terms of their clinical relevance.

3.1.4. Vaccine Efficacy in Your Population

The relative immunogenicity of the vaccination should also be taken into account. Vaccines vary in their efficacy, and there is some evidence that this may affect their susceptibility to psychosocial factors such as stress. For example, studies using the trivalent influenza vaccine often find that only one strain is influenced by psychosocial factors (11, 20). It has also been argued that strains which evoke robust antibody responses, i.e., are more immunogenic, are less susceptible to psychosocial influence whereas less antigenic strains are more vulnerable to such effects (1); as mentioned previously, this has also been observed in the context of acute stress and antibody response to vaccination. As well as choosing an appropriate vaccination for your cohort, this issue can also be addressed by changing the vaccine dose (40); this technique could be used to conduct a more systematic examination of the relationship between vaccine immunogenicity and susceptibility to stress. In sum, these various theoretical and clinical implications, and your own research priorities, should be considered when the choice of vaccination is made, in order to maximize the eventual impact of the study findings.

3.2. Timing of Assessment and Antibody Subclass

3.2.1. Baseline Assessments

One of the key benefits of the vaccination model, compared to examining the response to naturalistic infection, is the ability to measure the antibody status at baseline, prior to antigen exposure, and then again post-vaccination in order to assess the magnitude of the response over a set period. The baseline measurement allows the researcher to adjust for previous exposure to the antigen; as discussed above, this is crucial as pre-vaccination antibody levels are a good predictors of the subsequent response.

3.2.2. Initial Antibody Responses

The amount of time between vaccination and follow-up assessment will, again, depend on the priorities of the study. Immunoglobulin G, the main antibody subclass generated by vaccination, typically peaks at 4–6 weeks post-vaccination; this has been the focus of the majority of PNI studies. However, a novel vaccine will also elicit a primary immune response, generating immunoglobulin (Ig) M which peaks at around 1 week post-vaccination. IgM plays a key role in clearance of infection by activating the complement cascade, and promoting an efficient neutralizing IgG response (41). Recent research has demonstrated that social support is positively associated with the IgM (9) response to the polyvalent pneumococcal polysaccharide vaccine. In addition, chronic self-regulatory failure, in which individuals see themselves as failing to make progress towards their goals, has been shown to be associated with the IgM, but not the IgG, response to influenza vaccination (42); the clinical implications of such a finding for this viral antigen is less clear, and these issues warrant further attention in a wider range of vaccines.

3.2.3. Maintenance of Antibody Protection

As well as early and peak responses, it is important to assess the maintenance of antibody levels over time. When vaccinating patients, it is assumed that the vaccine will provide long lasting protection against the appropriate disease. In fact, there is considerable individual variation in the extent to which antibody levels are sustained, and there are preliminary indications that psychosocial factors may be associated with this maintenance. For example, a study of two cohorts of students vaccinated against hepatitis B, either within the last year or earlier than that, only found associations between antibody levels and psychological stress in those participants vaccinated more than a year ago (37). Similarly, a study comparing pneumococcal vaccine efficacy between caregivers and controls found group differences at 3 and 6 months post-vaccination, but not at 2 weeks or 1 month (43). By assessing early, peak, and long term antibody levels, the impact of psychosocial processes on different aspects of immune protection can be investigated.

3.3. Outcome Measures

The choice of assay is a more practical consideration that can impact on the costs and labor involved in measuring the antibody levels.

3.3.1. Ways of Measuring Antibody Levels

Hemagglutination Inhibition Assay

A common and economical method for assessing the response to influenza vaccine is the hemagglutination inhibition (HAI) assay. Influenza virus particles are able to bind erythrocytes together into a lattice-like structure, via a surface protein known as hemagglutinin; specific antibodies inhibit this process. This assay compares the ability of a range of serum dilutions to inhibit the hemagglutination. The highest dilution of serum that prevents hemagglutination is the antibody titer; for example, a serum antibody titer of 40 means that hemagglutination was blocked at a dilution of 1:40, but not at further dilutions. The HAI assay is a clinically relevant, widely accepted tool for assessing antibody levels to influenza vaccination. These are relatively simple assays that do not need specialist equipment beyond that of a standard laboratory. However, the HAI assay is unable to distinguish between different antibody subclasses, and must be conducted separately for each vaccine strain of interest.

Enzyme-Linked Immunosorbent Assay

An enzyme-linked immunosorbent assay (ELISA) is a common method used to assess specific antibody levels against a variety of vaccinations. The relevant antigen is adhered to the base of the small plastic wells of a microtiter plate and the serum samples added. Any specific antibody binds to the antigen and the rest of the serum is then washed away. Through a series of chemical reactions, a color response is generated; the greater the antibody concentration, the deeper the color. This assay is simple to perform, and can be adapted to measure different antibody subclasses. However, as with the HAI assay, antibodies against only one antigen can be assessed at a time. As vaccines such as influenza and pneumococcal contain multiple antigens, assessment of the antibody response to each strain can be time consuming.

Luminex

A more recent technological development are multiplex systems, such as Luminex, which allow simultaneous assessment of the antibody response to multiple antigens. Instead of adhering the antigen to the base of a microtiter plate, the system uses up to 100 sets of microscopic color-coded beads; each set can be associated with a different antigen. A "cocktail" of relevant beads can be mixed with the serum, whereby any specific antibodies will adhere to the appropriate beads. Captured antibodies are detected using a biotinylated detection antibody and streptavidin–phycoerythrin (S–PE); again, this can be modified to assess either IgG or IgM levels. The sample is passed through the dual laser analyzer; one laser identifies the bead, and therefore the antigen, and the other determines the magnitude of the PE-derived signal which is in direct proportion to the amount of analyte bound. Multiple standard curves then allow this information to be translated into a specific antibody level for each of the separate antigens contained in the vaccine. As psychosocial effects have largely been found with polyvalent vaccinations where a number of similar acting antigenic strains are administered in one vaccine, this type of technology is likely to be crucial in comparing the relative susceptibility of different strains.

3.3.2. Alternatives to Antibody Response

Although antibody levels have been the most common way to assess vaccine efficacy, both in PNI and the wider immunology arena, there remain some concerns about how well they reflect clinical protection against infection (21). There are a number of propositions of alternate measures that could be considered, although the technology for some of the latter techniques remains in its infancy.

Serum Bactericidal Antibody Assay

For vaccines against bacterial antigens, a serum bactericidal antibody (SBA) assay can be performed. In this assay, serial dilutions of human sera are incubated with appropriate bacterial target cells and complement. Activation of the antibody-dependent classical complement pathway ultimately results in lysis of the target cell. The SBA titer for each serum is expressed as the reciprocal serum dilution yielding 50 % killing as compared to the number of target cells present before incubation with serum and complement (44). SBA activity has been shown to highly correlate with immunity to meningococcal disease (45). Although the only study to use this assay in this context found no associations with psychosocial factors (46), the clinical relevance of the measure would argue that future studies should consider incorporating this sort of approach.

Markers of Cellular Immunity

Although antibody levels are a key determinant of protection against viruses such as influenza, the involvement of the cellular immune system is also important in clearing the infection. As such, markers of cellular immunity are likely to be a useful outcome measure for PNI research. One example is the assessment of ex vivo production of Granzyme B in response to influenza virus following vaccination, which has been shown to predict risk of influenza infection (47). Similarly, flow cytometry techniques are being developed that could be used to assess cytokine responses induced by vaccines, and to determine which aspects of the response best predict vaccine efficacy (21, 48). PNI researchers will need to keep abreast of these developments in order to ensure that we continue to use the most advanced immunological methods available.

4. Conclusion

Antibody response to vaccination is a useful measure of in vivo immune function for PNI research. There is now a relatively large literature demonstrating that these markers are associated with a wide range of psychosocial factors, and preliminary evidence that they are amenable to psychological intervention. The multitude of methodological options to consider may be initially intimidating, but this variety also provides the researcher with many opportunities to tailor the studies to reflect their particular research priorities. These strategic methodological choices enable further investigation of underlying mechanisms of these relationships, and exploration of the role of psychosocial interventions in augmenting antibody response to vaccination. The results of these studies are likely to have important implications both for improving vaccine efficacy and as a marker of a more generalized improvement in immune system function.

References

1. Cohen S, Miller GE, Rabin BS (2001) Psychological stress and antibody response to immunization: a critical review of the human literature. Psychosom Med 63:7–18
2. Burns VE, Gallagher S (2010) Antibody response to vaccination as a marker of in vivo immune function in psychophysiological research. Neurosci Biobehav Rev 35:122–126
3. Vedhara K, Fox JD, Wang ECY (1999) The measurement of stress-related immune dysfunction in psychoneuroimmunology. Neurosci Biobehav Rev 23:699–715
4. Ader R (2006) Psychoneuroimmunology. Academic, New York
5. Segerstrom SC, Miller GE (2004) Psychological stress and the human immune system: a meta-analytic study of 30 years of inquiry. Psychol Bull 130:601–630
6. Glaser R, Kiecolt-Glaser JK (2005) Stress-induced immune dysfunction: implications for health. Nat Rev Immunol 5:243–251
7. Phillips AC, Carroll D, Burns VE et al (2005) Neuroticism, cortisol reactivity, and antibody response to vaccination. Psychophysiology 42:232–238
8. Pressman SD, Cohen S, Miller GE et al (2005) Loneliness, social network size, and immune response to influenza vaccination in college freshmen. Health Psychol 24:297–306
9. Gallagher S, Phillips AC, Ferraro AJ et al (2008) Social support is positively associated with the immunoglobulin M response to vaccination with pneumococcal polysaccharides. Biol Psychol 78:211–215
10. Gallagher S, Phillips AC, Ferraro AJ et al (2008) Psychosocial factors are associated with the antibody response to both thymus-dependent and thymus-independent vaccines. Brain Behav Immun 22:456–460
11. Phillips AC, Burns VE, Carroll D et al (2005) The association between life events, social support, and antibody status following thymus-dependent and thymus-independent vaccinations in healthy young adults. Brain Behav Immun 19:325–333
12. Marsland AL, Cohen S, Rabin BS et al (2006) Trait positive affect and antibody response to hepatitis B vaccination. Brain Behav Immun 20:261–269
13. Edwards KM, Burns VE, Reynolds T et al (2005) Acute stress exposure prior to influenza vaccination enhances antibody response in women. Brain Behav Immun 20:159–168
14. Davidson RJ, Kabat-Zinn J, Schumacher J et al (2003) Alterations in brain and immune function produced by mindfulness meditation. Psychosom Med 65:564–570
15. Vedhara K, Bennett PD, Clark S et al (2003) Enhancement of antibody responses to influenza vaccination in the elderly following a cognitive-behavioural stress management intervention. Psychother Psychosom 72:245–252
16. Roitt IM, Delves PJ (2001) Essential immunology. Blackwell, Oxford
17. Felten DL, Felten SY, Carlson SL et al (1985) Noradrenergic and peptidergic innervation of lymphoid tissue. J Immunol 135:755–765
18. Sanders VM, Straub RH (2001) Norepinephrine, the beta-adrenergic receptor, and immunity. Brain Behav Immun 16:290–332
19. Nance DM, Sanders VM (2007) Autonomic innervation and regulation of the immune system (1987–2007). Brain Behav Immun 21:736–745
20. Miller GE, Cohen S, Pressman S et al (2004) Psychological stress and antibody response to influenza vaccination: when is the critical period for stress, and how does it get inside the body? Psychosom Med 66:215–223
21. Bolton DL, Roederer M (2009) Flow cytometry and the future of vaccine development. Expert Rev Vaccines 8:779–789
22. Couch RB, Kasel JA (1983) Immunity to influenza in man. Annu Rev Microbiol 37:529–549
23. Hannoun C, Megas F, Piercy J (2004) Immunogenicity and protective efficacy of influenza vaccination. Virus Res 103:133–138

24. Hadler SC, Francis DP, Maynard JE et al (1986) Long-term immunogenicity and efficacy of hepatitis B vaccine in homosexual men. N Engl J Med 315:209–214
25. Grubeck-Loebenstein B (2010) Fading immune protection in old age: vaccination in the elderly. J Comp Pathol 142(suppl 1): S116–S119
26. Dhabhar FS, McEwen B (1999) Enhancing versus suppressive effects of stress hormones on skin immune function. Proc Natl Acad Sci USA 96:1059–1064
27. Edwards KM, Burns VE, Carroll D et al (2007) The acute stress-induced immunoenhancement hypothesis. Exerc Sport Sci Rev 35:150–155
28. Edwards KM, Burns VE, Adkins AE et al (2008) Meningococcal A vaccination response is enhanced by acute stress in men. Psychosom Med 70:147–151
29. Graham NMH, Douglas RM, Ryan P (1986) Stress and acute respiratory infection. Am J Epidemiol 124:389–401
30. Meyer RJ, Haggerty RJ (1962) Streptococcal infection in families: factors altering individual susceptibility. Pediatrics 29:539–549
31. Cohen S, Doyle WJ, Skoner DP (1999) Psychological stress, cytokine production, and severity of upper respiratory illness. Psychosom Med 61:175–180
32. Cohen S, Tyrrell DAJ, Smith AP (1991) Psychological stress and susceptibility to the common cold. N Eng J Med 325:606–612
33. Christian LM (2011) Psychoneuroimmunology in pregnancy: immune pathways linking stress with maternal health, adverse birth outcomes, and fetal development. Neurosci Biobehav Rev 36(1):350–361
34. Gallagher S, Phillips AC, Drayson MT et al (2009) Caregiving for children with developmental disabilities is associated with a poor antibody response to influenza vaccination. Psychosom Med 71:341–344
35. Gallagher S, Phillips AC, Drayson MT et al (2009) Parental caregivers of children with developmental disabilities mount a poor antibody response to pneumococcal vaccination. Brain Behav Immun 23:338–346
36. Govaert TME, Thijs CT, Masurel N et al (1994) The efficacy of influenza vaccination in elderly individuals. JAMA 272:1661–1665
37. Burns VE, Carroll D, Ring C et al (2002) Stress, coping, and hepatitis B antibody status. Psychosom Med 64:287–293
38. Smith TP, Kennedy SL, Fleshner M (2004) Influence of age and physical activity on the primary in vivo antibody and T cell-mediated responses in men. J Appl Physiol 97:491–498
39. Smith AJ, Bennett B, Vollmer-Conna U et al (2002) The effect of distress on the development of a primary immune response. Psychosom Med 64:166-Abstract
40. Edwards KM, Campbell JP, Ring C et al (2010) Exercise intensity does not influence the efficacy of eccentric exercise as a behavioural adjuvant to vaccination. Brain Behav Immun 24:623–630
41. Baumgarth N, Herman OC, Jager GC et al (2000) B-1 and B-2 cell-derived immunoglobulin M antibodies are nonredundant components of the protective response to influenza virus infection. J Exp Med 192:271–280
42. Strauman TJ, Coe CL, McCrudden MC et al (2008) Individual differences in self-regulatory failure and menstrual dysfunction predict upper respiratory infection symptoms and antibody response to flu immunization. Brain Behav Immun 22:769–780
43. Glaser R, Sheridan JF, Malarkey W et al (2000) Chronic stress modulates the immune response to a pneumococcal pneumonia vaccine. Psychosom Med 62:804–807
44. Maslanka SE, Gheesling LL, Libutti DE et al (1997) Standardization and a multilaboratory comparison of *Neisseria meningitidis* Serogroup A and C serum bactericidal assays. Clin Diag Lab Immunol 4:156–167
45. Goldschneider I, Gotschlich EC, Artenstein MS (1969) Human immunity to the meningococcus. I. The role of humoral antibodies. J Exp Med 129:1307–1326
46. Burns VE, Drayson M, Carroll D et al (2002) Antibody status following meningitis C conjugate vaccination is predicted by perceived stress and psychological well-being. Brain Behav Immun 16:173
47. McElhaney JE, Ewen C, Zhou X et al (2009) Granzyme B: correlates with protection and enhanced CTL response to influenza vaccination in older adults. Vaccine 27:2418–2425
48. Lash GE, Pinto LA (2010) Multiplex cytokine analysis technologies. Expert Rev Vaccines 9:1231–1237

Chapter 20

Translational Bioinformatics in Psychoneuroimmunology: Methods and Applications

Qing Yan

Abstract

Translational bioinformatics plays an indispensable role in transforming psychoneuroimmunology (PNI) into personalized medicine. It provides a powerful method to bridge the gaps between various knowledge domains in PNI and systems biology. Translational bioinformatics methods at various systems levels can facilitate pattern recognition, and expedite and validate the discovery of systemic biomarkers to allow their incorporation into clinical trials and outcome assessments. Analysis of the correlations between genotypes and phenotypes including the behavioral-based profiles will contribute to the transition from the disease-based medicine to human-centered medicine. Translational bioinformatics would also enable the establishment of predictive models for patient responses to diseases, vaccines, and drugs. In PNI research, the development of systems biology models such as those of the neurons would play a critical role. Methods based on data integration, data mining, and knowledge representation are essential elements in building health information systems such as electronic health records and computerized decision support systems. Data integration of genes, pathophysiology, and behaviors are needed for a broad range of PNI studies. Knowledge discovery approaches such as network-based systems biology methods are valuable in studying the cross-talks among pathways in various brain regions involved in disorders such as Alzheimer's disease.

Key words: Bioinformatics, Computers, Data integration, Data mining, Databases, Decision support, Personalized medicine, Psychoneuroimmunology, Systems biology, Translational medicine

1. The Role of Translational Bioinformatics in Psychoneuro-immunology

With the rapid development pace in scientific discoveries and information technology, biomedicine is reaching a revolutionary tipping point that could lead to better understanding of health and more effective preventive and therapeutic strategies for diseases. To achieve the optimal health and wellness, multidimensional factors need to be identified, including those from the behavioral, social, and biological aspects (1). Stronger interdisciplinary collaborations would be needed

Qing Yan (ed.), *Psychoneuroimmunology: Methods and Protocols*, Methods in Molecular Biology, vol. 934,
DOI 10.1007/978-1-62703-071-7_20, © Springer Science+Business Media, LLC 2012

to establish the biobehavioral-social-ecologic models of multilevel systems including the molecular, cellular, physiological, psychological, and environmental levels (see Chapter 1).

Studies in psychoneuroimmunology (PNI) may provide a platform for the collaboration between different disciplines including psychology, psychiatry, neurobiology, immunology, and informatics. Systems biology is also an interdisciplinary field across many knowledge domains including genomics, proteomics, physiology and pathology, pharmacology and toxicology, as well as clinical medicine (2). Systems biology is a promising field that studies the interactions among biological elements for the thorough understanding of diseases at the various systems levels toward personalized and systems medicine (3). With the new approaches in analyzing biomedical systems, studies in PNI and systems biology may offer novel preventive and therapeutic strategies.

However, one of the most significant obstacles in the practice of personalized and systems medicine is the translation of scientific discoveries into better therapeutic outcomes. A critical factor in the successful translation from the "bench" to the "bedside" is the access, management, and analysis of integrated data within and across functional domains (4). For example, most of clinical and basic research data are currently stored in disparate and separate systems, it is often difficult for clinicians and researchers to access and share these data (5). Furthermore, inefficient workflow management in clinics and laboratories has created many obstacles for decision making and outcomes assessments.

With the current shift of research strategies from reductionist-driven approaches to systematic approaches for extracting information from the whole system to develop hypotheses, informatics support is becoming indispensable (6, 7). For example, many approaches have been used for the elucidation of associated genes and potential biomarkers in patients with schizophrenia (8). These approaches include the analyses of relevant metabolomics, transcriptomics, proteomics, protein–protein interactions, neuronal cell cultures, as well as behavioral studies. Such approaches have generated a huge amount of data that need powerful data analysis and systems biology methods to analyze the complexity of the brain and behavior to develop systems models for better therapeutics (8).

With such demands, it is urgent to develop novel technologies for effective data management and integration, data sharing and exchanging, knowledge discovery and representation, as well as decision support. Bioinformatics uses computational approaches to solve problems and improve the communication, management, understanding, and analysis of biomedical information (9). Bioinformatics methods will be valuable to enable the effective collaboration among experts including both scientists and clinicians.

For instance, informatics models have been suggested to help psychiatric studies by establishing better theories that may integrate psychiatry with neuroscience, and by enabling better testing of complex hypotheses against complex data via their powerful analytical methods (10).

Specifically, translational bioinformatics can provide a powerful method to bridge the gaps between various knowledge domains in PNI and systems biology, as well as the gaps between the basic research findings and clinical outcomes in translational medicine. As defined by the American Medical Informatics Association (AMIA), translational bioinformatics is "the development of storage, analytic, and interpretive methods to optimize the transformation of increasingly voluminous biomedical data, and genomic data, into proactive, predictive, preventive, and participatory health" (11).

Translational bioinformatics in PNI studies needs to integrate multiple disciplines including general bioinformatics, neuroinformatics, immunoinformatics, health and medical informatics, public health, as well as translational medicine. Neuroinformatics and immunoinformatics have now become independent fields with rich contents. Discussion of these two fields is beyond the scope and length of this chapter. This chapter will focus on general translational bioinformatics methods and their applications in PNI studies, especially in behavioral studies and personalized medicine.

Translational bioinformatics may improve the integration of clinical and laboratory data streams for a better management of workflows for more efficient utilizations of healthcare resources with lower costs (7). Applications such as electronic health records (EHRs) and knowledge representation tools may facilitate the share of information and help solve the system interoperability problems. Such applications will also allow the establishment, implementation, and compliance of various biomedical standards in PNI studies.

More importantly, translational bioinformatics can promote the practice of personalized and systems medicine with its decision support functions based on the methods of data integration, data mining, and knowledge discovery (7). These methods can help with the reduction of clinical risks and the promotion of patient satisfaction. For example, computer-based information systems have been considered the most cost-effective and promising strategy for preventing adverse therapeutic events and overcoming therapeutic resistance (12). Such approaches will empower scientists and clinicians to design personalized strategies to bring the right interventions with the right dosages to the right people at the right time. By improving communications among multidisciplinary groups in PNI, better collaborations would allow more accurate diagnosis and the optimal outcomes.

2. Translational Bioinformatics Methods in PNI and Personalized Medicine

2.1. Systemic Profiles, Patient Subgroups, and Systems Models in PNI

To achieve the goal of personalized medicine, informatics tools are especially useful for the prediction of substantial disease subpopulations. Translational bioinformatics can facilitate pattern recognition, and expedite and validate the discovery of biomarkers to allow their incorporation into clinical trial design and outcome assessments (7). These are important steps for understanding the mechanisms of patient responses to diseases and therapeutics (13). Specifically, the analysis of high throughput (HTP) data, the establishment of patient systemic profiles, and the informatics modeling of molecular or higher level systems would enable profound and novel insights into the mechanisms of health and diseases.

For example, because genome-wide association studies (GWAS) have been unsuccessful in identifying risk variants in neuropsychiatric disorders including schizophrenia, behavioral informatics for analyzing multivariable behavioral profiles has been proposed (14). Behavioral profiles can be used as phenotypes instead of traditional "subtypes" of a disease. Behavioral profiles are an integrative and quantitative abstraction of the emotional characteristics, personality, and neurocognitive functions of each individual patient (14). Based on the systemic behavioral profile, patient subgroups can be identified for the further investigation of genetic risk factors. The associations between different neuropsychiatric diseases such as schizophrenia and bipolar disorder that share similar clinical features can also be discovered. In addition, the applications of such systemic behavioral profiles may enable more powerful statistical analysis for exploring the correlations at various systems levels. Analysis of behavioral profile-based phenotypes will make significant contributions to the transition from the single-measure and disease-based medicine to human-centered medicine.

By integrating and analyzing complex data, translational bioinformatics can also help establish predictive models for the simulation of interrelationships and interactions among the components of the system (2). According to the systems biology paradigm, interactions at various levels such as cellular networks are considered as dynamic and self-organizing events in the whole system. Such models can in turn help predict the behavior of the whole system, such as patient responses to vaccines or drugs. Translational bioinformatics would enable the identification of systems-based biomarkers, as well as the understanding of systemic structure–function, genotype–phenotype, and gene–environment correlations (7).

For example, in the field of psychiatric research, the development of systems biology models such as those of the neurons would play a critical role for a better understanding of mental disorders (15). Understanding the structural and functional complexity of the brain has become the main challenge in studying mental disorders from a system's point of view. Some theoretical quantitative models have been used for computer simulation to describe disorders including addiction (15). Systems modeling approaches can be used for studying systemic behaviors, signaling pathways, as well as neuronal networks dynamics and circuits such as the prefrontal cortical working memory circuits that are involved in schizophrenia (15). Such approaches may be very useful for the elucidation of spatio-temporal interactions in the PNI systems (i.e., the nervous, immune, and endocrine systems) to develop novel and effective interventions (15). Based on the identification of patient's systemic profiles and patient subgroups, translational bioinformatics can help establish the predictive and systems models in order to achieve more accurate diagnosis, prognosis, and the optimal therapy.

2.2. Translational Bioinformatics Methods at Various Systems Levels

Different bioinformatics methods can be used for PNI studies at various systems levels. At the molecular level, the genetic features can be explored, such as the structures, functions, the connections between them, as well as the effects of structural alterations on functional activities. To study genetic structural features, approaches can be used include the exploration of sequence similarities, patterns, and motifs, as well as structures in two- and three-dimensions (2D and 3D). Phylogenetic analysis by making phylogenetic trees can be used to study the evolution of the genes. Specifically, bioinformatics programs such as BLAST (16) and CLUSTAL (17) can be applied for finding structural and functional changes over time (see Table 1). The tools PROSITE (18) and UniProt (19) are helpful for studying genetic motifs, patterns, and gene families. The 2D and 3D structural modeling such as using PredictProtein (20) and PDB (21) can help understand the protein–protein and protein–drug interactions (see Table 1). To study genetic variations such as single nucleotide polymorphisms (SNPs), the International HapMap Project is helpful for GWAS of patterns and disease associations (22, 23). Another tool for the analysis of SNPs is the dbSNP (24) (see Table 1).

At the cellular level, many bioinformatics programs can be used for studying the interactions and pathways, such as GenMAPP (25), Kyoto Encyclopedia of Genes and Genomes (KEGG) (26), HPRD (27), Reactome (28), and BioGRID (29) (see Table 1). The analyses at higher levels including the tissue and organism levels are important for studying the genotype–phenotype correlations for understanding diseases and drug responses, such as by using OMIM (30) (see Table 1). The program of Gene Expression Omnibus (GEO) (31) can be used together with experimental approaches such as HTP technologies and next-generation sequencing techniques. Furthermore, neuroinformatics and immunoinformatics tools can also be applied in PNI studies (see Table 1).

For example, computational methods for candidate gene selection and prioritization have been used based on the similarity

Table 1
Translational bioinformatics resources for PNI studies[a]

Name	URL	Applications
BLAST	http://www.ncbi.nlm.nih.gov/BLAST/	Sequence comparisons
CLUSTAL	http://www.clustal.org/	Sequence alignments
PROSITE	http://www.expasy.org/prosite/	Finding motifs in a sequence
UniProt	http://www.uniprot.org/	Protein information
PredictProtein	http://www.predictprotein.org/	Protein 2D structure prediction
Protein Data Bank (PDB)	http://www.pdb.org	Structural data
International HapMap Project	http://snp.cshl.org/	Sequence variations, maps
dbSNP	http://www.ncbi.nlm.nih.gov/SNP/	NCBI's database of SNPs
GenMAPP	http://www.genmapp.org/	Pathway tools
KEGG	http://www.genome.jp/kegg/pathway.html	Pathway databases, tools
HPRD	http://www.hprd.org/	Pathways and networks
Reactome	http://www.reactome.org/	Pathways
BioGRID	http://www.thebiogrid.org/	Interaction datasets
Online Mendelian Inheritance in Man (OMIM)	http://www.ncbi.nlm.nih.gov/omim	A catalog of human genes and genetic disorders
Gene Expression Omnibus (GEO)	http://www.ncbi.nlm.nih.gov/geo/	Gene expression and array database
Microarray Informatics at EBI	http://www.ebi.ac.uk/microarray/	Microarray data analyses
NHGRI Microarray Project	http://research.nhgri.nih.gov/microarray/	Microarray databases, tools
The Neuroinformatics Portal	http://www.pharmtao.com/neuroinformatics	Neuroinformatics resources
The Immunoinformatics Portal	http://www.pharmtao.com/immunoinformatics	Immunoinformatics resources
Unified modeling language (UML)	http://www.uml.org/	An object-oriented modeling language
Gene Ontology (GO)	http://www.geneontology.org/	Genetic ontology
G2Cdb	http://www.genes2cognition.org	A neuroscience database of synapse proteins
Phenowiki	www.Phenowiki.org	A knowledge base for neuropsychiatric research

(continued)

Table 1 (continued)

Name	URL	Applications
Systems Biology Markup Language (SBML)	http://sbml.org/Main_Page	For building systems biology models
Systematized Nomenclature of Medicine—Clinical Terms (SNOMED-CT)	http://www.nlm.nih.gov/research/umls/Snomed/snomed_main.html	A comprehensive clinical terminology
International Classification of Disease (ICD)	http://www.who.int/classifications/icd/en/	Classifications of diseases
Logical Observation Identifiers Names and Codes (LOINC)	http://loinc.org/	Universal codes to identify clinical observations
Digital Imaging and Communication in Medicine (DICOM)	http://medical.nema.org/	A standard for information in medical imaging
Health Level Seven (HL7)	http://www.hl7.org/	Standards for interoperability
Unified Medical Language System (UMLS)	http://www.nlm.nih.gov/research/umls/	Terminology, classification and coding standards
The Health Insurance Portability and Accountability Act (HIPAA)	http://www.hhs.gov/ocr/privacy	About patient privacy, security, and relevant rules
Healthcare Information and Management Systems (HIMSS)	http://www.himss.org/ASP/index.asp	Information technology (IT) and systems for healthcare
The Translational Bioinformatics Portal (TBP)	http://bioinformatics.pharmtao.com	A collection of translational bioinformatics resources

[a]The sites were accessed December, 2011

analysis with known disease genes, the functional genetic annotations, and the analysis of pertinent sequence motifs or signatures. The application of such approaches in analyzing X-linked mental retardation (XLMR) resulted in a ranked list of candidate genes related to the development of mental retardation, such as the genes APLN, MAGED4, and UXT (32). Short sequence patterns and motifs were analyzed to differentiate XLMR from non-XLMR genes. Such approaches that combine gene annotation, sequence motif analysis, and gene prediction methods are very useful for identifying candidate genes in PNI research.

In another example, by screening transcriptome data from the GEO program associated with anxiety- and depression-like phenotypes, potential biomarkers were found for anxiety (33). These candidate markers include the dysfunction of carbohydrate metabolism, tight junction, and the phosphatidylinositol signaling pathways. In depression, features found included the dysfunction of gap junction, gonadotropin-releasing hormone signaling, and ubiquitin-mediated proteolysis pathways (33). Both anxiety and depression had features of dysfunctions of VEGF signaling, long-term potentiation, and the glycolysis pathway (33). These examples have demonstrated the usefulness of the translational bioinformatics methods and the applications of the tools in PNI.

3. Translational Biomedical Informatics for Decision Support in PNI

3.1. Data Management and Data Integration

Data are often complicated with various factors such as time, heterogeneous sources, and individuals. Data integration is an important step for the identification of biomarkers and for creating predictive models of interactions. Because PNI contains knowledge from multiple domains, the data integration process is especially important. Data and workflow integration can help improve time and economic efficiency, allow further data mining, and benefit clinical outcomes. Data integration is critical not only for providing data sharing and access, but also for pattern analysis, knowledge discovery, and decision support (9).

Specifically, data integration is a process that removes errors, resolves inconsistencies in the representation of data, standardizes names and values, and integrates common values together (7). It is an "evolution" process from "untreated" crude format to the ready-to-use information. At the beginning of this process, data are identified, collected, and chosen by screening all available sources and selecting the ones that can best meet the requirements. For PNI studies, different types of data from various knowledge domains need to be selected and collected, such as nucleotide and amino acid sequence information, expression data, protein–protein interaction data, as well as behavioral data. Data sources can be from high-throughput experiments, clinical practice, as well as electronic systems. For example, a Web-based computer-assisted interviewing (CAI) system has been found useful for collecting data from those with mental disorders to provide valuable and quickly accessible data for better clinical decision making (34).

Data are hardly clean. Based on concept extraction and modeling methods such as using the Unified Modeling Language (UML) (35), the selected data need to be cleansed, validated, curated, updated, and structuralized. Because biomedical data have a feature of volatility, i.e., the contents in the database may grow and change over time, updates are needed frequently. Selected data may have different formats from disparate sources. Common values in data need to be integrated together with a consistent and unified format. Redundancies and inconsistencies are common problems with biomedical data and need to be resolved (7). For example, one gene may have many different names, such as TAP1, ABC17, and ABCB2, which all refer to the same gene "transporter 1, ATP-binding cassette, sub-family B (MDR/TAP)" but may have different entries. Such redundancies and inconsistencies need to be solved by using genetic nomenclatures such as the Gene Ontology (GO) (see Table 1).

For genomic studies, data merging techniques are usually used. That is, various datasets can be concatenated in a database by cross-referencing the sequence identifiers. Another method is to integrate multiple layers of data into one mathematical model, such as by using a kernel-based integration framework (36). In such an approach, data can be selected based on the relevant features from all available sources, and integrated in a machine learning-based model.

Databases that integrate various data of genes, proteins, pathophysiology, anatomy, and behaviors are needed for a broad range of PNI studies. One approach is to develop a general Web-based data infrastructure. For example, G2Cdb is a neuroscience database focusing on the role of synapse proteins in physiology and diseases ((37), also see Table 1). The database contains data from proteomic mass spectroscopy of signaling pathways. Using automated text-mining and human curation methods, the database extracted information from published neurobiological studies relevant to synaptic signaling electrophysiology and diseases influenced by mutations in synaptic genes (37). Such datasets may be useful for correlating genotypes in the brain-signaling with phenotypes in diseases.

Based on the human genome project, significant amount of data and knowledge have been collected at the genomic level. However, higher-level knowledge bases that connect genotypes and phenotypes are underdeveloped, such as those for the complex neuropsychiatric symptoms, cognitive functions, and neural systems phenotypes. Some efforts have been made to bridge such gaps, such as a knowledge base for neuropsychiatric research ((38), also see Table 1). The knowledge base focuses on the features of specific cognitive tasks and prioritizes endophenotypes for translational research. Such integrative databases or knowledge bases can help with the analysis of genome-wide expression microarray datasets by using methods such as variance analysis, correlation analysis, and functional annotation tools (39).

Some advanced computational techniques can also be very beneficial. For instance, a data warehouse can be useful to provide a unified platform for data curation (5). Data warehousing is the technique to combine and integrate data from different sources into a common format. It is a collection of subject-oriented databases, and designed exclusively for decision support purposes (30). Further developments of the bioinformatics capability are still needed to provide adequate support for the rapidly increasing data and knowledge in PNI and other biomedical fields.

3.2. Data Standardization, Ontology, and Knowledge Representation

Standardization techniques including semantic mapping are needed for better communication and data exchanging in both laboratory and clinical settings. Standardization is valuable for solving the interoperability problems among heterogeneous scientific and clinical systems. Such approaches are necessary for decision support in biomarker discovery and making predictive models.

Extensive biomedical and technical standards can be used for translational bioinformatics applications in PNI, including those for genomic data, imaging data, and clinical data. For example, for clinical data, standards such as Systematized Nomenclature of Medicine—Clinical Terms (SNOMED CT) and the International Classification of Disease (ICD) are often used (see Table 1). For laboratory data, the universal codes to identify laboratory observations (LOINC) can be used. For imaging data such as the neuroimaging analyses, Digital Imaging and Communications in Medicine (DICOM) is useful. For genomic data, nomenclature references including the GO can be applied (see Table 1). For building genetic pathways and systems biology models, the Systems Biology Markup Language (SBML) can be useful (40). Some organizations such as HL7 also provide standards for solving interoperability problems (see Table 1). One integrative platform, the Unified Medical Language System (UMLS) integrates various terminology and coding sources and serves as a reference system (see Table 1).

Besides cleaning and standardization, another important step for data integration and decision support is data structuralizing. Structured data and information enables rapid and efficient access and retrieval, as well as automated processing (41). It would also facilitate the integration with general information systems such as EHRs. Structured information and knowledge presentation methods such as using ontologies may reduce the complexity of text processing and improve searching performance.

Data integration and knowledge representation are essential elements in building computerized decision support systems (CDSS) to be used by researchers, clinicians, and the general public. Knowledge representation refers to the expression of knowledge in a format that can be explained and reasoned with by humans and machines (42). Knowledge representation can be achieved via data modeling and the building of multidimensional databases (35). As a useful method, ontology studies concept definitions in a domain and the associations among the concepts. For example, documents can be pre-indexed by a conceptual hierarchy to facilitate concept-based search (43). Ontologies have been used to represent clinical guidelines and biomedical facts. These approaches can help transform biomedical data into useful information for decision support in clinical practice.

Ontology-based computational network model can be used for analyzing large-scale genetic association data for complex diseases and phenotypes (44). Such models can embrace knowledge from various levels including molecules, cellular pathways, complex behavioral phenotypes, and environmental factors. By representing complex scientific theories, these models can be used to support interdisciplinary research and facilitate meta-analysis in PNI. Such approaches will enable the analysis of potential interactions and disease risk factors, and support causal modeling (44).

For example, EHRs usually contain rich data sources for translational studies in personalized medicine. Phenotypic data of patients can be collected in a systematic manner. The structured record data from EHRs can be used for generating fine-grained patient stratification and disease statistics. For instance, using ontology methods such as one based on the ICD standard, records from a psychiatric hospital were used for the identification of disease correlations to be mapped to systems biology frameworks (45). In another example, cognitively motivated methodology has been applied for the simulation of expert ability to support diagnostic hypotheses. Using semantic distance measures, diagnostically meaningful clusters can be modeled as geometric structures within the semantic space that relate psychiatric terms (46).

3.3. Data Mining, Neural Networks, and Knowledge Discovery

Based on the collected and integrated data, knowledge discovery approaches such as data mining and machine learning methods can be used for the discovery of meaningful patterns, associations, interactions, and clinical rules to build systems biology models (7). Data mining methods include clustering, decision trees, genetic algorithms, artificial neural networks (ANN), Bayesian networks, and various statistical methods (7). The detailed description of each of the methods is beyond the scope and length of this chapter. This section focuses on their applications in PNI and relevant studies.

For instance, translational bioinformatics and systems biology analyses have been found useful for elucidating the systemic mechanisms in inflammation. Dynamic mathematical modeling methods such as agent-based modeling (ABM) and equation-based modeling (EBM) have been used for such analysis (47). Immunoinformatics tools based on ANN methods can be applied for analyzing structural and functional patterns of the immune system (48). Furthermore, text mining and natural language processing (NLP) techniques can be useful for better searching and retrieval of health information (49). The clustering of expression data at both the gene and protein levels can help identify biomarkers and candidate targets (7).

Some methods can be used specifically for personalized medicine. For example, dynamic p-technique (DPT) is a useful statistical method for finding associations in dynamic constructs in a single person or small group of individuals over time. Its applications in a pediatric psychology area have demonstrated its usefulness because of its power in modeling repeated observations from small samples (50). Using statistical methods, GWAS can be used for the study of genotype–phenotype correlations based on data-driven rather than hypothesis-driven approaches. Combined with informatics methods, the studies of structural genetic variation and the approaches targeting rare genetic variation using the whole-genome "deep" sequencing technologies may provide better understanding of genetic epidemiology (51). These new methods including epigenetic studies and gene–gene interactions in complex networks using systems biology approaches have great potentials to lead to novel treatments.

One systems biology approach to study complex diseases is via the understanding of simple nonlinear interactions of a very small number of variables (52). For example, circuit diagrams may be used to illustrate the macro-anatomic structures and links of the brain associated with major depression and other mental problems (52). Computational models can be especially useful for modeling inter- and intracellular molecular networks such as the complex systems of synapses involved in the mental disorders (53).

An important challenge in systems biology is the quantification of experimentally induced changes in biological pathways such as multiple metabolic pathways. The algorithm based on the Generalized Singular Value Decomposition (GSVD) has been found useful for analyzing pairs of networks for studying changed metabolic pathways from those found in the database of KEGG (54). Such an approach can be applied for analyzing differences in clusters, such as in the quantification of the changes in metabolic pathways between two groups in the studies of schizophrenia.

In another example, a network-based systems biology approach has been found valuable in studying the cross-talks among pathways in various brain regions involved in Alzheimer's disease (AD) (55). By building a network of pathways, the associations among AD pathways and the neighbor pathways can be systematically studied and visually illustrated. By using such approaches, the neighbor pathways of AD have been found important in the AD progression (55).

3.4. Clinical Applications of Biomedical Decision Support Systems

Decision support systems (DSSs) based on translational bioinformatics can be incorporated into EHR systems and other clinical information systems. Here decision support includes information management, diagnostic decisions, as well as providing patient-specific recommendations for prevention and treatment (42). In addition, effective decision support means better communication and documentation, more efficient workflow, and more convenient literature and resource retrieval.

The goal of such decision support is to bring the "right knowledge to the right people in the right form at the right time" (56). Workflow integration is a critical component toward the success of decision support (42). A widely used methodology for modeling the workflow and decision support processes is a standard object-oriented modeling language, the UML (35, 42). By using a methodology specifically designed for biomedical sciences, UML can be applied for the modeling of biomedical knowledge to facilitate concept extraction as well as sharing of knowledge (35).

The analysis of the decision making process of human experts has been considered useful for personalized care in psychiatric rehabilitation by matching diverse treatment options to individually unique profiles (57). Computerized clinical decision support systems (CDSSs) that integrate databases, domain ontology, and problem-solving algorithms can be applied for personalized psychiatric rehabilitation and optimized outcome. CDSSs have been demonstrated valuable in improving medication safety such as by analyzing clinical relevance of drug interactions (58).

For example, a CDSS and a multidimensional classification system containing the Operational Classification of Drug Interactions (ORCA) were used in analyzing 359,207 cross-sectional prescriptions in a large sample of psychiatric patients (58). Danger interaction alerts were issued by the CDSS, which were further analyzed by ORCA reclassification. A total of 151 contraindicated and 4,099 provisionally contraindicated prescriptions were identified, with detailed categorical information on recommended management and risks related to interactions (58). Such approaches may provide efficient solutions for identifying drug interactions in large prescription datasets to decrease potentially harmful drug interactions.

EHR systems with large volumes of patient data can be used for Comparative Effectiveness Research (CER). CER may help identify the effectiveness and risks of different treatment options based on data from patient subsets with similar medical conditions (59). However, the data in EHR system are usually not ready for rapid explanation of therapeutic outcomes. Decision support tools can be very useful to help with the clinical decision-making process and personalized patient care. For example, visual analytics tools have been found effective for CER-based clinical decision support, especially in the analyses of the effectiveness and risks of different treatment options for different patient subgroups (59).

In addition, DSSs can also be used for improving consumer decisions and behavioral interventions. For example, DSS is a sustainable method for supporting the decision process of both consumers and providers by improving communications and promoting involvement for better health outcomes (60). Such systems may help clients develop their own care plans and discuss with their case managers. In addition, DSSs such as a Web-based system have been found useful for promoting the motivation to quit smoking and for cessation treatment in patients with severe mental illnesses (61). Computerized administration of the mental health-related questionnaires may support efficient outcomes assessment, adaptable research network, and promotion of clinical impact in community mental health agencies (62). For example, a computer mouse-tracking method for evaluating mental processes in psychological tasks in real time may enable the measurements of spatial attraction, complexity, velocity, and acceleration (63).

In fact, computer-assisted behavioral therapies have been suggested as a small revolution in mental health care as they may provide a new and cost-effective method for individuals with psychiatric disorders (64). This approach may allow access to psychiatric care by many individuals with the extension of the time and expertise of clinicians. Computer-aided psychotherapy (CP) systems have been found effective in improving common mental health problems (65). For example, cognitive-behavioral therapy (CBT) is an effective non-pharmacological intervention for mental disorders including anxiety and depression. Because of treatment availability and cost, many patients with mental problems are unable to get help. Computer-assisted CBT (cCBT) can be applied to help solve such difficulties (66). For better outcomes using such therapies, it is still necessary to identify more effective approaches and to manage possible adverse effects. In addition, more consistent standards for methodological quality will be needed (67).

4. Conclusion and Future Perspectives

In order to allow the smooth practice of translational bioinformatics, societal and ethical issues should also be addressed. For example, the networks such as the Electronic Medical Records and Genomics Network (eMERGE) have emphasized the relevant ethical, social, legal, and policy issues (68). The Genetic Information Nondiscrimination Act (GINA) was established to "protect Americans against discrimination based on their genetic information when it comes to health insurance and employment" (69). The Health Insurance Portability and Accountability Act (HIPAA) (70) needs to be complied for the protection of patient privacy and confidentiality (see Table 1).

An enhanced capacity in translational bioinformatics may accelerate the revolutionary process toward personalized and systems medicine. Such developments may also create an environment for applying evidence-based principles from behavioral medicine (71). The Health Information Technology for Economic and Clinical Health Act of 2009 may help support this evolution. For example, data analyses by using informatics tools have been suggested to accelerate the discoveries in psycho-oncology and treatment of cancer by changing the behavioral settings (71). In addition, the goal of Human Connectome Project (HCP) is to collect and analyze connectivity data as well as neuroimaging, behavioral, and genetic data from more than 1,000 healthy adults (72). The project tries to provide a resource for neuroscience studies for the understanding of the brain functions in different individuals. The HCP consortium is building an informatics platform and workbench for data management, data sharing, systematic data analysis and data mining, as well as data visualization (72). The platform will use standard data formats with application programming interfaces (APIs) for data utilization and integration of applications (72).

In summary, translational bioinformatics plays an essential role in transforming PNI into personalized medicine. It would enable the identification of biomarkers based on systemic analyses. It can improve the understanding of correlations between genotypes and phenotypes to establish patient systemic profiles such as behavioral profiles. It would also enable novel insights into the interactions and interrelationships among different parts in a whole system to establish predictive models for patient responses to diseases, vaccines, and drugs. In addition, translational bioinformatics methods based on data integration, data mining, and knowledge representation can provide decision support for both researchers and clinicians. These approaches are crucial for understanding PNI mechanisms at systems levels, and for the development of personalized and optimal treatment strategies. Specifically, translational bioinformatics may contribute significantly to the development of health information systems including EHRs. Such systems should be able to collect and manage both clinical and genetic data, as well as to support data analyses and decision making. However, currently commonly accepted EHR programs with these features are still in demand. Further developments are needed in translational bioinformatics to meet these requests.

References

1. Mabry PL, Olster DH, Morgan GD et al (2008) Interdisciplinarity and systems science to improve population health: a view from the NIH Office of Behavioral and Social Sciences Research. Am J Prev Med 35(2 suppl):S211–S224
2. Yan Q (2008) The integration of personalized and systems medicine: bioinformatics support for pharmacogenomics and drug discovery. Methods Mol Biol 448:1–19
3. Yan Q (2005) Pharmacogenomics and systems biology of membrane transporters. Mol Biotechnol 29:75–88
4. Madhavan S, Zenklusen JC et al (2009) Rembrandt: helping personalized medicine become a reality through integrative translational research. Mol Cancer Res 7:157–167
5. Wang X, Liu L, Fackenthal J et al (2009) Translational integrity and continuity: personalized biomedical data integration. J Biomed Inform 42:100–112
6. Gebicke-Haerter PJ (2008) Systems biology in molecular psychiatry. Pharmacopsychiatry 41(suppl 1):S19–S27
7. Yan Q (2010) Translational bioinformatics and systems biology approaches for personalized medicine. Methods Mol Biol 662:167–178
8. Giegling I, Hartmann AM, Genius J, Benninghoff J, Möller H-J, Rujescu D (2008) Systems biology and complex neurobehavioral traits. Pharmacopsychiatry 41(suppl 1):S32–S36
9. Yan Q (2003) Bioinformatics and data integration in membrane transporter studies. Methods Mol Biol 227:37–60
10. Huys QJM, Moutoussis M, Williams J (2011) Are computational models of any use to psychiatry? Neural Netw 24:544–551
11. American Medical Informatics Association (AMIA). Available from http://www.amia.org/applications-informatics/translational-bioinformatics. Accessed Nov 2011

12. Yan Q (2000) Preventing adverse drug events (ADEs): the role of computer information systems. Drug Inf J 34:1247–1260
13. Radulovic D, Jelveh S et al (2004) Informatics platform for global proteomic profiling and biomarker discovery using liquid chromatography-tandem mass spectrometry. Mol Cell Proteomics 3:984–997
14. Bloss CS, Schiabor KM, Schork NJ (2010) Human behavioral informatics in genetic studies of neuropsychiatric disease: multivariate profile-based analysis. Brain Res Bull 83:177–188
15. Tretter F, Albus M (2008) Systems biology and psychiatry—modeling molecular and cellular networks of mental disorders. Pharmacopsychiatry 41(suppl 1):S2–S18
16. Altschul SF, Gish W, Miller W et al (1990) Basic local alignment search tool. J Mol Biol 215(3):403–410
17. Larkin MA, Blackshields G, Brown NP et al (2007) Clustal W and Clustal X version 2.0. Bioinformatics 23:2947–2948
18. Sigrist CJA, Cerutti L, de Castro E et al (2010) PROSITE, a protein domain database for functional characterization and annotation. Nucleic Acids Res 38(Database issue):D161–D166
19. The UniProt Consortium (2010) The Universal Protein Resource (UniProt) in 2010. Nucleic Acids Res 38(Database issue):D142–D148
20. Rost B, Yachdav G, Liu J (2004) The PredictProtein server. Nucleic Acids Res 32(Web Server issue):W321–W326
21. Rose PW, Beran B, Bi C et al (2011) The RCSB Protein Data Bank: redesigned web site and web services. Nucleic Acids Res 39(Database issue):D392–D401
22. Frazer KA, Ballinger DG, Cox DR et al (2007) A second generation human haplotype map of over 3.1 million SNPs. Nature 449:851–861
23. Manolio TA, Brooks LD, Collins FS (2008) A HapMap harvest of insights into the genetics of common disease. J Clin Invest 118:1590–1605
24. Sherry ST, Ward MH, Kholodov M et al (2001) dbSNP: the NCBI database of genetic variation. Nucleic Acids Res 29:308–311
25. Salomonis N, Hanspers K, Zambon AC et al (2007) GenMAPP 2: new features and resources for pathway analysis. BMC Bioinformatics 8:217
26. Kanehisa M, Goto S, Hattori M et al (2006) From genomics to chemical genomics: new developments in KEGG. Nucleic Acids Res 34(Database issue):D354–D357
27. Keshava Prasad TS, Goel R, Kandasamy K et al (2009) Human protein reference database—2009 update. Nucleic Acids Res 37(Database issue):D767–D772
28. Croft D, O'Kelly G, Wu G et al (2011) Reactome: a database of reactions, pathways and biological processes. Nucleic Acids Res 39(Database issue):D691–D697
29. Stark C, Breitkreutz B-J, Chatr-Aryamontri A et al (2011) The BioGRID interaction database: 2011 update. Nucleic Acids Res 39(Database issue):D698–D704
30. Hamosh A, Scott AF, Amberger JS et al (2005) Online Mendelian Inheritance in Man (OMIM), a knowledgebase of human genes and genetic disorders. Nucleic Acids Res 33(Database issue):D514–D517
31. Barrett T, Edgar R (2006) Gene expression omnibus: microarray data storage, submission, retrieval, and analysis. Methods Enzymol 411:352–369
32. Lombard Z, Park C, Makova KD et al (2011) A computational approach to candidate gene prioritization for X-linked mental retardation using annotation-based binary filtering and motif-based linear discriminatory analysis. Biol Direct 6:30
33. Gormanns P, Mueller NS, Ditzen C et al (2011) Phenome-transcriptome correlation unravels anxiety and depression related pathways. J Psychiatr Res 45:973–979
34. Wolford G, Rosenberg SD, Rosenberg HJ et al (2008) A clinical trial comparing interviewer and computer-assisted assessment among clients with severe mental illness. Psychiatr Serv 59:769–775
35. Yan Q (2010) Bioinformatics for transporter pharmacogenomics and systems biology: data integration and modeling with UML. Methods Mol Biol 637:23–45
36. Daemen A, Gevaert O, Ojeda F et al (2009) A kernel-based integration of genome-wide data for clinical decision support. Genome Med 1:39
37. Croning MDR, Marshall MC, McLaren P et al (2009) G2Cdb: the genes to cognition database. Nucleic Acids Res 37(Database issue):D846–D851
38. Sabb FW, Bearden CE, Glahn DC et al (2008) A collaborative knowledge base for cognitive phenomics. Mol Psychiatry 13:350–360
39. Kim S, Webster MJ (2010) The stanley neuropathology consortium integrative database: a novel, web-based tool for exploring neuropathological markers in psychiatric disorders and the biological processes associated with abnormalities of those markers. Neuropsychopharmacology 35:473–482
40. Hucka M, Finney A, Bornstein BJ et al (2004) Evolving a lingua franca and associated software infrastructure for computational systems biology: the Systems Biology Markup Language (SBML) project. Syst Biol (Stevenage) 1:41–53

41. Rassinoux AM (2008) Decision support, knowledge representation and management: structuring knowledge for better access. Findings from the yearbook 2008 section on decision support, knowledge representation and management. Yearb Med Inform 2008:80–82
42. Peleg M, Tu S (2006) Decision support, knowledge representation and management in medicine. Yearb Med Inform 2006:72–80
43. Moskovitch R, Martins SB, Behiri E et al (2007) A comparative evaluation of full-text, concept-based, and context-sensitive search. J Am Med Inform Assoc 14:164–174
44. Thomas PD, Mi H, Swan GE et al (2009) A systems biology network model for genetic association studies of nicotine addiction and treatment. Pharmacogenet Genomics 19:538–551
45. Roque FS, Jensen PB, Schmock H et al (2011) Using electronic patient records to discover disease correlations and stratify patient cohorts. PLoS Comput Biol 7:e1002141
46. Cohen T, Blatter B, Patel V (2008) Simulating expert clinical comprehension: adapting latent semantic analysis to accurately extract clinical concepts from psychiatric narrative. J Biomed Inform 41:1070–1087
47. Vodovotz Y, An G (2010) Systems biology and inflammation. Methods Mol Biol 662:181–201
48. Yan Q (2010) Immunoinformatics and systems biology methods for personalized medicine. Methods Mol Biol 662:203–220
49. Cohen AM, Hersh WR (2005) A survey of current work in biomedical text mining. Brief Bioinform 6:57–71
50. Nelson TD, Aylward BS, Rausch JR (2011) Dynamic p-technique for modeling patterns of data: applications to pediatric psychology research. J Pediatr Psychol 36:959–968
51. Rudan I (2010) New technologies provide insights into genetic basis of psychiatric disorders and explain their co-morbidity. Psychiatr Danub 22:190–192
52. Tretter F, Gebicke-Haerter PJ, an der Heiden U et al (2011) Affective disorders as complex dynamic diseases—a perspective from systems biology. Pharmacopsychiatry 44(suppl 1):S2–S8
53. Tretter F (2010) Mental illness, synapses and the brain–behavioral disorders by a system of molecules within a system of neurons? Pharmacopsychiatry 43(suppl 1):S9–S20
54. Xiao X, Dawson N, Macintyre L et al (2011) Exploring metabolic pathway disruption in the subchronic phencyclidine model of schizophrenia with the Generalized Singular Value Decomposition. BMC Syst Biol 5:72
55. Liu Z-P, Wang Y, Zhang X-S et al (2010) Identifying dysfunctional crosstalk of pathways in various regions of Alzheimer's disease brains. BMC Syst Biol 4(suppl 2):S11
56. Schreiber G, Akkermans H, Anjewierden A et al (2000) Knowledge engineering and management: the common KADS methodology. The MIT Press, Cambridge, MA
57. Spaulding W, Deogun J (2011) A pathway to personalization of integrated treatment: informatics and decision science in psychiatric rehabilitation. Schizophr Bull 37(suppl 2):S129–S137
58. Haueis P, Greil W, Huber M et al (2011) Evaluation of drug interactions in a large sample of psychiatric inpatients: a data interface for mass analysis with clinical decision support software. Clin Pharmacol Ther 90:588–596
59. Mane KK, Bizon C, Schmitt C et al (2012) VisualDecisionLinc: a visual analytics approach for comparative effectiveness-based clinical decision support in psychiatry. J Biomed Inform 45(1):101–106
60. Woltmann EM, Wilkniss SM, Teachout A et al (2011) Trial of an electronic decision support system to facilitate shared decision making in community mental health. Psychiatr Serv 62:54–60
61. Brunette MF, Ferron JC, McHugo GJ et al (2011) An electronic decision support system to motivate people with severe mental illnesses to quit smoking. Psychiatr Serv 62:360–366
62. Goldstein LA, Connolly Gibbons MB, Thompson SM et al (2011) Outcome assessment via handheld computer in community mental health: consumer satisfaction and reliability. J Behav Health Serv Res 38:414–423
63. Freeman JB, Ambady N (2010) MouseTracker: software for studying real-time mental processing using a computer mouse-tracking method. Behav Res Methods 42:226–241
64. Carroll KM, Rounsaville BJ (2010) Computer-assisted therapy in psychiatry: be brave-it's a new world. Curr Psychiatry Rep 12:426–432
65. Marks I, Cavanagh K (2009) Computer-aided psychological treatments: evolving issues. Annu Rev Clin Psychol 5:121–141
66. Stuhlmiller C, Tolchard B (2009) Computer-assisted CBT for depression & anxiety: increasing accessibility to evidence-based mental health treatment. J Psychosoc Nurs Ment Health Serv 47:32–39
67. Kiluk BD, Sugarman DE, Nich C et al (2011) A methodological analysis of randomized clinical trials of computer-assisted therapies for psychiatric disorders: toward improved standards for an emerging field. Am J Psychiatry 168:790–799
68. The eMERGE Network. Available from https://www.mc.vanderbilt.edu/victr/dcc/projects/acc/index.php/Main_Page. Accessed Oct 2011

69. National Human Genome Research Institute. Available from http://www.genome.gov/24519851. Accessed Oct 2011
70. The Health Insurance Portability and Accountability Act (HIPAA). Available from http://www.hhs.gov/ocr/privacy/. Accessed Oct 2011
71. Hesse BW, Suls JM (2011) Informatics-enabled behavioral medicine in oncology. Cancer J 17:222–230
72. Marcus DS, Harwell J, Olsen T et al (2011) Informatics and data mining tools and strategies for the human connectome project. Front Neuroinform 5:4

INDEX

Qing Yan (ed.), *Psychoneuroimmunology: Methods and Protocols*, Methods in Molecular Biology, vol. 934, DOI 10.1007/978-1-62703-071-7,

D

E

F

G

H

I

K

L

M

N

T

U

V

W

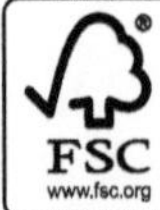

MIX
Papier aus verantwortungsvollen Quellen
Paper from responsible sources
FSC® C105338

If you have any concerns about our products, you can contact us on
ProductSafety@springernature.com

In case Publisher is established outside the EU, the EU authorized representative is:
Springer Nature Customer Service Center GmbH
Europaplatz 3, 69115 Heidelberg, Germany

Printed by Libri Plureos GmbH
in Hamburg, Germany